Clinical Nutrition
in Paediatric Disorders

Clinical Nutrition in Paediatric Disorders

DONALD BENTLEY, MB ChB, DCH, MSc, MRCP

Consultant Paediatrician, Ealing Hospital, Southall, Middlesex; Honorary Senior Lecturer, Royal Postgraduate Medical School and Honorary Consultant Paediatrician, Hammersmith Hospital, London; Examiner, Diploma in Child Health to the Royal College of Physicians

MARGARET LAWSON, MSc, SRD

Senior Lecturer in Nutrition and Course Tutor in Dietetics, Department of Applied Chemistry and Life Sciences, The Polytechnic of North London

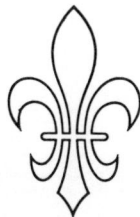

BAILLIERE TINDALL
London Philadelphia Sydney Tokyo Toronto

Baillière Tindall
W.B. Saunders   24—28 Oval Road
London NW1 7DX

West Washington Square
Philadelphia, PA 19105, USA

1 Goldthorne Avenue
Toronto, Ontario M8Z 5T9,
Canada

ABP Australia Ltd
44—50 Waterloo Road
North Ryde, NSW 2113,
Australia

Harcourt Brace Jovanovich Japan Inc.
Ichibancho Central Building,
22—1 Ichibancho
Chiyoda-ku, Tokyo 102, Japan

© 1988 Baillière Tindall

First published 1988

British Library Cataloguing in Publication Data
Bentley, D.
    Clinical nutrition in paediatric disorders.
    1.   Children. Paediatrics. Diseases.
Therapy, Diet
I. Title   II. Lawson, M.
615.8'54

ISBN 0-7020-1245-9

Typeset by Setrite Typesetters
Printed in Great Britain by Thomson Litho Ltd, East Kilbride, Scotland

Contents

Contents

Contents

Foreword

This textbook, entitled *Clinical Nutrition in Paediatric Disorders*, is a valuable reference source for paediatricians, family practice physicians, nutritionists caring for children, and paediatricians in training or students with a paediatric interest. Unlike many textbooks of this magnitude dealing with clinical nutrition, this book is written entirely by two authors, Dr Donald Bentley, a seasoned Clinical Academician with enormous personal experience in nutrition and gastroenterology, and Ms Margaret Lawson, a Nutritionist with both practical and theoretical experience in paediatric nutrition. In fact, it was my privilege to have contributed in some way to Dr Bentley's formal training in paediatric gastroenterology and nutrition during his stay in Boston in the early seventies. As a textbook of limited authorship, the book provides in-depth coverage of major clinical nutrition problems in paediatrics, and underscores the importance of nutrition in the care of complex gastrointestinal problems. Instead of a collection of chapters written by multiple authors about their personal research interests, this book involves an important theme and has a continuity of approach which allows for ease of reading and access as a reference source.

The text itself comprises eighteen chapters and seven appendices. Section 1 considers normal paediatric nutrition and generalized malnutrition, as well as approaches to the nutritional management of the normal, healthy growing infant and child, and the child with protein—calorie malnutrition. Section 2 presents a detailed approach to the pathophysiology of nutritional deficiencies in hepatobiliary and gastrointestinal disorders, including malabsorptive syndromes, pancreatic insufficiency, including cystic fibrosis, liver diseases and inborn errors in metabolism. The final section deals with selective, non-enteric disorders requiring modified diets which have been controversial in the paediatric literature over the years. The authors discuss the unique nutritional problems with cardiac and renal diseases and the complicated management of diabetes mellitus, concluding with an important perspective on the controversial psychonutritional disorders which comprise a significant time in most clinical practice of paediatrics. Of particular importance are the appendices which provide an invaluable reference for normal growth and development, nutritional data for unique problems in paediatrics such as prematurity, as well as approaches to diseases, use of intravenous nutrients and further reference of manufacturers and their products.

All in all this textbook should be strongly considered by any physician or student-physician dealing with infants and children in which nutrition is considered to be an important part of their approach to practice. My congratulations to Dr Bentley and Ms Lawson on the enormous effort to provide a practical textbook dealing with nutrition in paediatrics.

PROFESSOR W. ALLAN WALKER
Harvard Medical School, Combined Program in Pediatric Gastroenterology and Nutrition at The Children's Hospital and Massachusetts General Hospital, Boston, MA 02115, USA

To my beloved wife Elaine and our children Russell Daniel, Melissa Sarah, Elliott Saul, Davina Shula for their tireless support and to my mother Marie for her faith and forebearance.

DB

A knowledge of dietetics is practically one of the most helpful things in the field of medicine, because of the constant need for food, which is never ending, during health as well as during illness.

De Alimentorum Virtutibus
Maimonides 1135—1204

Preface

Many paediatricians, particularly those who do not have access to expert dietetic advice, will recognize the need for practical guidance on the nutritional management of paediatric disorders. Paediatricians faced with such problems as acute enteritis and steatorrhoea can readily get caught up in the irrational ritual of switching milk formulae. Our experience in less developed countries has convinced us that there are many who are unsure of the rationale for specific feeds or diets or, indeed, rehydration solutions used in therapeutic regimens. In addition, parents are often tempted, almost empirically, to blame the milk product or dietary constituent for any enteric or allergic reaction. Such situations are avoidable.

This textbook, prepared jointly by a practising clinician and a paediatric nutritionist, covers a range of childhood disorders where nutritional management plays an important role in therapy. We have not confined the text to dietetic topics because this approach would be too limiting for the general paediatrician. For each condition described, there is first an introduction on pathogenesis and diagnosis and then more extensive sections on the clinical and dietetic management.

Although we have endeavoured to emphasize basic diagnostic techniques, we have mentioned more sophisticated methods where appropriate because yesterday's research tool is often tomorrow's standard marker of disease. Some paediatricians have ready access to enzymologists and nuclear physicists, but many are not so fortunate. As our colleagues are to be found in very dissimilar environments, we have stressed fundamental clinical features and aims of investigation throughout rather than more exotic research findings. One aim has been to pay particular attention to the well-tried regimens of management while directing the reader's attention to recent advances in pharmacology and nutrition. This balanced approach will, we believe, be of most use to paediatricians faced with problems in everyday practice.

We would be grateful to receive any comments about the contents of this textbook.

DONALD BENTLEY
MARGARET LAWSON

Acknowledgements

We have had much encouragement and advice from colleagues both at Ealing and Hammersmith Hospitals from the time we conceived the idea of this book until the manuscript completed its prolonged if not protracted gestation. In particular we wish to thank Drs M.J. Brueton and B. Sandhu of Westminster and Charing Cross Hospital Medical School, Dr E.A. Hughes of the Royal Postgraduate Medical School, Dr J. Brostoff of the Middlesex Hospital Medical School and Judy Bayliss of London. Also we would like to express our gratitude to Dr P.J. Aggett of the University of Aberdeen for his many helpful comments. We are most grateful to Mrs J. Poller, Postgraduate Centre Administrator at Ealing Hospital for her skills as a librarian and to Mrs S. Azzopardi for her secretarial assistance. We are indebted to Mr J. Lukeman, District Pharmacist and his staff of the Drug Information Unit at Ealing Hospital for compiling pharmaceutical and nutritional data. Finally, we wish to acknowledge the assistance and support received from Nicholas Dunton (formerly of Baillière Tindall), Katharine Hinton and Alison Campbell of Baillière Tindall, and Jane Sugarman, our committed subeditor.

Section 1

NORMAL NUTRITION, DEFICIENCY STATES AND INCREASED DIETARY REQUIREMENTS

1

Normal Dietary Requirements, Recommendations and Deficiency Diseases

Many international bodies publish recommendations for all or some essential nutrients; variations between the recommended dietary allowances (RDAs) can be attributed to a number of factors, but comparison between various sets of RDAs is difficult because the age groupings used are not standardized. The theoretical aspects of normal infant and child requirements and recommended dietary allowances (RDAs) are to be found in other publications (Fomon, 1974; Lifshitz, 1980; Suskind, 1981; Ziegler *et al.*, 1981; McLaren and Burman, 1982; Walker and Watkins, 1985).

There are four main reasons for the varying nutrient intake recommended: the quality of the diet and nutrient bioavailability in the normal foods eaten in a particular region will affect requirements. Protein quality is important — breast milk and egg protein have a protein score of 100 because they contain a balance of amino acids that closely approximates to human requirements. Most recommendations assume a lower score for a mixed diet, but if only proteins of a poor nutritional quality are available, then total protein requirements will be higher; the form in which folate and iron are present in the diet and the proportions of trace elements such as zinc and copper will affect absorption.

Environmental factors may need to be considered: the ambient temperature will marginally affect energy needs and exposure to sunlight will alter vitamin D requirements.

Physical and social aspects of a community may also have an influence: the age at which children undergo the adolescent growth spurt, the onset of menarche and the age at which childbearing begins will affect the requirements for all nutrients.

Levels of requirement can be set at the lowest intake which will prevent clinical signs of deficiency, the physiological minimum, which will maintain normal metabolism and growth, or a level of intake which will give maximum values in function tests and/or tissue saturation. The USA recommendations for vitamin C are appreciably higher than those for most other regions as tissue saturation was felt to be desirable.

In addition, RDAs usually ensure that the requirements of the majority of the population are met. Some countries, such as the USA, include a larger safety margin; other bodies such as FAO/WHO have a smaller one so that the requirements of some people will be above the recommendations. The FAO/WHO values can therefore be considered as minimum intakes for normal growth and development, while those of the UK and USA represent desirable intakes for the paediatric population.

It is important to remember that the RDAs are designed for groups not individuals. A normal child may have a requirement that is considerably above or below the RDA for his age or size. This is particularly true for energy, where recommendations are based on the average intakes of children omitting the normal safety margin.

Appendices I.1–I.6 give the RDA for most nutrients known to be essential for three organizations: FAO/WHO/UNU (WHO, 1974; FAO, 1985), the UK (DHSS, 1980) and the USA (National Academy of Sciences, 1980). Data on the requirements for some nutrients are felt to be insufficiently precise as a basis on which to make recommendations and the USA has issued an estimated safe and adequate daily intake for these nutrients (Appendix I.7). An upper limit has also been suggested for some minerals because adverse effects can occur at levels not greatly in excess of the estimated requirements.

Because the whole of an infant's nutritional requirements must be met by one food, standards for the composition of such formulae have been suggested by several bodies (*see* Anon, 1987a). The recommendations of FAO/WHO (WHO, 1976), the American Academy of Pediatrics (1976)

3

and the UK (DHSS, 1980, 1987) are given in Appendices II.1 and II.11.

Recommendations refer to starter formulae used for healthy full-term infants under the age of 6 months. The sick infant may well have an amended requirement for some nutrients, and these variations are covered in the sections dealing with the specific disorder. The requirement for the majority of nutrients will remain unaltered, and any special formula must meet the total requirements of the infant. The standards for normal formulae given here should provide a reference base for all feeds designed to be the sole source of nutrients.

Vitamins are chemical compounds present in various animal and plant sources in minute quantities. Although vitamins are to be found in diminutive concentrations, they play an essential role in metabolic processes and the overall maintenance of good nutrition. Disorders of vitamins include deficiency, toxicity and also biochemical dependency states. Benton and Roberts (1988) have shown in a modest sample of British schoolchildren that the administration over 8 months of a multivitamin/mineral supplement resulted in an increase in non-verbal intelligence. The investigators did not categorically implicate any specific nutrient deficiency, but suggest that thiamine has a role in the aetiology of psychological dysfunction. A condition of optimal health inevitably relates to the presence of trace elements and these cannot be synthesized. Almost every inorganic mineral and indeed heavy metal is to be found in human tissues. Trace elements have many roles and interact with enzymes and biological membranes. Elements can be classified into an essential (macro) trace group with a concentration above 0.005% of the body weight (e.g. calcium and magnesium) and another group where the essential (micro) trace element content is less than 0.005% of the body weight (e.g. iron, iodine, copper).

Fat-soluble vitamins

Vitamin A

This fat-soluble vitamin is an essential nutrient which is stored in the liver. Hormone like in function, vitamin A aids night vision, the wellbeing of the cell membrane, maintenance of bone growth, integrity of mucus secretion and spermatogenesis (Fell, 1970). Avitaminosis A causes growth failure, skin and corneal disease.

Symptoms

Major symptoms of deficiency include: night blindness; xerophthalmia (dry cornea); keratomalacia (dryness, ulceration leading to perforation of cornea).

Vitamin A deficiency is often seen in children suffering from protein−energy malnutrition (PEM) in countries such as Brazil, India, Indonesia and the Middle East.

Intoxication can occur from too much fish liver oil or excess vitamin preparations. 'Food faddists' are also at risk of intoxication from a high intake of carrots or pumpkins.

Sources

Retinol (vitamin A_1) is present in the livers of fish and most land vertebrates, dairy produce, eggs and meat.

Laboratory diagnosis

The plasma vitamin A level is below 200 µg/ml and the plasma retinol binding protein is less than 20 µg/ml.

Prophylaxis

75 µg/day or 9 µg/kg per day in first year of life.
120 µg/day from 12 to 36 months (Fomon, 1974).

Vitamin D

Vitamin D compounds derive from sterols and are responsible for the absorption of calcium and phosphate from the gastrointestinal tract. Vitamin D_3 (cholecalciferol), a hormone, is formed from 7-dehydrocholesterol by the action of ultraviolet light on the skin.

Vitamin D_3 is transported to the liver and hydroxylated at the 25-position to 25-hydroxycholecalciferol ($25(OH)D_3$). $25(OH)D_3$ is hydroxylated by the renal enzyme 1α-hydroxylase to 1,25-dihydroxycholecalciferol ($1,25(OH)_2D_3$). Parathyroid hormone controls this enzyme.

$25(OH)D_3$ enhances bone reabsorption and the uptake of gastrointestinal calcium thereby elevating serum calcium.

The term vitamin D as such would be recognized by many as a misnomer because it is known that vitamin D is part of an elaborate endocrine system that is not limited to the regulation of bone and mineral metabolism, but has a fundamental and diverse role in controlling cellular proliferation and differentiation (Anon, 1987b). Indeed there are positive receptors for $1,25(OH)_2D_3$ in many human cancer cell lines. Receptors for 1,25-dihydroxycholecalciferol are not found solely in the intestine and skin but are widespread, being present in numerous potential target-organs such as the brain, liver, kidney and skin.

Rickets

Deficiency of vitamin D in the growing child leads to rickets (Fig. 1.1), a metabolic disorder especially common in England during the time of the Industrial Revolution because of poor nutrition, arising from both financial and educational poverty as well as the result of a hazy, smoggy atmosphere with little exposure to sunlight (ultraviolet radiation). Adequate sunshine is not the entire explanation because rickets was

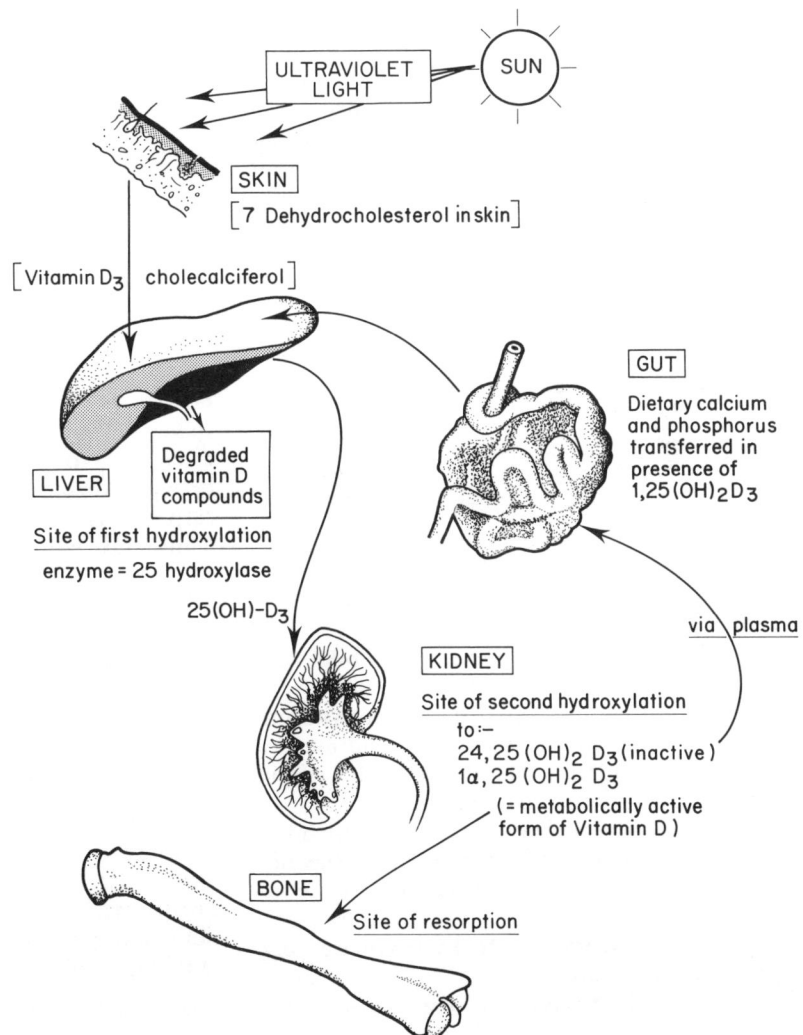

Fig. 1.1 Vitamin D is derived from the diet and from the effect of ultraviolet light on the skin. It is hydroxylated in the liver $(25(OH)D_3)$ and undergoes a second hydroxylation in the kidney to the biologically active form $(1\alpha,25(OH)_2D_3 = 1,25$-dihydroxycholecalciferol). $1,25(OH_2)D_3$ acts on the gut and bone to increase gut absorption and bone resorption. $24,25(OH)_2D_3 = 24,25$-dihydroxycholecalciferol. (Courtesy of Professor P. Byrne.)

common in the 1940s in southern California (Lawson, 1981) and today in India (Raghuramulu and Reddy, 1980). Furthermore, from October to March no ultraviolet light reaches the earth's surface in the UK and consequently vitamin D is not formed in the skin during that period. Skin synthesis is the major source of this vitamin and tanning prevents further formation. With the development of vitamin D fortified milks and milk products rickets has decreased in incidence. Human milk contains almost 20 times more of this vitamin than unmodified whole cow's milk.

Rickets was described in Asian immigrants in Glasgow, Scotland in 1956 (Arneil and Crosbie, 1963). An estimate of the incidence of clinically overt rickets among UK Asians 0–16 years old, for 1977, was 4 cases per 1000 in London and 10 per 1000 in the Midlands and the north of England. Rickets seemed to increase from 1960 to 1973 and then decreased (Goel *et al.*, 1981). Pregnant Asian women with osteomalacia risk having infants with neonatal convulsions and rickets and need adequate supplements of vitamin D throughout pregnancy and lactation. Typically, rickets is seen in breast-fed premature babies and is especially prevalent in those born to Asian mothers in the UK. Rickets has also been described in the fetus (Russell and Hill, 1974). Adolescent Asian rickets, characteristically in children 8–14 years old, may present with gross genu valgum (knock-knees) and aching joints.

Causes.

1. Inadequate exposure to sunlight.
2. Inadequate vitamin D intake.
3. Malabsorption of vitamin D (fat soluble), e.g. coeliac disease, short bowel syndrome, bacterial overgrowth in bowel, deficiency of bile salts, Shwachman's syndrome, cystic fibrosis.
4. Increased enzyme activity: anticonvulsants (phenobarbitone and/or phenytoin) will increase metabolic degradation of $25(OH)D_3$ by stimulating hepatic microsomal enzymes.
5. Decreased enzyme activity: vitamin D-dependent rickets (pseudovitamin D deficiency; deficiency of the renal enzyme 25-hydroxyvitamin D 1α-hydroxylase).
6. Acquired deficiency of 1α-hydroxylase, e.g. chronic renal failure.
7. Failure of 25-hydroxylation, e.g. chronic liver failure.

8. Fanconi's syndrome—phosphaturia: the principal component of the disorder leads to hypophosphataemic rickets.

Early manifestations of rickets.

1. Craniotabes (skull feels like a 'ping-pong' ball).
2. Frontal bossing and thickening of skull ('hot cross bun' appearance).
3. Rachitic rosary (enlarged costochondral junctions).
4. Widening of epiphyses at wrists (Fig. 1.2).

Manifestations of advanced rickets.

1. Craniotabes.
2. Large fontanelle with delayed closure.
3. Soft, widely separated sutures.
4. Enlarged costochondral junctions.
5. Dental defects (delayed eruption, poor enamel).
6. Sternal protrusion ('pigeon chest').
7. Depression along lower border of chest at level of insertion of diaphragm (Harrison's sulcus).
8. Scoliosis/kyphosis/lumbar lordosis.
9. Bow-legs, knock-knees (genu valgum).
10. Waddling gait secondary to femoral bowing.
11. Weak muscles and hypotonia.
12. Non-musculoskeletal features include fretfulness, sweating and a coincidental iron-deficiency anaemia.

Diagnosis. Diagnosis is radiological. In active rickets (Fig. 1.2), note cupping and fraying of distal ends of radius and ulna, increased distance between distal ends of forearm bones and metacarpals. The table and base of the skull are demineralized.

Biochemical findings.

1. Increased plasma alkaline phosphatase (of bone origin).
2. Phosphate normal or reduced.
3. Calcium normal or reduced.
4. Serum PTH normal or increased.
5. Generalized aminoaciduria.

Reactive secondary hyperparathyroidism can complicate interpretation of biochemical diagnostic data.

Treatment. Adequate amounts of dietary calcium and phosphate should be ensured. Vitamin D therapy should be instituted:

Mild rickets: 40 µg/day vitamin D.
Advanced rickets: 125 µg/day vitamin D.

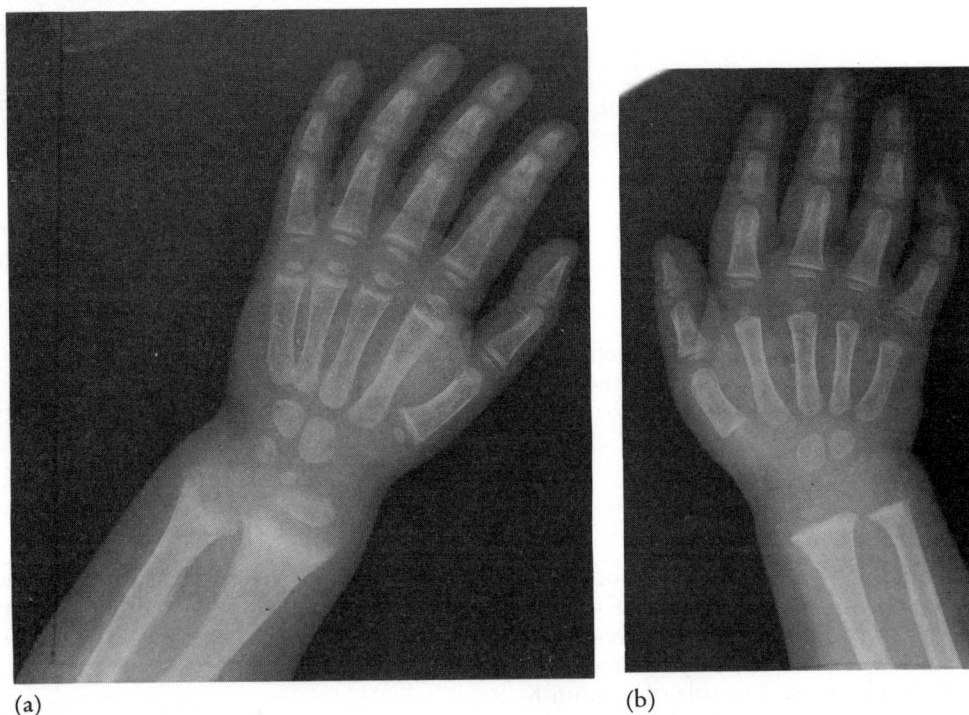

Fig. 1.2 (a) X-ray showing rickets. The lower ends of the radius and ulna are widened, cupped and indistinct — the 'frothing champagne glass' appearance. (b) X-ray of a normal child aged 18 months for comparison. (By courtesy of Dr AMK Thomas.)

Once rickets is treated give 15 mg in a single dose or over 24 hours or 125–250 µg/day for 6–8 weeks.

Prophylaxis. Daily intake of 10 µg a day. Those with renal failure, liver failure or bowel malabsorption should receive 50–125 µg a day. Patients with cystic fibrosis should receive 10–20 µg a day.

Vitamin E (tocopherols)

This fat-soluble vitamin has a major role as an intracellular antioxidant maintaining the stability of membranes. Biological membranes contain phospholipids and in the presence of oxygen are auto-oxidizable (or peroxidizable). Vitamin E is an effective antioxidant in that it inhibits the combination of a compound with oxygen. Low-birth-weight babies and those of less than 36 weeks' gestation are particularly susceptible to haemolytic anaemia provoked by vitamin E deficiency. As the level of polyunsaturated fatty acids (PUFAs) increases, vitamin E requirements rise. In addition a high iron intake (e.g. iron-supplemented formulae)

increases the risk of vitamin E deficiency and of a haemolytic anaemia developing. Therefore, specialized formulae for low-birth-weight babies containing in excess of 1 mg iron/100 kcal must have adequate amounts of both PUFAs and an absorbable form of vitamin E (American Academy of Pediatrics, 1976). There is conflicting evidence regarding the role of tocopherol in the prevention or amelioration of retrolental fibroplasia and bronchopulmonary dysplasia in premature babies.

Secondary vitamin E deficiency may be seen in malabsorption from any cause especially in steatorrhoea from pancreatic insufficiency. Neurological signs associated with vitamin E deficiency have been noted. Children with steatorrhoea for other reasons (e.g. biliary atresia) fail to absorb vitamin E.

Diagnosis

Erythrocytes are excessively fragile in the presence of hydrogen peroxide and between 30 and 100% of the red blood cells will haemolyse. In vitamin E deficiency, serum tocopherol is less than 5 mg/l.

Prophylaxis

1. Pre-term babies: 5—25 mg/kg per day.
2. Term babies: vitamin E/PUFA ratio of 0.4 mg: 1 g.

Satisfactory plasma concentrations of α-tocopherol (1 mg/100 ml) will be achieved by this ratio (Lewis, 1969).

Therapy

In pre-term infants with vitamin E deficiency, 75—100 mg daily in divided oral doses should be given. In cases of malabsorption, water-miscible preparations (0.75—1.5 g) can be given.

Vitamin K

Vitamin K is a fat-soluble methylnaphthoquinone derivative. The chief source of vitamin K_1 (phylloquinone) is from the diet — mainly green plants — while vitamin K_2 (menaquinone) is synthesized by gastrointestinal bacteria. The role of vitamin K_1 is the maintenance of normal levels of prothrombin (factor II) and the vitamin K-dependent clotting factors VII, IX and X. This vitamin requires bile salts for its absorption from the small bowel after which it is stored in the liver.

In children bacteria are the main source of this vitamin, while in adults vitamin K is obtained from the diet. The estimated newborn requirements are 0.5—1.0 μg/kg per day.

Haemorrhagic disease of the newborn

This self-limiting disease has an incidence of 1 in 200—400 births (Greer *et al.*, 1988). It presents from days 1 to 5, but not within the first 24 hours or beyond day 5 in a term baby. It is much more common in breast-fed babies than in a baby on formula suggesting that breast feeding is a predisposing factor.
Presentation. There is often excessive bleeding from the umbilical cord or bruising but the most common newborn manifestation is melaena.

Causes of vitamin K deficiency in the newborn

The fetus lacks the prothrombin precursor prothrombinogen. In the newborn fat absorption is impaired, particularly if the baby is immature. Sterility of the intestinal tract prevents vitamin K

synthesis (a theory disputed by Keenan *et al.*, 1971).

Breast milk is deficient in vitamin K (15 μg/l), whereas cows' milk contains 60 μg/l.

Diagnosis

The prothrombin and partial thromboplastin time (PT/PTT) are prolonged and levels of factors II, VII, IX and X are low.

Treatment

The initial treatment is vitamin K_1 1 mg intravenously. If PT has not improved in 6 hours repeat.

Prophylaxis

All newborns (pre-term or term) should receive vitamin K_1 0.5—1.0 mg i.m. or 1.0—2.0 mg orally. There is no risk of haemolysis as might occur with larger doses of a synthetic analogue.

Water-soluble vitamins

The water-soluble vitamins include the vitamin B complex made up of vitamin B_1 (thiamine), vitamin B_2 (riboflavin), niacin or nicotinic acid and nicotinamide (vitamin B_3), pantothenic acid (vitamin B_5), biotin (a coenzyme), vitamin B_6 (pyridoxine) and vitamin B_{12} (cyanocobalamin); vitamin C (ascorbic acid); folic acid (pteroylglutamic acid).

Vitamin B$_1$ (thiamine)

Co-carboxylase (thiamine pyrophosphate) which is the phosphorylated, active form of thiamine plays a major role in two enzymatic activities (decarboxylation of α-ketoacids and transketolase reactions). Dietary sources are many and include rice husks, cereal grains, yeast, liver, eggs and milk. Human milk is relatively low in vitamin B_1 (16 μg/ml) compared to cows' milk (42 μg/ml). In the endemic form, the deficiency disease is confined to rice-eating populations. Isolated disorders of this vitamin may occur but it is more often associated with decreased riboflavin and niacin.

Thiamine deficiency

Certain foods such as shellfish, raw carp or herring contain thiamine-destroying enzymes (thiaminases) which may considerably reduce the vitamin B_1 content of food. Infantile beriberi has been reported in many countries but with improved nutritional education the prevalence is declining. This deficiency disorder can present as polyneuritis, cardiomegaly with heart failure and/or aphonia. Most infants with beriberi have been breast fed and their mothers were on low thiamine diets. A diet of milled rice will result in a poor thiamine intake.

A diagnosis of thiamine deficiency should be suspected where there is starvation and/or malnutrition and can be confirmed by finding a very reduced urine thiamine level, i.e. less than 15 μg/24 hours (normal = 40−100 μg/24 hours). Another diagnostic laboratory technique is the estimation of erythrocyte transketolase activity with and without added thiamine pyrophosphate.

Prevention. Adding premix rice to milled rice or encouraging the use of undermilled rice will be effective. Recommended daily intake of vitamin B_1 is: infants, 0.5 mg; children, 0.7 mg.

Treatment. Beriberi will usually respond rapidly (24−72 hours) to treatment but motor weakness may last for 1−3 months. The treatment is oral thiamine 5 mg/day (once) or 10 mg intravenously twice a day for seriously ill children.

Vitamin B_2 (riboflavin)

Riboflavin has an important biochemical role and is incorporated into flavoproteins and many enzyme systems (e.g. flavin mononucleotide, FMN; flavin adenine dinucleotide, FAD). FMN and FAD are both electron carriers found in oxidation systems.

Dietary sources are milk products, eggs, meats, fruits and green leafy vegetables. Vitamin B_2 is not destroyed by ordinary cooking in an acid medium.

Deficiency

Riboflavin deficiency may be a result of malabsorption or a decreased intake. Dietary deficiency is most likely in the spring and the summer months. Ariboflavinosis causes a scaly skin, especially of the face. The areas of greatest skin involvement relate to sites of the sebaceous glands. Cheilosis (swollen and cracked lips), angular stomatitis and lesions at mucocutaneous junctions (anus and vagina) and a distinct eye condition are responsible for the label of oro-oculogenital syndrome.

The ophthalmic features include photophobia and corneal vascularization. The tongue is not only painful but may have a magenta colour.

Diagnosis. This can be confirmed by determining the 24-hour urinary excretion of riboflavin. Normal value for adults exceeds 100 μg/24 hours and a deficiency would be characterized by a concentration of less than 50 μg/24 hours. Assay of erythrocyte glutathione reductase with and without FAD can establish the diagnosis.

Treatment. Children need 1 mg three times a day for several weeks, and infants 0.5 mg twice a day. Response to therapy is usually prompt.

Niacin

Nicotinic acid and nicotinamide are both referred to as niacin (vitamin B_3). Nicotinamide can be formed from nicotinic acid, and some nicotinic acid is synthesized from tryptophan. Niacin is incorporated into nicotinamide adenine dinucleotide (NAD) and nicotinamide adenine dinucleotide phosphate (NADP). It can be seen that nicotinamide is a constituent of important coenzymes needed for oxidation−reduction reactions (including high energy phosphate compounds).

Dietary sources include liver, yeast, white meat, poultry, peanuts and legumes. Milk and eggs are good sources of tryptophan and subsequently niacin.

Deficiency

Foods with a high leucine content (e.g. corn and millet) interfere with the conversion of tryptophan to niacin. Furthermore, nicotinic acid is present in corn in a bound state as niacytin. Evidently corn- or millet-consuming communities are at risk of developing niacin deficiency. Patients receiving isoniazid for tuberculosis can acquire pellagra because the medication competes with pyridoxal phosphate and vitamin B_6 is required for the transformation of tryptophan to niacin. In Hartnup's disease, a rare inherited metabolic disorder involving the transport of amino acids, a deficiency state can arise and large amounts of monoamino monocarboxylic acids are recovered in the urine.

Clinical features. Niacin deficiency leads to pellagra which shows pathognomonic skin changes. Niacin deficiency is characterized by the three (or four) Ds: dermatitis, diarrhoea, dementia and death (if untreated). The skin lesions are seen on areas exposed to light and become erythematous: later keratosis and brown pigmentation are commonly seen.

Diagnosis. Normal excretion of N'-methylnicotinamide is usually 4–6 mg/day and values less than 3 mg/day suggest niacin deficiency. In pellagra, urinary N'-methylnicotinamide is 0.5–0.8 mg/day.

Treatment. Oral nicotinamide 50–100 mg/day or parenteral therapy with 5 mg three or even five times a day.

Pantothenic acid

Pantothenic acid (vitamin B_5) is a component of coenzyme A (CoA) and as such is a central molecule in metabolism. In its active form, as acetyl-coenzyme A, it is involved in the citrate cycle (tricarboxylate cycle or Kreb's cycle).

Pantothenic acid is found in nearly all naturally occurring foods.

Deficiency. Pantothenate deficiency rarely occurs in adults except under extreme conditions (e.g. famine) and there is no evidence, as yet, that it is seen in infants or children.

Biotin

Biotin is a carrier of activated carbon dioxide and enables pyruvate to be carboxylated. Pyruvate carboxylase is important not only in gluconeogenesis, but plays a critical role in maintaining the level of the citrate cycle intermediates. Avidin, a specific protein in egg albumin, inhibits the enzymes of carboxylation because of its affinity for biotin.

Gastrointestinal bacteria produce biotin. Dietary sources include liver, egg yolk, milk, yeast extract and meat.

Deficiency

This can occur in those who consume large quantities of raw eggs for several months. There have been several case reports of biotin deficiency associated with total parenteral nutrition, particularly where there is altered bowel flora secondary to the use of antibiotics (Mock *et al.*, 1981; Gillis *et al.*, 1982).

Clinical features. The features include a rash resembling seborrhoeic dermatitis, lassitude, muscular pain and eventually anorexia.

Diagnosis. The symptoms are relatively non-specific, but the values for whole blood levels are known: 820–2700 pg/ml and urinary excretion is normally 14–100 µg/day.

Treatment. The treatment is oral biotin 85 µg/day for 4–6 years old (Zlotkin *et al.*, 1985), and 30 µg/kg per day for infants (in total parenteral nutrition).

Vitamin B_6 (pyridoxine)

Pyridoxine occurs in three closely related compounds: pyridoxine, pyridoxal and pyridoxamine. The prosthetic group of all transaminases is pyridoxal phosphate which is derived from pyridoxine (vitamin B_6). During transamination, pyridoxal phosphate acts as a coenzyme and is transiently converted to pyridoxamine phosphate.

High levels are found in liver, vegetables, fruits, wholegrain cereals and meats. Milling of wheat can remove 80–90% of vitamin B_6.

Deficiency

Hyperactivity and convulsions have occurred in infants who were inadvertently fed an inaccurately prepared milk formula with a much reduced pyridoxine content. Symptoms were aggravated by an increased protein intake but the convulsions responded to 5 or 10 mg of pyridoxine. One hypothesis is that γ-aminobutyric acid (GABA) inhibits synaptic transmission in the brain and, when at a reduced level due to pyridoxine deficiency, the threshold for irritability is lowered. Pyridoxine deficiency is seen in slow inactivators of isoniazid. Isoniazid is an antagonist of vitamin B_6.

Clinical features. Clinical characteristics include non-specific features such as insomnia, weakness, depression, cheilosis, stomatitis, dermatitis, peripheral neuropathy and seizures.

Diagnosis. The diagnosis should be considered in infants with convulsive disorders, microcytic–hypochromic anaemias unresponsive to iron, severe catabolic states, anorexia nervosa or food faddism.

Laboratory diagnosis. In pyridoxine deficiency the following are observed

1. Plasma pyridoxine <25 ng/ml.
2. Urinary excretion <10 µg pyridoxine/mg creatinine.
3. Urinary excretion 0.2 mg/day 4-pyridoxic acid.
4. Tryptophan load test — 50 mg/kg — maximum

of 2 g shows increased urinary excretion of xanthenuric acid (>10 mg/day).

Treatment. For convulsive disorders infants should be given 10 mg of pyridoxine intravenously or 10 mg/day for 1–2 weeks. Large doses of pyridoxine are not toxic to man but the synthetic analogue deoxypyridoxine is highly poisonous.

Vitamin B_{12} (cobalamin)

Megaloblastic anaemia arising from vitamin B_{12} deficiency is rare in childhood because, in normal circumstances, the fetus has built up a store sufficient to last for the first year of life. This vitamin is the largest of all vitamins (molecular weight of 1355) and is essential for a number of biochemical reactions including purine and pyrimidine metabolism as well as methionine and DNA synthesis.

Sources

The average daily content of vitamin B_{12} in breast milk is about 0.3 μg which is the amount suggested by the Food and Nutrition Board of the American National Research Council as the recommended dietary allowance for infants up to the age of 1 year with 1 μg for children 1–3 years, 1.5 μg for 4–6 years and 2 μg for those 7–10 years. As little as 0.1 μg of vitamin B_{12} will result in an haematological improvement. Sterilizing milk can reduce the vitamin B_{12} content by more than 75%.

A normal Western-style diet usually contains 5–10 μg/day. This water-soluble vitamin is synthesized by microorganisms and that is the sole source of the vitamin in animal foods. The highest concentrations are found in the liver (1 μg/g), kidney, shellfish and muscle meats. Human milk has a content of only 0.1 μg/100 g.

Deficiency states — inadequate ingestion

Strict vegetarians (those who abstain from meat, fowl, seafood, eggs, milk and dairy products) will develop vitamin B_{12} deficiency slowly over a period of years. However, a deficit will not develop if they are not strict vegetarians, i.e. if they are ovolactovegetarians (consumers of eggs and milk as well as vegetables) or if they ingest seaweed or vitamin B_{12}-fortified foods such as soybean milks or cereals. Vitamin B_{12} deficiency can occur in infants who are exclusively breast fed by strict vegetarian mothers not on supplements (Johnston,

1984). Followers of atypical or 'alternate' lifestyles (e.g. Zen macrobiotic diets) may have children at risk of developing particular nutritional disorders during certain phases of their dietary regimen and deaths have occurred.

Impaired absorption

There are both active and passive mechanisms for vitamin B_{12} absorption. The former method is dependent on gastric intrinsic factor and intact receptors in the terminal ileum. The site of passive absorption is the small intestine where pharmacological vitamin B_{12} preparations are taken-up in the mucosa. Adequate ileal absorption also requires normal pancreatic exocrine secretions.

Inadequate vitamin B_{12} absorption may be due to an absence of intrinsic factor (IF) in gastric parietal cells. In hereditary absence of IF, megaloblastic anaemia will develop by the age of about 3 years, when fetal stores will have become depleted. If hypothyroidism is associated with gastric damage, circulating antibodies to both parietal cells and IF may appear. Antibody to parietal cells confirms gastric mucosa damage but antibody to IF signals the presence of pernicious anaemia.

IF may be congenitally defective and therefore prevent the formation of a IF–Vitamin B_{12} complex. Megaloblastic anaemia can be secondary to small intestinal diseases (coeliac enteropathy, Crohn's regional enteritis, tuberculosis, lymphosarcoma of the ileum etc.). Medication such as neomycin and *p*-aminosalicylate if used for months can impede vitamin B_{12} absorption.

Intestinal parasites or bacteria can compete for available vitamin B_{12}, e.g. the fish tapeworm (*Diphyllobothrium latum*) is found in raw freshwater fish in Scandinavia, Japan, the Great Lake regions of Canada and America. Small bowel bacterial overgrowth, in the 'blind loop' or 'stagnant bowel' syndrome is associated with anatomical abnormalities of the small intestine such as diverticula, anastomoses and strictures. In the rare congenital autosomal recessive Imerslund–Gräsbeck syndrome (Gräsbeck *et al.*, 1960; Imerslund, 1960), there is defective transmembrane intestinal transport of vitamin B_{12} with benign proteinuria.

Defective transport and metabolism

Abnormalities of transcobalamin II: this is a very rare congenital but serious and potentially fatal disease because transcobalamin II is responsible for delivering vitamin B_{12} to the bone marrow and other tissues.

Transcobalamin I carries nearly all the vitamin B_{12} in the serum and binds it avidly before it is released. Absence of this globulin has been reported.

Vitamin B_{12} deficiency can be the result of a specific inability to form adenosylcobalamin or methylcobalamin (vitamin B_{12} responsive methylmalonic aciduria and vitamin B_{12} non-responsive methylmalonic aciduria, respectively).

Clinical manifestations

The onset of vitamin B_{12} deficiency is insidious. Pallor, apathy and fatigability are early symptoms and recurrent glossitis is common. Paraesthesiae are not rare even in the absence of an actual neuropathy. Episodic diarrhoea may become evident. The skin develops a 'lemon yellow' coloration. Signs of spinal cord degeneration are unusual and do not appear in folic acid deficiency.

Diagnosis

The blood smear and bone marrow film show a macrocytic megaloblastic anaemia. In vitamin B_{12} deficiency, the serum level is < 100 pg/ml (presence of antibiotics in patients may influence the microbiological assays). Vitamin B_{12} absorption tests will show if uptake is defective.

The Schilling test is used for the differential diagnosis of megaloblastic anaemias. The test involves giving oral radioactive vitamin B_{12} (0.5–2.0 µg) followed in 2 hours by an intramuscular injection of 1000 µg of non-radioactive vitamin B_{12} to saturate the vitamin B_{12}-binding protein and allow the oral radioactive vitamin to be excreted in the urine. Normal subjects excrete 10–35% of the administered dose and those with severe vitamin B_{12} malabsorption less than 3%. The Schilling test measures both the availability of IF and the intestinal phase of absorption. In pernicious anaemia the defect is compensated for by the addition of IF and vitamin B_{12} is then absorbed (Lanzkowsky, 1978). Assays for IF (in gastric juice) and antibodies for IF and parietal cells offer additional diagnostic techniques.

Treatment. This is 25–100 µg of vitamin B_{12} as the initial therapy (injection) followed by monthly injections of 50–100 µg.

Vitamin C (ascorbic acid)

Deficiency of this water-soluble vitamin results in scurvy, in which hydroxylation of collagen is impaired and as a result normal fibres cannot be formed, thereby producing skin lesions and fragile blood vessels. A vivid description of scurvy was given by Jacques Cartier in 1536 when his men were exploring the Saint Lawrence River:

'some did lose all their strength, and could not stand on their feet . . . . Others also had their skins spotted with spots of blood . . . . Their mouths became stinking, their gums so rotten that all the flesh did fall off, even to the roots of the teeth.'

Historically, long sea voyages in the sixteenth and seventeenth centuries were associated with ascorbic acid deficiency because of poor nutrition. In 1753, James Lind (1716–1794) who had been a naval surgeon published *A Treatise of the Scurvy* and demonstrated how fresh fruit or lemon juice could prevent the disease.

Vitamin C functions as a strong reducing agent and has multiple biochemical functions in man, such as the oxidation of phenylalanine, conversion of folic to folinic acid and cholesterol to bile acids. Ascorbic acid will destroy vitamin B_{12}. The average dietary intake is 50–150 mg/day and this results in a plasma level of 1.2 mg/100 ml.

Dietary sources are fresh fruits, vegetables and raw liver. Cooking results in the loss of much vitamin C. It is destroyed by both heat and oxidation.

Pasteurized and boiled milk contain little vitamin C. Food faddism and famine are important causes of scurvy. Infantile scurvy has appeared in infants fed exclusively cows' milk for 7–12 months (cows' milk contains 2 mg/100 ml; compare breast milk: 4–7 mg/100 ml).

Clinical features of deficiency

Haemorrhages beneath the long-bone periosteum, usually at the knees and ankles, cause painful and tender swellings. The child is irritable and lies still ('pseudoparalysis'), because slight movement causes pain and the thighs are positioned in abduction in the 'pithed frog position'. The costochondral junctions are prominent forming a rosary from subluxation of the sternum. This is dissimilar to the rosary in rickets in which there is expansion of the rib ends. Also haemorrhages may appear in the skin, the gums become spongy and swollen but are less affected than in adults. X-rays show a characteristic dense line of calcification at the metaphysis. The bones have a 'ground-glass' appearance and the epiphyses have a pencil outline or a ringed white margin. In advanced scurvy, red cells are found in the urine.

Diagnosis. In vitamin C deficiency the serum level is less than 0.2 mg/100 ml but plasma levels vary widely. In the buffy coat of centrifuged peripheral blood, the concentration is about 30 mg/100 ml. The ascorbic acid saturation test is based on the principle that, if the patient is not deficient, any vitamin C given will be excreted and recovered from the urine.

Treatment. Vitamin C 25 mg is given four times a day for 4–5 days then 25 mg twice a day until healing occurs. Large doses of vitamin C can interfere with vitamin B_{12} absorption.

Prevention. Vitamin C 30 mg/day for infants and 40–50 mg/day for pre-school children.

Folic acid (pteroylglutamic acid)

Folic acid (folate) deficiency is the commonest cause of megaloblastic anaemia in childhood and it is the parent compound of the structurally related folates. Tetrahydrofolate derivatives act as coenzymes and serve as donors of one-carbon units in a variety of biosyntheses such as amino acid and nucleotide metabolism. Folic acid is present in many plants and animal tissues. Foods with the highest folate concentrations include liver, kidney, nuts, fresh green and yellow leafy vegetables and legumes. Liver is a very rich source (300 µg/100 g).

Body stores of folate at birth are small and can be rapidly depleted (Vanier and Tyas, 1966) as a result of growth especially in small prematures. The maintenance dose to prevent deficiency in prematures is 0.05–0.1 mg/day.

Deficiency

The infant's needs for folic acid are only just met by human or cows' milk both of which are poor sources and contain about 54 µg/l (Ford and Scott, 1968). However, goats' milk has an even lower content and can cause 'goats' milk anaemia'. Boiling milk reduces the folate by about 50%. Unlike vitamin B_{12}, which is not easily destroyed, folate is removed by oxidative processes especially cooking. The central nervous system of the developing fetus needs folate.

Primary causes. Malnutrition, food faddism, use of goats' milk, boiling of folate foods etc.

Secondary causes. Malabsorption due to reduced surface area of small bowel and/or mucosal damage, e.g. coeliac disease, tropical sprue or extensive resection of the small bowel. Some anticonvulsants (diphenylhydantoins) block the absorption of folate, but large doses of folic acid, if given, antagonize the anticonvulsant drugs and cause more seizures.

Increased folate needs. Infants with nutritional problems, especially the prematures and those who have had haemolytic anaemia, will need extra folic acid. Various types of infection are associated with folate deficiency especially if of a chronic nature such as pulmonary tuberculosis. Malignancy because of rapidly growing tissues will increase the need for folic acid. Folate analogues, such as methotrexate, pyrimethamine and trimethoprim interfere with the conversion of dihydrofolate to the active form.

Clinical features. Anaemia, glossitis, splenomegaly (in one-third), leucopenia, thrombocytopenia, and mental changes such as irritability are some of the characteristics.

Diagnosis. Megaloblasts are present in both the bone marrow and the buffy coat of centrifuged peripheral blood. A reduced red cell folate (normal 160–640 ng/ml) is a better measure of the deficiency disorder than a low plasma folate (normal 6–21 ng/ml), because the latter reflects recent dietary sources of folate over the previous 3 weeks.

Therapy. Folic acid (pterolyglutamic acid) 0.5–1.0 mg daily.

Minerals and trace elements

Many minerals and some trace elements are known or are suspected of having an important role in nutrition (Table 1.1) (Aggett, 1985):

1. Calcium/phosphorus: 99% of total body calcium is in bone.
2. Chromium: optimizes glucose tolerance.
3. Copper: essential for many enzymes, e.g. oxidases.
4. Iodine: required for thyroid hormones.
5. Iron: haemoglobin contains 60–70% and myoglobin 10% of body iron.
6. Magnesium: found in bone and acts as a cofactor in oxidative phosphorylation.

Table 1.1 Functions and sources of minerals

Element	Functions	Dietary sources in the UK	
		Good	Poor
Calcium	Part of skeleton, mainly in the form of hydroxyapatite $3Ca_3(PO_4)_2$, $Ca(OH)_2$ Found inside and outside body cells, and bound to membranes Triggers muscle contraction Activates enzymes, e.g. phosphorylase (glycolysis),prothrombin (blood clotting)	Milk, cheese, yoghourt Small fish eaten with bones Eggs Pulses, nuts and chocolate White flour (added)	Butter, double cream White fish Meat Most fruits and vegetables Rice, sugar, fats and oils
Magnesium	Forms part of bone Found mainly inside body cells, within mitochondria Cofactor for enzymes concerned with energy transfer	Green vegetables Pulses, nuts and chocolate Wholemeal cereals Fish and shellfish	Fruits, Sugar, fats and oils White flours and rice
Phosphorus	Forms part of bone, as hydroxyapatite Found inside and outside body cells and part of membranes Part of nucleic acids DNA and RNA Part of ADP−ATP energy transporting system within cell Component of phospholipids (transport of lipids) Involved in maintainence of acid−base balance	Similar foods to calcium Added to foods during processing	Butter, double cream Fruits Rice, sugar, fats and oils
Sodium	Some found in bone Found in extracellular fluid Regulates acid−base balance of extracellular fluid Maintains osmotic pressure of extracellular fluid Involved in transmission of nerve impulses Alters cell membrane permeability, e.g. glucose absorption by gut and uptake by cells, relaxation of muscle fibres	Table salt Added to foods during processing Milk, cheese and eggs	Fruits and vegetables Cereals Fish and meat Sugar, fats and oils
Potassium	Found mainly inside body cells Small amount in extracellular fluid Regulates acid−base balance of intracellular fluid Maintains osmotic pressure of intracellular fluid Influences muscle activity, particularly cardiac muscle	Fruits and vegetables, Wholemeal cereals Milk, cheese and eggs Meat and fish Pulses and nuts	Sugar, fats and oils Rice Butter

Table 1.1 *(Contd)*

Element	Functions	Dietary sources in the UK	
		Good	Poor
Chloride	Found in intra- and extracellular fluid Part of hydrochloric acid in stomach Maintains acid–base balance in blood Maintains osmotic pressure of intra- and extracellular fluid	Similar foods to sodium	As for sodium
Iron	High concentrations in liver, spleen and bone marrow Part of blood haemoglobin and muscle myoglobin Important in storage and transport of iron Part of enzyme systems, e.g. xanthine oxidase (uric acid metabolism), lysyl hydroxylase (collagen synthesis)	Liver and red meats Eggs Pulses and chocolate Whole grain cereals White bread and breakfast cereals (added)	Milk and cheese Fish Non-leafy vegetables Rice and fruits Sugar, fats and oils

Table 1.2 Functions and sources of trace elements

Element	Functions	Dietary sources in the UK	
		Good	Poor
Copper	High concentrations in liver, brain, kidney and heart Part of plasma protein ceruloplasmin — many functions, e.g. incorporation of iron into transferrin Part of several enzymes, e.g. cytochrome oxidase (energy transfer in cells)	Green vegetables Fish and shellfish Liver Pulses, nuts, chocolate	Non-leafy vegetables Meat and milk Sugar, fats and oils Refined cereals
Zinc	High concentrations in liver, kidney, heart and muscle Part of 200 enzymes Necessary for normal growth and sexual maturation Important for tissue repair Involved in protein and fatty acid metabolism Necessary for entry of glucose into cells and glycolysis Stabilizes intracellular membranes	Oyster and shellfish Meats Whole grain cereals Nuts	Fruits and non-leafy vegetables Sugars, fats and oils Refined cereals

Table 1.2 (*Contd*)

Element	Functions	Dietary sources in the UK	
		Good	Poor
Manganese	High concentrations in liver, pancreas, kidney, heart Part of some enzymes, e.g. pyruvate decarboxylase (glycolysis) Activates several enzymes, e.g. glycosyl transferase (polysaccharide synthesis)	Tea Pulses and nuts Whole grain cereals	Milk Meats Refined cereals Sugar, fats and oils
Chromium	Widely distributed throughout tissues Potentiates insulin activity — 'glucose tolerance factor' Involved in lipid (cholesterol) metabolism	Brewer's yeast and beer Egg yolk	Milk White meats
Selenium	Higher concentrations in liver, kidney and heart Part of enzymes, e.g. glutathione peroxidase (protects cell membrane from oxidation) Interacts with vitamin E	Wholemeal cereals Liver Meat and fish	Refined cereals Sugar, fats and oils Milk Vegetables and fruit
Molybdenum	Distributed throughout soft tissues Part of enzymes, e.g. xanthine oxidase (uric acid and iron metabolism) Interacts with sulphur metabolism	Wholemeal cereals Pulses Vegetables (dependent on soil levels)	Refined cereals Sugar, fats and oils
Iodine	Concentrated in thyroid gland; also in ovaries and parotids Part of thyroid hormones — thyroxine and triiodothyronine Thyroid hormones control rate of cell metabolism Connected with metabolism and integrity of connective tissue	Fish and shellfish Meat and eggs Dairy products Vegetables (dependent on soil levels)	Fruits Cereals Sugar, fats and oils
Cobalt	Part of vitamin B_{12}	Green vegetables Live and kidney	Dairy products Refined cereals

7. Manganese: activates many enzyme systems, e.g. hydroxylases, kinases.
8. Zinc: required by a great many enzymes, e.g. superoxide dismutase, alkaline phosphatase.
9. In addition, sodium, potassium and chloride are needed for maintenance of water balance.

The following trace elements are also necessary:

1. Cobalt (as cobalamin): in vitamin B_{12}.
2. Selenium: antioxidant in intracellular defence.
3. Molybdenum: for sulphur and purine metabolism.
4. Fluorine: in dentine formation.

It is likely that this list will be expanded as the understanding of the role trace elements play in biosynthesis develops. Other trace elements which could be essential include: arsenic, boron, bromine, lithium, nickel, silicone, tin and vanadium. Two-thirds of the mineral content of the term newborn is acquired in the last 3 months of gestation.

Zinc

Adequate zinc is essential for normal development and there are many zinc-dependent enzyme systems, e.g. thymidine kinase and carbonic anhydrase. Zinc depletion may cause congenital malformations of the central nervous system. This metal is required for keratogenesis, osteogenesis, development of the immune system and sexual maturation (Hambidge, 1976).

The zinc content of the fetus increases by approximately 300 μg/kg per day during the last 4 months of gestation (Shaw, 1973).

Treatment of deficiency

Treatment should be given with 0.5—1.0 mg Zn/kg daily. For those on prolonged intravenous feeding the rate should be 50 μg/kg daily. Excessive zinc can cause copper deficiency.

Copper

Copper also has an important function within numerous enzyme systems, e.g. cytochrome oxidase. Deficiency of copper will lead to microcytic hypochromic anaemia which is not responsive to iron therapy and which has a skeletal pathology not dissimilar to scurvy or non-accidental injury. Copper-containing ferroxidases, including ceruloplasmin, are required for the oxidation of ferrous salts in the intestinal mucosa and body stores of the reticuloendothelial system to a ferric state. The chief global causes of copper depletion are: malnutrition; malabsorption; diarrhoea; prematurity.

Term infants are not at risk of encountering copper deficiency because of their adequate stores. Cows' milk is a poor source of dietary copper and has less than half the copper content of human milk (Appendix II.10).

Other features of copper deficiency are skin/hair depigmentation, dermatitis, anorexia, dilated superficial veins, diarrhoea, failure to thrive, apnoea, hypotonia and psychomotor retardation.

The recommended daily intake for prophylaxis in low-birth-weight infants is 50—90 μg/kg per day (Cordano, 1978).

Menkes' steely-hair or kinky-hair syndrome is a rare X-linked recessive metabolic disorder due to impaired gastrointestinal transport of copper (Danks *et al.*, 1973) which, in the absence of early diagnosis and treatment, eventually results in severe neurological deterioration and death. The characteristic sign is the secondary growth of hair which lacks lustre and breaks off easily leaving stubble that feels like 'steely' hair. In addition to this the facies are said to be characteristic, the eyebrows are 'tangled' and the upper lip is in the shape of 'Cupid's bow'. Other clinical features are hypothermia, poor feeding, frequent infections, transient jaundice, seizures and death before the age of 3 years.

Chromium

Chromium deficiency is seen in protein—energy malnutrition and can be corrected by a single dose of 250 μg chromium salt. An impaired glucose tolerance test may be the only clue to the diagnosis. Chromium is a cofactor for and forms a complex with insulin. Daily requirements are 2 μg/kg.

2

Dehydration and Enteritis

Diarrhoea consists of the discharge of undigested food in a fluid state; [such as] when the heat does not digest the food, nor convert it into its proper chyme, but leaves its work half finished. For it is liquid and wants consistence from not being completely elaborated, and from no part of the digestive process having been properly done, except the commencement.

Aretaeus; The Cappadocian
(Second–third century AD)

.... Too much stress can be put on poverty as a prime cause of diseases and malnutrition, but poverty of knowledge and initiative is, in nearly every case, as important as poverty of material possessions. .... Williams and Jelliffe, 1972.

Intestinal infections are not only a major cause of childhood fatalities in less developed communities, they are also responsible for a significant morbidity in Europe, North and South America and Scandinavia (McLaren and Cutting, 1986). Some very simple environmental and educational measures, especially the promotion of breast feeding, would do much to lower the global incidence of enteritis (Bellanti, 1983). Prevention of diarrhoeal disease will achieve more than that which can be accomplished through treatment. A major WHO policy is aimed at an expanded measles immunization programme. There is a significant mortality in children with dysentery following measles. New and improved vaccines are proposed against rotavirus and cholera. In countries with endemic cholera, the latter would have a major impact. The provision of safe and uncontaminated water supplies, better sanitation and improved hygiene all play a role in combating childhood diarrhoea. The simple measure of adequate hand washing will reduce the secondary attack rate of diarrhoea within a family by 85% (Ebrahim, 1987).

There are a number of factors which have a protective role against acute intestinal infections.

1. Gastric acid is bactericidal.
2. Reduced gastric emptying results in greater exposure to an acid environment.
3. Small bowel motility — rapid peristalsis is a protective ('flushing action') in that it shortens the contact time between the intestinal mucosa and the organisms or toxins. For this reason opiates, codeine and diphenoxylate are contra-indicated in therapy.
4. Indigenous flora compete with the pathogens for available nutrients. — Lactoferrin, the iron-carrying protein in human milk, plays an important role in reducing infections in breast-fed infants by preventing *E. coli* multiplication.
5. Immune system of the intestine (Thomas and Jewell, 1979; Stites *et al.*, 1984): secretory IgA is a rich source of specific antibody and it is this dimer of IgA which offers the prime means of immunological protection of the gut. Intestinal lysozymes can lyse particular bacteria. Aggregated intestinal lymphoid tissue, intestinal mucus which restricts bacterial adherence to the mucosa, macrophages, complement, bile and short-chain fatty acids are all involved in the pathogenesis of enteritis.
6. Breast milk contains both humoral and cellular agents.

Pathophysiology

The virulence of an organism will influence the severity of the clinical illness. Acute bacterial intestinal infections are caused by either the production of a toxin and/or the organism invading the mucosa (*see* p. 20). Some organisms, e.g. staphylococci, can elaborate a toxin which is then ingested and is itself pathogenic rather than the actual microbe. Alternatively, the toxin is formed after ingestion (e.g. *E. coli* — ETEC, *see under* Bacterial infections).

Transport of water and electrolytes

The net flow of water across the intestine represents the difference between undirectional flux from the lumen to the interstitial fluid and the opposite flux into the bowel lumen. This is a passive phenomenon accompanying solute movement. Intestinal mucosal cells are bound together by tight junctions at their apical borders and, if water is absorbed, most of it must pass through the tight junctions. Glucose and sodium share a common receptor site on the microvilli of the membranes and are transferred into the intercellular spaces. Sodium movement into the cell is either coupled with chloride or solute absorption.

Watery diarrhoea can be the consequence of toxins which activate cAMP (cyclic 3′:5′-adenosine monophosphate) or cGMP (cyclic 3′:5′-guanosine monophosphate). These biochemical messengers inhibit sodium chloride co-transport into the cell and induce chloride secretion into the bowel lumen, (Booth and Harries, 1984).

Mechanisms of diarrhoea

Diarrhoea can arise from destruction of the epithelial cells of the villi which then prevents water and electrolyte absorption. Alternatively, enteritis can be caused by a toxin stimulating an active secretory process, as shown, for example, in cholera. Absorptive processes are located on epithelial cells and secretory processes in the crypts of Lieberkühn. cAMP is formed from ATP (adenosine triphosphate) by the action of the membrane-bound enzyme adenylate cyclase. cAMP influences a wide range of cellular processes (Stryer, 1975). Toxins increase the adenylate cyclase activity of the mucosal membranes leading to elevated levels of cAMP. As a result, cAMP stimulates chloride secretion in the crypts and inhibits absorption of sodium chloride in the villi. Vasoactive intestinal polypeptide (VIP), prostaglandins, deconjugated bile acids and hydroxy fatty acids are all able to stimulate mucosal cAMP. It is not only cholera toxin that raises intracellular levels of adenylate cyclase; *Escherichia coli*-induced (heat labile enterotoxin) diarrhoea is mediated in a similar manner (Figs 2.1–2.3).

Non-cAMP mechanisms, i.e. the enzyme

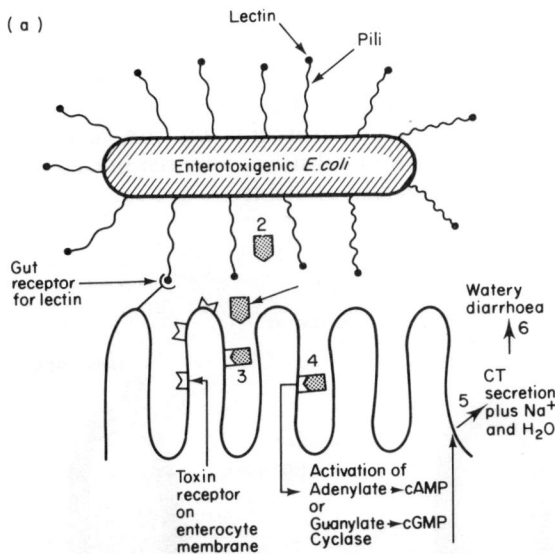

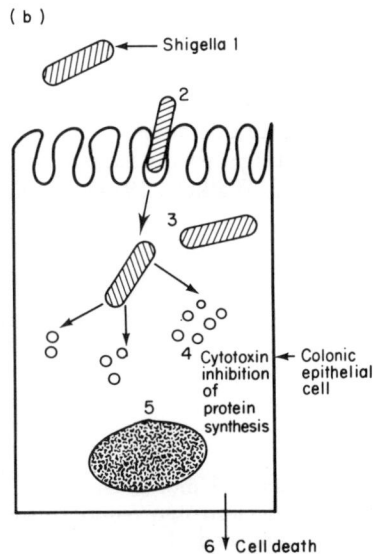

Fig. 2.1 (a) Pathogenesis of watery diarrhoea due to enterotoxigenic *E. coli* (ETEC). These organisms (1) attach to the intestinal epithelium by a lectin (specific sugar-binding protein) on filamentous appendages known as pili, which interact directly with a receptor on the microvillus membrane; (2) then secrete a toxin(s) which binds to another specific intestinal receptor (3), which activates intracellular enzymes (4) to produce second messengers (cAMP and cGMP). These open chloride channels in the apical membrane (5) resulting in secretion of chloride and sodium ions and water, finally resulting in (6) watery diarrhoea. (b) Pathogenesis of shigella dysentery. (1) *Shigella* sp. multiplies within the intestinal lumen and directly invades (2) the apical membrane of epithelial cells of the colon. Following intracellular multiplication (3), the organism produces a potent cytotoxin (4) which is a powerful inhibitor of protein synthesis (5). This ultimately leads to cell death (6), epithelial cell loss and ulceration. (By permission of Dr MJG Farthing (1987) and the Medical Tribune Group.)

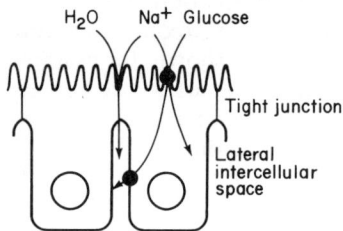

Fig. 2.2 Enterocytes showing receptor sites to glucose-coupled sodium transport. (Modified after Turnberg LA, 1978, Water and electrolyte metabolism, in *Scientific Foundations of Gastroenterology*, W Sircus and AN Smith, eds, WB Saunders, Philadelphia.)

guanylate cyclase will increase cellular levels of the ribonucleotide guanosine monophosphate. Guanosine cyclase is stimulated by the heat-stable (ST) enterotoxin of enterotoxigenic E. coli (ETEC).

Normally, the concentration of sodium in the enterocyte is lower than within the bowel lumen as a result of an electrochemical gradient which is maintained by sodium–potassium ATPase. This enzyme is located on the basolateral membrane and is responsible for the 'sodium pump'. Sodium–potassium ATPase can be inhibited by deoxycholate, the latter being formed when anaerobic bacteria deconjugate bile acids.

For further reading into mechanisms of diarrhoea see Gryboski and Walker (1983), Walker-Smith and McNeish (1986), Silverman and Roy (1983), Lebenthal (1984), Bellanti (1983), and Francis (1986, 1987).

Bacterial infections

Vibrio cholerae

In cholera there is an acute secretory diarrhoea that can rapidly cause severe dehydration because of the vast stool volume (5–15 l/day). The stools have a sodium content of 125 mmol/l and are described as 'rice-water', because they contain no solid material. Contaminated water and food are the major sources of this toxin-producing organism. The organism is readily destroyed by gastric acid and is more common in conditions of hypochlorhydria.

Sodium–solute–coupled 'cotransportive' absorptive mechanism remains intact and oral rehydration with a salt/glucose preparation is feasible and the preferred option in the absence of circulatory collapse. Tetracyclines can accelerate the disappearance of stool vibrios and diminish both the volume and duration of the diarrhoea.

Diagnosis. Stool microscopy will not reveal any cells. Special stool culture is essential but facilities may not be readily available.

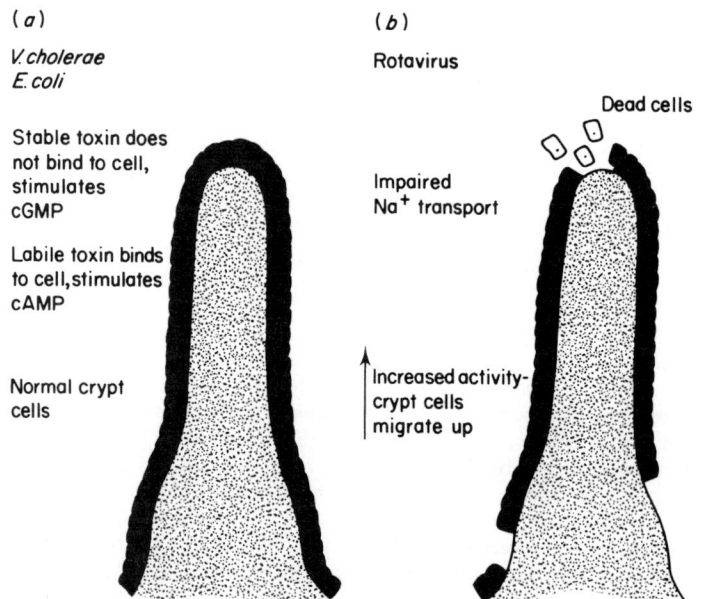

Fig. 2.3 (a) Normal cell morphology. Water and electrolyte secretions are stimulated by cAMP and cGMP. (b) Cells of villi damaged by rotavirus infection. Epithelial cells are disrupted and replaced by immature crypt cells in which there is defective electrolyte transport. The impaired sodium transport of immature cells combined with the decreased activity of ATPase contributes to malabsorption. (From Gryboski and Walker, 1983.)

Escherichia coli

Diarrhoea from *E. coli* can cause outbreaks in
nurseries and is an important source of acute enteritis
in non-industrialized countries. This organism plays
a major role in traveller's diarrhoea. *E. coli* enteritis
is very rare in breast-fed infants. Most enteroinvasive
E. coli serotypes are different from those identified
in enteropathogenic and enterotoxigenic infections.

	Enteropathogenic (EPEC)	Enterotoxigenic (ETEC)	Enteroinvasive (EIC)
Site	duodenum + jejunum	duodenum + jejunum	large bowel
Toxin	?	+ (ST and/or LT)	?
Invasive	0	0	+

ST = heat stable
LT = heat labile toxin

Management. The principle of treatment is to replace lost water and electrolytes. Antibiotics are
not normally indicated. Good cross-barrier nursing
techniques are essential to avoid transmission of
the organism to other babies and infants.

Shigellosis

One type of shigellosis is known as bacillary dysentery because the stools contain blood, mucus
and pus (*Shigella shiga*). Transmission is by person-
to-person or food/water contamination. Flies can
transmit this microbe, but only man is the host,
unlike salmonellosis. Antibiotics are only used in
those who are seriously ill. Shigellosis involves the
colon and is a self-limiting disease.

Other important organisms causing enteritis are:
Salmonella sp., *Yersinia enterocolitica* (previously
known as *Pasteurella pseudotuberculosis*) which
because of its associated severe abdominal pain and
fever can pose as acute appendicitis. Campylobacter
enteritis has only relatively recently come to the
attention of paediatricians, although it was well
known to veterinary surgeons. This acute bowel
disease can mimic both inflammatory disease of
the colon and even obstruction (Bentley *et al.*,
1985).

Salmonellosis is usually transmitted through food,
such as meat, milk, shellfish and eggs. Domestic
pets must always be considered as a source of the
pathogen especially if a tortoise is in the household,
but cats, dogs and parakeets can also act as reser-
voirs. In salmonellosis, septicaemia and severe
neurological signs can be the dominant features.

Viral gastroenteritis

Viruses are a very common cause of acute enteritis,
particularly the rotavirus (formerly known as reo-,
orbi- or duovirus). Rotavirus was identified from
biopsied duodenal mucosa by Bishop in Australia
(Bishop *et al.*, 1973). In the developed world group
F adenoviruses (serotypes 40 and 41) are the commonest virus after rotaviruses to cause infantile
gastroenteritis (Wood, 1988). There are many other
virus particles which can cause acute intestinal
disease such as adenovirus, astrovirus, calicivirus
and parvovirus-like particles (Norwalk agent).
Electron microscopy has enabled a rapid diagnosis
to be made but the ELISA technique (enzyme-
linked immunosorbent assay, e.g. 'Rotazyme' by
Abbott Laboratories, Illinois) permits quick
identification without sophisticated microscopes
and is said to be more sensitive than electron
microscopy (Kovacs *et al.*, 1987). The electron
microscope allows many viruses with a characteristic
morphology to be recognized (e.g. astrovirus —
'star-like'; rota — 'wheel-like'; corona — 'crown-
like' etc.)

Rotavirus infections peak in winter. No specific
therapy is needed but hydration must be
adequate.

Fifty per cent of those infants or children with
rotavirus enteritis have glucose malabsorption.

Other agents with a similar size to Norwalk
agent are Hawaiian and Montgomery County
(MC) particles.

Mechanisms of the diarrhoea

Immature crypt cells migrate to the tips of the villi
and, because they function abnormally, cannot
absorb water and electrolytes.

Parasitic infections

Protozoa — giardiasis

Giardia lamblia is a protozoon which was discovered

by Leeuwenhoek in 1681 in his own stool. Person-to-person transmission and water contamination represent the main sources. To diagnose giardiasis, a number of fresh stools have to be examined; however, microscopy of a specimen of duodenal fluid is a more rewarding technique. Small bowel biopsy tissue not invariably shows the trophozoites upon haematoxylin and eosin stain. Formerly, metronidazole (35–50 mg/kg per day for 10 days — although 3 days is usually successful) was the favoured treatment, but quinacrine (6 mg/kg per day — maximum 300 mg/day — for 5 days) has many advocates.

Other infections that must be considered include amoebiasis, which often mirrors inflammatory bowel disease. *Strongyloides stercoralis* may be asymptomatic but can cause malabsorption and examination of fresh duodenal fluid is one of the best means of diagnosis. Treatment is with thiobendazole 25 mg/kg, twice a day for 3 days. The other major nematode (roundworm) is *Ascaris lumbricoides*. Important cestodes (tapeworms) are *Taenia saginata* and *T. solium* (beef and pork tapeworms), *Hymenolepis nana* (commonest tapeworm in the USA), *Diphyllobothrium latum* (fish tapeworm) and *Echinococcus granulosus* and *E. multilocularis* (hydatid disease). *Candida albicans*, a normal inhabitant of the human small bowel, is the commonest fungus to cause gastrointestinal disease especially in the immunologically compromised.

Diarrhoea with or without vomiting can readily lead to a state of dehydration (Fig. 2.4). A malnourished infant will be less able to tolerate an episode of acute enteritis than a previously healthy child. The severity and prevalence of dehydration is greater in the less developed countries than in the industrialized nations. Babies and infants within an impoverished home, exposed to poor sanitation, ignorance of hygiene, polluted water supplies and possible infestation, are very vulnerable to a variety of pathogens in their environment.

Acute dehydration

This term includes isotonic, hypotonic and hypertonic dehydration — a classification which depends upon the proportions of water and sodium loss and the sodium concentration in the plasma and extracellular fluid. It is important to define the cause and extent of dehydration because this will influence both the choice of fluid and the rate of replacement. The most accurate method of assessing the degree of dehydration is to estimate acute weight loss which will equal the amount of fluid lost. Where a recent pre-illness weight is unknown or cannot be determined from the child's birth weight centile and present age, then the clinical signs should be assessed (Fig. 2.5). In the first instance the aim must always be to correct dehydration by the oral route because this is more physiological and safer than parenteral methods.

Choice of intravenous fluids

In the presence of circulatory collapse with severe dehydration, intravenous therapy is indicated. There is a considerable variety of electrolyte solutions that can be used for the resuscitation of acutely dehydrated infants (*see* Appendix II.15). In hypovolaemia, the intravascular compartment must be expanded and blood, plasma or plasma expanders have less of a short-term impact than electrolyte

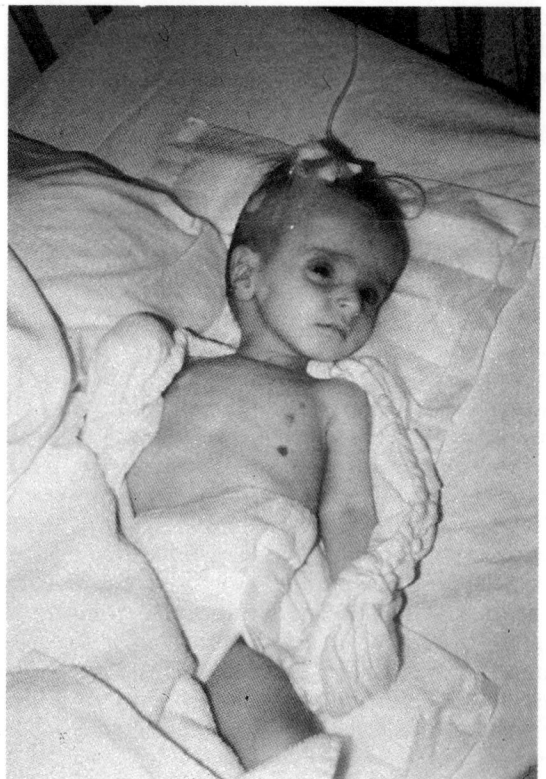

Fig. 2.4 A severely dehydrated child — note tribal 'therapeutic' burns.

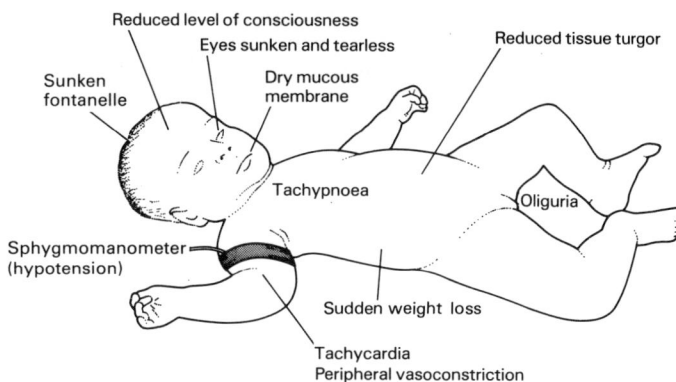

Fig. 2.5 The clinical signs of acute dehydration syndrome.

preparations. Electrolyte solutions are commonly at hand; the following alternatives are suggested:

1. Sodium chloride (0.9%) in 5% glucose.
2. Sodium chloride (0.9%) without glucose (particularly indicated in diabetic ketoacidosis).
3. Lactate Ringer's solution (Hartmann's solution is similar).
4. Dextran 70 (plasma expander) (molecular weight 70 000).
5. Human plasma protein fraction (HPPF) 4.3%.
6. Human albumin 20% ('salt poor').
7. Blood.

Physiological saline has a high sodium content and a low pH (6.1) when contrasted with plasma (pH 7.35−7.45). Optimal use of physiological saline is in the presence of acute fluid loss.

Ringer's solution: this preparation has an ionic composition resembling plasma but can cause lactic acidosis — the pH is 6.5. Dextran is a synthetic colloid made up of inert polysaccharides with an average molecular weight of 40 000 (Dextran 400) or 7000 (Dextran 70). Smaller molecules enter the renal tubules and can cause acute tubular necrosis in the presence of impaired renal blood flow (Yates, 1987).

Albumin solutions are held in the plasma space and depending upon their oncotic activity draw fluid into the microcirculation. Albumin preparations are free from hepatitis B virus and human immunodeficiency virus (HIV). The use of albumin is inappropriate for hypovolaemic shock unless there is also albumin deficiency.

Do not use 0.18% sodium chloride in 4% glucose (hypotonic, therefore sodium is too low) or Darrow's solution (potassium too high, 36 mmol/l).

Isotonic dehydration (= sodium of 131−149 mmol/l)

This problem occurs when equal proportions of water and sodium are lost causing a reduction of the extracellular fluid and subsequently a drop in the glomerular filtration with a resulting rise in urea. For clinical features *see* p. 29.

Causes

Enteritis, diabetes mellitus, intestinal obstruction and heat exhaustion are the usual causes.

Management

Mild dehydration (5% weight loss or less than 50 ml/kg) can be managed with oral fluids only in the absence of persistent vomiting. Moderate dehydration is where the loss is about 10% of the body weight or 100 ml/kg. In severe dehydration there is a 15% fall in body weight. Prior to treatment, where feasible, the pH, volume and osmolality of body fluids and intra- and extracellular alterations of electrolytes and water should be ascertained (Table 2.1).

Intravenous regimen

During the first 4 hours fluid should be infused rapidly (10−40 ml/kg per hour) and during the subsequent 8 hours at a rate of 6−15 ml/kg per hour depending upon the severity of the dehydration. Table 2.1 gives details of suggested infusion rates.

Table 2.1 Isotonic dehydration: rate and volume of intravenous infusion

Severity (loss of body weight)	Deficit (ml/kg)	0−1 hours (ml/kg)	2−3 hours (ml/kg)	4−8 (or 9) hours (ml/kg)	8 (or 9)−24 hours (ml/kg)
Mild (5%)	50	10 (10 ml/kg per h)	20 (6 ml/kg per h)	25 (4 h at 6 ml/kg per h)	100 (16 h at 6 ml/kg per h)
Moderate (10%)	100	20 (20 ml/kg per h)	30 (10 ml/kg per h)	50 (5 h at 10 ml/kg per h)	90 (15 h at 6 ml/kg per h)
Severe (15%)	150	30−40 (30−40 ml/kg per h)	45 (15 ml/kg per h)	75 (5 h at 15 ml/kg per h)	90 (15 h at 6 ml/kg per h)

From J.A. Black (1979) *Paediatric Emergencies*, p. 97, London, Butterworths, with permission.

Hypertonic (hypernatraemic) dehydration
(plasma sodium ⩾ 150 mmol/l)

This occurs when the greater proportion of the loss is water rather than sodium and the body water is maldistributed. The high osmolality of plasma and extracellular fluid (ECF) draws water from cells causing intracellular dehydration and shrinkage which, in the case of brain cells, may produce cerebral haemorrhage and fits. Seizures following rehydration are probably caused by re-entry of water into brain cells when the osmolality of the plasma and ECF is lowered. For a helpful review of this topic *see* Paneth (1980).

Recognition

The skin turgor is dough like and the anterior fontanelle may be bulging rather than sunken. Irritability, stupor and hyperventilation may be evident. The diagnosis may easily be missed in obese infants.

Causes

High solute loads in feeds, enteritis with high sodium intake, salicylate toxicity, hyperventilation, prolonged fever, water deprivation, extensive burns, hyperosmolar enema solutions and prematurity (which is characterized by immature renal function and a relatively large body surface area to weight) can all be causes.

In the UK, high solute milks were replaced by safer feeds of low solute content from the mid-1970s and guidelines were issued by the Department of Health and Social Security. Guidelines have been issued by many bodies including the American Academy of Pediatrics, Committee on Nutrition, the Codex Alimentarius Commission of the Food and Agriculture Organization and the World Health Organisation, and the European Society of Paediatric Gastroenterology and Nutrition, regarding the desired composition and marketing of infant milks/feeds.

Management

The first step is to assess the infant's pre-illness weight. Knowing the birth weight and present age, the approximate weight can be calculated from the centile lines of growth charts. Expected weight (or predicted) minus actual weight = fluid loss.

The keynote of management in hypernatraemia is to allow a slow and very gradual fall in plasma sodium — 15 mmol/l per day. Failure to follow this principle will provoke seizures. Shock and hypotension are uncommon and rapid expansion of the plasma volume is rarely needed. Although hyperglycaemia may be present (because of a co-existing acidosis), insulin is contraindicated because it might provoke cerebral oedema by adjusting the blood glucose too rapidly.

Replacement

Phase I   (0–4 hours): initial deficit usually 50 ml/kg — half of this loss (25 ml/kg every 4 hours or 6 ml/kg per hour) should be replaced.

Phase II   (4–8 hours): replace remaining deficit of 25 ml/kg over 4 hours (= 6 ml/kg per hour).

Phase III (8–24 hours): if hypernatraemia persists use 0.45% sodium chloride in 2.5% glucose.

Choice of fluid

This topic is controversial. In the presence of shock use plasma in the initial 4-hour period, otherwise 0.9% sodium chloride without glucose.

Hypotonic (hyponatraemia) dehydration
(plasma sodium ≤ 130 mmol/l)

Hypotonic dehydration arises when the sodium loss exceeds that of water. It is not uncommon in malnourished infants who develop gastroenteritis and has recently been reported in well nourished infants in the USA (Finberg, 1986). Because of a reduction of extracellular fluid and plasma volume shock develops rapidly after a short illness with diarrhoea. This form of dehydration is accompanied by a fall in plasma osmolality.

Causes

Acute adrenal failure, cystic fibrosis, heat exhaustion and gastroenteritis can be responsible for this condition.

Management

Phase I   If shocked give isotonic saline (0.9% sodium chloride) in 5% glucose at 20 ml/kg per hour. Where severely shocked and hypotensive give plasma 10–20 ml/kg per hour.

Phase II   (4–8 hours): if plasma sodium ≤ 130 mmol/l, continue with 0.9% sodium chloride in 5% glucose or 0.45% sodium chloride in 2.5% glucose if plasma sodium is normal.

Do not give potassium if there is evidence of hypoadrenalism. If hyponatraemia persists and hyperkalaemia (in the absence of potassium supplements) is present, consider the need for a salt-retaining steroid and a diagnosis of congenital adrenal hyperplasia.

Oral rehydration fluids

It was reported in *The Lancet* (1983) that the annual world supply of 40 million sachets for oral rehydration therapy was sufficient for only 2% of acute diarrhoeal episodes. This contrasts with 170 million packages distributed in 1984 and held responsible for saving the lives of half a million children every year (Morley, 1985) (Fig. 2.6). Less developed countries producing oral rehydration salts are listed in Table 2.2.

Whenever possible rehydration should be by the oral route. Studies have shown that oral regimens are safe and effective (Tamer et al., 1985) in all but the most severely shocked or dehydrated child, although treatment of the dehydrated neonate is less well documented. Infants who are vomiting can be successfully treated with half-hourly feeds of a very small volume providing that vomiting is not severe. Oral clear fluids should contain sodium, potassium, carbohydrate and base ions. However, the quantity and balance of ingredients is ill-defined. The World Health Organisation has recommended the adoption of a universal salt mixture (WHO ORS) for adults and children with diarrhoea (for compiled data *see* WHO, 1980). The composition of the recommended mixture is given in Table 2.3. This recommendation is not accepted by all paediatricians, some of whom feel that various formulae should be available for different types of enteritis. However, a standard ORS does simplify universal management (Tripp and Candy, 1984). For well-nourished infants a solution with a lower sodium concentration of 40/50 mmol/l for maintenance and 75 mmol/l to correct a deficit has been advocated, and a trial comparing two rehydration fluids with 90 and 75 mmol/l sodium has shown them to be equally effective (Pizarro et al., 1987). In two multicentre trials in London, in which the rotavirus was the commonest pathogen, electrolyte solutions of differing sodium content were compared for efficacy (Sandhu, 1987a, b). The compounds studied were WHO formula (sodium 90 mmol/l), and the commercial preparations Dioralyte (Armour

Table 2.2 Less developed countries producing oral rehydration salts

Region	Country
Africa	Burundi
	Ethiopia
	Kenya
	Lesotho
	Mozambique
	Burkina-Faso*
	Zaire
Americas	Argentina
	Brazil
	Colombia
	Costa Rica
	Dominican Republic
	El Salvador
	Haiti
	Honduras
	Mexico
	Paraguay
	Peru
	Venezuela
Eastern Mediterranean	Afghanistan
	Egypt
	Iran (Islamic Republic of)
	Pakistan
	Syrian Arab Republic
	Tunisia
Europe	Morocco
South-east Asia	Bangladesh*
	Burma
	India
	Indonesia
	Nepal
	Mongolia*
	Thailand
Western Pacific	China*
	Kampuchea*
	Malaysia
	Philippines
	Republic of Korea

* Indicates a cottage industry approach.
Source: WHO/CDD/84. 10 World Heath Organisation, Geneva, 1984.

Pharmaceutical Co. Ltd; 35 mmol/l), Rehidrat (Searle Pharmaceuticals; 50 mmol/l) and a specially prepared glycine/glucose solution (50 mmol/l). No significant difference was observed in the duration

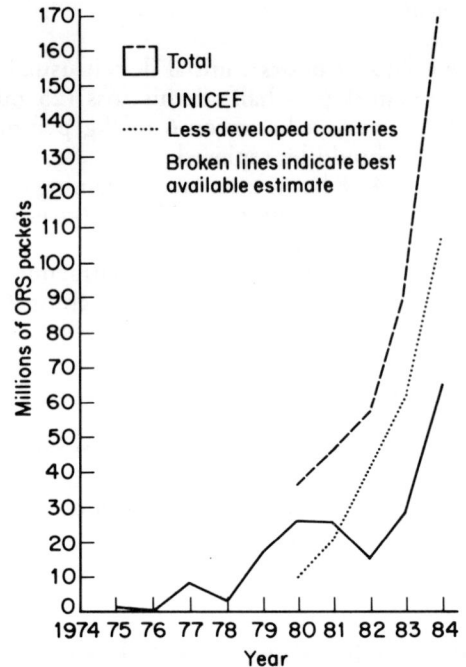

Fig. 2.6 Global supply of oral rehydration salts (WHO/UNICEF formula). (Note: figures exclude commercial production. In addition to the above figures, an estimated 10 million packets are supplied by other international and bilateral aid agencies.) (Source: UNICEF, 1985, *The State of the World's Children Report*, published by Oxford University Press.)

Table 2.3 WHO recommendations for a universal oral rehydration solution

	Concn (mmol/l)
Glucose	111
Sodium	90
Potassium	20
Bicarbonate	30

Osmolality = 330 mosmol/kg water.

of postadmission diarrhoea, hospital stay or percentage weight gain. In rotavirus enteritis, the stool content of sodium is 37 mmol/l compared to 90 mmol/l in cholera and 53 mmol/l in enterotoxigenic *E. coli*. Hence a standard solution is irrational but expedient.

Sodium and carbohydrate

There is active co-transport of sodium and organic

molecules such as glucose and amino acids across the gut wall; sodium and glucose are absorbed in equimolecular amounts. For this to happen the concentration of both should be between 56 and 140 mmol/l. When the sodium content of the gut lumen is below normal, active secretion of sodium takes place, even in the presence of glucose. At concentrations above 160 mmol/l glucose and sodium absorption are decreased.

Malabsorption of lactose, sucrose and glucose in diarrhoeal states is well documented. In rotavirus infections (Fig. 2.7) poor absorption of glucose is common and the inclusion of high concentrations of glucose, in excess of 50 g/l (185 mmol/l), can exacerbate glucose malabsorption by causing an osmotic diarrhoea. In addition, malabsorption of carbohydrate worsens acidosis owing to hydrogen ion production from the fermentation of unabsorbed carbohydrate by gut flora.

It has been suggested that use of the WHO recommendation of 90 mmol/l of sodium can lead to hypernatraemia but this arises from solutions containing substantially more than the 111 mmol/l of glucose. Carbohydrates other than glucose can facilitate sodium absorption. Sucrose has the theoretical advantage of containing the same amount of energy as glucose with only half its osmolality; glucose polymers facilitate sodium absorption and also have a low osmolality. However, it is in the lumen of the small intestine that sucrose is hydrolysed to release equimolecular amounts of glucose and fructose, thus doubling the osmolality. The inclusion of high concentrations of polymer in oral rehydration fluids has been shown to cause deleterious effects in acute diarrhoea. Glucose appears to be the carbohydrate of choice yet sucrose can provide a useful and cheaper alternative. Fructose is not recommended because of its high cost and contribution to a state of metabolic acidosis. The

amino acid glycine stimulates sodium-coupled water absorption from the gut, independently from glucose, but is of no benefit when added to an oral rehydration solution containing sodium 60 mmol/l (Vesikari and Isolauri, 1986).

In the 5% of infants with severe glucose malabsorption, it is usually necessary to resort to intravenous fluids. However, other organic molecules such as peptides will also facilitate sodium absorption. Providing that a normal blood glucose level can be maintained, a solution containing glucose 10 g/l (37 mmol/l) and a small amount (10 g/l) of a hydrolysed protein product such as Pregestimil (p. 256) or product 3232A (p. 266) can be tried as an alternative to intravenous feeding.

Potassium and anions

Malnourished children are likely to be suffering from a chronic deficit of potassium. A minimum of 1 mmol K^+/kg body weight daily should be included in a rehydrating preparation; however, many infants and children require far greater amounts. Acidosis is common in diarrhoeal states and the inclusion of a base such as bicarbonate, lactate, citrate or acetate should improve this; furthermore, bicarbonate helps sodium absorption. However, the addition of these substances will increase the cost and shorten the shelf-life of products. The usefulness of base precursors in all but the most severe states of acidosis has been questioned (Elliot *et al.*, 1987).

Administration of oral fluids

A minimum of 150 ml fluid/kg expected weight per 24 hours should be aimed for in hyponatraemic and normonatraemic dehydration (Table 2.4). If the solution is being fed by nasogastric tube, fluid balance should be carefully monitored, but if given by cup or bottle it is difficult to overhydrate.

There should be a difference in the concentration of a feed which is being used to replace a sodium deficit and one which is being used to maintain hydration. In hyponatraemic dehydration, it is suggested that the WHO solution is given for approximately 6 hours, then extra free water in the ratio of 2 volumes of rehydration mixture plus 1 volume boiled water.

It is particularly important that malnourished children receive an adequate sodium intake because of their deficit.

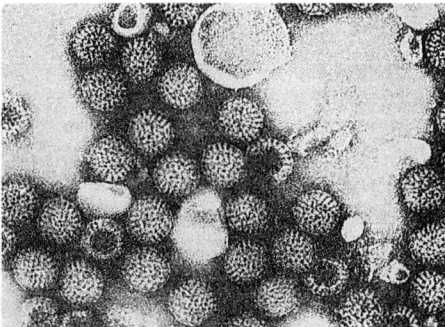

Fig. 2.7 Rotavirus particles in filtered human stool.

Table 2.4 Regimen for 5 kg child with hyponatraemia (expected weight 6 kg) using WHO oral rehydration salts*

		Sodium (mmol)	Potassium (mmol)
First 6 hours	240 ml ORS	21.6	4.8
Next 18 hours	480 ml ORS + 240 ml water	43.2	9.6
	Total	64.8	14.4
Per kg expected weight		10.8	2.4

* Fluid requirements 6 kg × 150 ml = 900 ml, i.e. approximately 240 ml every 6 hours. This can be given as 40 ml hourly or 20 ml half-hourly.

Table 2.5 Regimen for 5 kg child with hypernatraemia using WHO oral rehydration salts

Regimen	Sodium (mmol)	Potassium (mmol)
330 ml ORS 150 ml water	29.7	6.6
Per kg actual weight per 24 hours	5.9	1.32

Fluid requirements 5 kg × 100 ml per 24 hours approximately = 500 ml. Osmolality = 227 mosmol/kg water. This should be given as 20 ml hourly or 10 ml half-hourly.

In hypernatraemia, the replacement regimen should be much slower (Table 2.5). It is important that the fluid used should have a similar osmolality to normal plasma (i.e. 275–295 mosmol/kg). If breast feeding is to be continued then some breast milk can be given in both hypo- and hypernatraemia. After the first 6 hours of either regimen then an equal quantity of rehydration fluid and breast milk should prove satisfactory.

Oral rehydration mixtures

In the rural areas of less developed countries mothers and auxiliary health personnel can be trained to use oral rehydration therapy (Egemen and Bertan, 1980). Commercially prepared oral rehydration mixtures are marketed in the form of a powder, either in a pre-weighed sachet, or in a can. They are also available in a ready-to-feed (RTF) system. Appendix II.11 lists this type of preparation. Realimentation fluids and mixtures designed to be used as a temporary regimen between clear rehydration mixtures and full milk feeds are described in Appendix II.16.

Where possible the RTF system is preferable, but if powder has to be reconstituted it is important that the mother receives adequate instruction. Oral rehydration mixtures should be reconstituted with water not milk and the water must be boiled before the salts are added.

'Home remedies'

Although there are a number of commercial electrolyte products, many centres use a 'home-ready'

preparation rather than one specifically designed for rehydration. These solutions include clear soups, stock or bouillon cubes, coconut water, rice water, ground dry rice and water, carbonated soft drinks, honey and oral rehydration fluid, fruit juice and teas. None of these contains the optimum balance of carbohydrate, sodium, potassium and base to replace fluid loss.

A door-to-door half-hour training programme in Bangladesh resulted in 2.5 million women being taught individually how to prepare a home-made solution using salt (lobon) and molasses (gur). A subsequent survey revealed that 98% of the mothers understood how to use the ingredients correctly. Perhaps this impressive educational achievement related to the financial incentive given to the best trainers.

Great care must be taken to ensure that the mother is correctly taught. Wharton *et al.* (1988) remind clinicians of the inaccuracy in composition of home-made salt and sugar solutions. Often an empty baby-milk tin and measuring spoon will suffice as an improvised measure. Clean boiled water must be to hand. A recipe which supplies 85 mmol sodium and chloride and 111 mmol carbohydrate per litre can be prepared from the following: 5.0 g sodium chloride; 30.0 g glucose or sucrose; water to make up a volume of 1000 ml.

Ideally, the purpose-intended, double-ended spoon with one end for the salt measure and the other for sugar (Fig. 2.8) should be used. The spoon bears printed instructions. If a suitable measure for the sodium chloride cannot be devised then it should be pre-weighed and given to the mother. Fruit is a valuable source of potassium and can also be used to replace some of the carbohydrate.

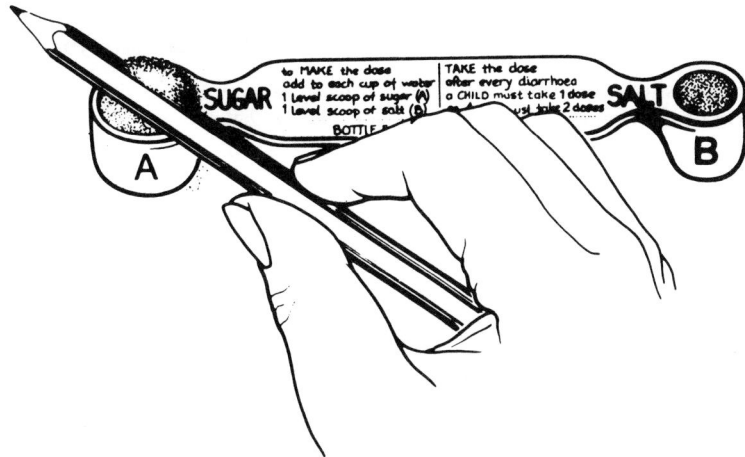

Fig. 2.8 Double-ended spoon for measuring sugar and salt in making up rehydration fluid.

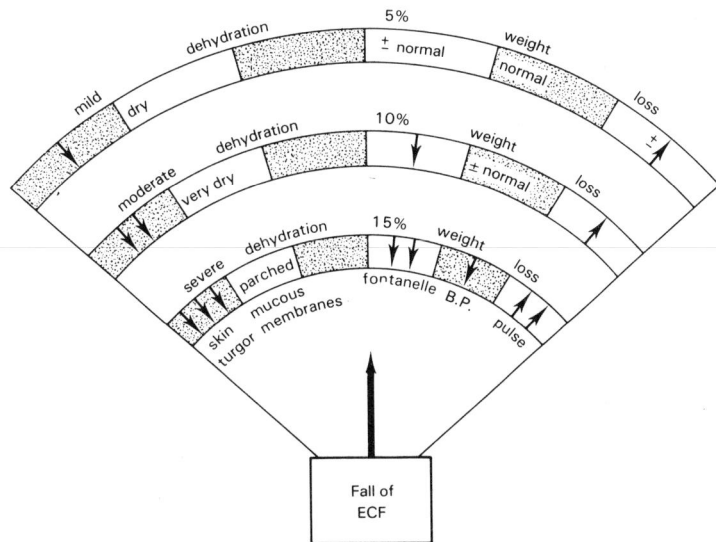

Fig. 2.9 Clinical signs in isotonic dehydration of different magnitude.

One small banana (50 g) will provide approximately 4.5 mmol potassium and 10 g carbohydrate. When constituting ORS it is very necessary, in non-industrialized countries, to be aware of the electrolyte composition of the local fresh water which will be influenced by various geological factors. Mir and Elzouki (1984) observed that in Benghazi, Libya the natural fresh water content of sodium was only 0.35–0.72 mmol/l in contrast to 25–56 mmol/l in the unboiled drinking water, which rose to 39–82 mmol/l when boiled. Mehta and Subramanian (1986) advocated that rice-based fluids, especially rice water, are superior to WHO glucose electrolyte solutions in treating infants under 6 months. Rice water has the advantage of a low osmolality (8.9 ± 3.4 mosmol/kg) but has a poor electrolyte content.

Introduction of solid food

The continued feeding of milk (apart from breast-milk) or solid foods in different situations can be either advantageous or disadvantageous. Even if the diarrhoea is chronic food should not be withheld unless an intolerance is suspected, because starvation exacerbates the depletion of small bowel and pancreatic enzymes. If dehydration is severe then withdrawing solid foods, which delay gastric emptying, may increase the rate of rehydration.

Dehydration and enteritis

A scheme showing clinical signs in isotonic dehydration of different magnitudes is given in Fig. 2.9. Vital signs will vary from the symptoms shown in Fig. 2.9 in hypotonic and hypertonic dehydration.

There are least two important clinical signs that are very dissimilar within the three main types of dehydration syndrome: the skin elasticity (turgor) and the child's mental state can be very distinct (Table 2.6).

The great tragedy about diarrhoea is not solely the appalling mortality and morbidity but the fact that it is both preventable and indeed treatable by relatively simple measures. An aggressive educational campaign publicizing the numerous advantages of breast feeding combined with improved sanitation and clean water supplies could make

Table 2.6 Clinical signs in the three types of dehydration syndrome

	Isotonic dehydration	Hypertonic dehydration	Hypotonic dehydration
Skin elasticity	Reduced	Thickened, 'dough like'	Much reduced
Mental state	Lethargy, confusion or stupor	Irritability and/or stupor [± convulsions]	Coma

dehydration as rare as the diseases now almost eradicated by immunization procedures. We must combat the Westernization influence of formula feeding in the less developed countries and endorse a holistic approach in child care practices.

3

Parenteral and Enteral Nutrition

Enteral nutrition

The practice of enteric nutrition is self-evidently more akin to the physiological norm than the parenteral route. In addition, total parenteral nutrition can be more hazardous (Jones and Silk, 1980), costly (Clark, 1977) and complex than enteral feeding. Specific advantages are to be had when alimentation is via the gastrointestinal tract. In essence, the maintenance or restoration of optimum bowel function enhances cellular proliferation and enzyme induction. Feeding also initiates the activity of non-luminal neuronal and hormonal factors which stimulate the bowel (Anon, 1987). There is considerable animal experimental work supporting this hypothesis. Only if the enteral route is precluded through inability to digest or absorb nutrients should parenteral feeding be planned.

Tube feeding

There are many indications for tube feeding. If oral supplements to food or a complete liquid diet (Appendix III. 6.) can be taken then that is preferable to a tube method. Moreover, there are psychological advantages in maintaining oral feeds. Reasons for failure of the oral route to satisfy nutrient requirements are given in Table 3.1.

Methods of tube feeding

Tubes can be sited at various positions in the upper gastrointestinal tract (Table 3.2). Each position is associated with different advantages and disadvantages. The nutrients can be infused by a bolus or an intermittent feeding regimen which confers the benefit of simulating a normal pattern and may contribute to gut recovery. If the child is conscious he will benefit from the frequent contact which feeding necessitates. Contraindications to bolus feeding include delayed gastric emptying, vomiting

and conditions where gastric distension may embarrass respiratory or cardiac function.

Alternatively, the tube feed can be given by continuous infusion. Enteral feeding pumps, though not as costly nor as complex as pumps for intravenous therapy, should conform to safety standards (Auty, 1988). There are potential hazards including deaths associated with this option. In young children, constant supervision is necessary to ensure the tube is not displaced because the infusate might then flow into the lungs. Constant infusions have the advantage of achieving a much higher fluid intake, less gastric distension and aspiration and improved absorption of nutrients. However, the uptake of some infused drugs, e.g. phenytoin, is depressed when given via constant infusion. Nocturnal infusions may cause less inconvenience and can be used as a supplement to the daytime diet, but medical and nursing surveillance is usually less intensive at such times.

Enteral feeding pumps, though not as costly nor as complex as pumps for intravenous therapy, should conform to safety standards (Auty, 1988).

Bowel endocrine response to feeding

When selecting the method of enteral nutrition it should be remembered that the gut hormone profile in pre-term infants is influenced by the feeding regimen. Postprandial responses are greater where there has been bolus feeding as opposed to continuous intragastric milk infusions. It is suggested that milk in the gut results in the release of a number of hormones inducing developmental changes in the bowel and pancreas (Aynsley-Green, 1983). Hormone responses to the first extrauterine feed are dissimilar in the pre-term and term infant as the term infant is primed to respond to the initial feed with metabolic and endocrine changes. It would seem that developmental changes arise in the final weeks of gestation which prepare the term baby for enteral feeding.

Table 3.1 Indications for tube feeding

Reasons for inadequate oral intake	Examples
Inability to suck and/or swallow	Prematurity, mental retardation, neurological disorders, trauma or surgery to mouth or throat
Impaired level of consciousness	Trauma, surgery, meningitis
Anorexia due to chronic disease	Renal failure, hepatic failure
Anorexia due to cytotoxic drug therapy	Leukaemia, solid tumours
Anorexia due to psychiatric disorders	Severe anorexia nervosa
Weakness due to chronic illness	Malnutrition, protracted diarrhoea
Exhaustion/breathlessness exacerbated by feeding	Cardiac insufficiency, chest infection
Increased nutrient requirements needing large fluid volumes and feeding throughout 24 hours	Pancreatic insufficiency, short bowel, burns, trauma, cystic fibrosis
Unpleasant tasting feeds — chemically defined diets	Malabsorption, short bowel syndrome, inborn errors of protein metabolism

Table 3.2 Delivery of tube feed

Method	Advantages	Disadvantages
Nasogastric tube	Ease of insertion and checking Bolus or continuous infusion	Gastric distension Risk of aspiration Discomfort in nasopharynx
Nasojejunal tube	No gastric distension Less risk of aspiration	Difficulty of insertion Needs radiographic check of position Risk of perforation Abdominal pain and diarrhoea unless continuous infusion Discomfort in nasopharynx Reflux of bile is facilitated
Gastrostomy	Wide tube—choice of feed preparations Patient unaware of tube Greater patient mobility	Surgical procedure Local skin irritation Risk of leak into peritoneum Gastric distension and aspiration
Fine needle jejunostomy	Patient unaware of tube No gastric distenstion Little risk of aspiration	Surgical procedure Tube liable to block Risk of perforation Must be constant infusion

Equipment for tube feeding

Feeding tubes are made from polyethylene, polyvinyl chloride, polyurethane or silicone rubber. Polyurethane and silicone tubes are soft, cause less discomfort and can remain *in situ* for several months. They have a small internal diameter and not all types of feeds can be used with these tubes. Also pumps are often required and insertion into the stomach is difficult. Usually it is difficult to aspirate from this type of product and the unweighted tube is easily dislodged by coughing.

Polyethylene and polyvinyl chloride tubes generally have a wider lumen and can be used for liquidized whole diets or home-prepared feeds. They are more suitable for bolus feeding than polyurethane or Silastic tubes although they, too, can be used for continuous infusion. Furthermore, they are easier to introduce than the softer tubes. However, they harden *in situ* and have been reported to cause gut perforation (Metz *et al.*, 1978) unless they are changed frequently. The use of the softer polyuretherane and Silastic variety is commoner than other types. For all tubes the position of the metallic tip after insertion should be confirmed radiologically. Alternatively, air can be injected and the end of the tube auscultated at the presumed site of the opening to ensure that the bronchi have not been cannulated.

Containers such as bags, bottles and gavage sets are available when tube feeding is by continuous infusion. Alternatively glass bottles can be sterilized to provide a less expensive system. All containers must be sterile when the feed is introduced and be changed every 4–6 hours in order to reduce the likelihood of introducing pathogens. Pumps are available to deliver the infusion at a predetermined rate. (For a review of pumps and tubes available *see* Courtney *et al.*, 1985.)

Products for tube feeding

Silk and Keohane (1982) classified enteral feeds into three categories: standard polymeric diets; 'chemically defined' diets; specifically formulated diets.

Chemically defined or elemental diets contain nutrients which require little or no digestion and hence are easily absorbed. Their use is discussed more fully in the section on p. 258. Specially formulated diets are those designed to overcome a specific problem in digestion such as lactose intolerance. Details of this type of feed are given in the appropriate section.

The standard polymeric diet has whole protein as the nitrogen source as opposed to amino acids and is appropriate where there is normal or near normal gastrointestinal function. Preparations suitable for tube feeding are of three types: normal food liquidized and sieved, reconstituted powder preparations which require the addition of water or milk and 'ready-to-feed' products. Liquidized food has the disadvantage that it is difficult to achieve a consistency that will pass through an enteric feeding tube. Home-prepared feeds will block fine polyurethane or Silastic tubes. Feeds of

this type are usually low in energy unless modular fat and carbohydrate are used; in addition, liquidized foods are likely to become contaminated either from the food or from unclean liquidizing equipment. For a child being fed at home via a gastrostomy there may be social and emotional benefits to the mother, child and family as a result of using home-prepared foods but, apart from this, they have a limited role in tube feeding.

Complete feeds, either ready-to-feed or reconstituted powders should contain the recommended dietary allowance (RDA) for all nutrients including vitamins, minerals and trace elements, yet it may be necessary to supplement if a small volume is given, as for a young child. Ready-to-feed powders have advantages over reconstituted feeds in that they are sterile and less liable to preparation errors by hospital staff or parents. Unfortunately, they are both expensive and bulky for transport and storage. Products used for enteral feeding are described in Appendix III. 1.

Modular products containing fat, protein or carbohydrate can be used to formulate an entire tube feed, thus allowing greater flexibility of content. Care should be taken to ensure that the vitamin, mineral and trace element requirements are fulfilled. Details of modular products are given in Appendices III.1 and III.2. Where specialized products are not available then a 'home-made' tube feed based on cows' milk can be used. The energy content is increased by the addition of fat and carbohydrate and a full vitamin supplement is necessary. It should also be noted that this type of feed is high in calcium (120 mg/100 ml) and sodium (2.17 mmol/ 100 ml). A tube feed based on milk is shown in Table 3.3.

Feeding different age groups

Under the age of 6 months, breast milk or a standard infant formula as described on p. 221 should be suitable. If nutrient requirements are high then it may be necessary to supplement with a modular preparation. After the age of 6 months, formulae fail to satisfy energy requirements if used as the sole source of nutrition. Between the ages of 6 months and 2 years a 'follow-on' formula (p. 221) with additional energy is most appropriate. The quantity of formula is determined by the fluid requirement and the energy deficit is calculated. Equal quantities of carbohydrate (preferably glucose polymer) and fat emulsion are added to make

Table 3.3 Enteral feed based on cows' milk (for a child age 5 years, weight 18.5 kg, RDA fluid 1550 ml, protein 42.0 g, energy 1550 kcal, 650 MJ)

	Protein (g)	Fat (g)	Carbohydrate (g)	Energy (kcal)	(MJ)
Milk 1550 ml	51	55.5	72.0	990	4.16
Fat emulsion 40 ml (or oil 20 ml)[a]	—	20.0	—	180	0.75
Glucose polymer 80 g (or sugar)	—	—	80.0	320	1.34
Totals	51	75.5	152.0	1490	6.25
Percentage solution		5%	10%		

[a] If vegetable oil is used in place of a fat emulsion then delivery must be by bolus and the feed should be vigorously shaken to disperse the fat.
In addition a supplement of the RDAs for vitamins A, D, C, thiamine (vitamin B_1) and pryidoxine (vitamin B_6) should be given, plus supplemental iron.

up any deficiency. Energy supplements can cause diarrhoea if they are introduced too rapidly or used in large quantities.

Most powder and ready-to-feed preparations are designed to meet adult requirements. However, they can be used for children over the age of 2 years. Adult preparations usually provide more than the RDA for protein and sodium but, provided these are monitored and vitamin and mineral deficits are supplemented, they provide an acceptable option. Examples of tube feeds suitable for various age groups are shown in Table 3.4.

Initiating tube feeding

It is important that enteral feeding is introduced gradually. If the child has not been fed for 24 hours or if there is any reason to suspect malabsorption or gut statis then feeding should commence slowly. Dextrose (5%) can be given for one to two feeds, then quarter- to half-strength preparations. If the patient is being fed intravenously then a gradual change increasing the volume of tube feeds and decreasing parenteral fluids can take place over about 4–5 days (*see* p. 272). In the absence of parenteral feeds the full fluid requirement should be established in about 2 days. Once the total fluid requirement of the half-strength dilution has been given, full-strength feeds can be gradually introduced over the next 2 days. Increasing both the volume and concentration of the feed on the same day is best avoided as this can provoke abdominal pain and diarrhoea.

Problems associated with tube feeding

The commonest problem is abdominal pain and diarrhoea due to too rapid an advancement of the regimen. If gastrointestinal symptoms do occur, return to half-strength feeds and decrease the fluid intake by 30%. Gradually increase the volume by 10% daily for 3 days then increase the concentration to three-quarters followed by full strength. If symptoms recur, check that the recipe of the final feed is not too concentrated and hyperosmolar. For young children, the carbohydrate concentration should not be above 10 g/100 ml (10%) and the fat content should not exceed 5 g/100 ml (5%). When this concentration is tolerated then further additions can be made.

Delayed gastric emptying may be due to decreased gut motility. Alternatively, it may be the result of the bolus feeding of an over-concentrated hyperosmolar feed. In such a case, a continuous infusion should be considered and the volume and concentration of feeds be decreased and gradually built up as suggested in the previous paragraph.

Overload of fluid and nutrients can occur if care is not taken in calculating the requirements of individual patients. RDAs for protein, fluid and sodium (Appendix I) should be particularly considered as raised blood urea will result from protein over-load, hypernatriuria from a high sodium intake and congestive cardiac failure can occur if there is a defect in glucose metabolism, as seen in burns and trauma or if the feed contains a high concentration of carbohydrate.

Blockage of the nasogastric tube occurs when it is inadequately rinsed after bolus feeding and this is more likely in the narrow lumen polyurethane or Silastic types. A thick viscous tube feed, one that contains discrete particles or a feed based on meat are the most likely to cause obstruction Home-prepared feeds, whether based on homogenized food or reconstituted powders are more likely to cause obstruction than a commercially prepared ready-to-feed system.

Oral supplements and liquidized diets

There are occasions when children are able to take fluids by mouth but are unable to eat sufficient solids to satisfy their needs. In such cases pleasant tasting liquids can be used either to replace the diet or to provide extra nutrients.

If the whole of the diet is to be replaced by liquids then it is important that a variety of taste, colour and temperature is offered, particularly for the older child. A mixture of sweet and savoury, milky and fruit based, hot, room temperature and chilled should be aimed for in order to accomplish maximum intake. Almost any food enjoyed by the child can be liquidized and used as a drink; sweet liquids can be frozen and made into an ice lolly or popsicle. Recipes for high-protein, high-energy savoury soups, milk shakes and fruit drinks are given on p. 244. Commercially prepared products which have a pleasant flavour are listed on p. 243. The principles of feeding are the same as described for tube feeding — the RDAs for protein, energy and fluid should be calculated and the amount of sodium, mineral, vitamins and trace elements noted in the diet.

High-energy, high-protein drinks can be given in addition to food in an anorexic child or where nutrient requirements are particularly high. Supplements should be given 1–2 hours before a meal; they need to be emptied fairly rapidly from the stomach and should not therefore be too hot or cold or have a high fat content in order to ensure the child retains his appetite.

Total parenteral nutrition

Total parenteral nutrition (TPN) has been one of the most innovative techniques to be introduced into paediatrics in the second half of this century. The first documented case of TPN was described in 1944 by Helfrick and Abelson although it is said that more than 300 years earlier (1665), Sir Christopher Wren gave alcohol intravenously to dogs. A major development in TPN was the demonstration that Beagle puppies grew and developed normally during a prolonged period of intravenous feeding using a central catheter (Dudrick *et al.*, 1968). Following the development of constant enteric feeding techniques, using elemental diets, TPN is now indicated less often than it has been. For an authoritative and helpful review detailing the indications and contraindications of TPN *see* Harries (1971) and Zlotkin *et al.* (1985); for working regimens *see* Panter-Brick (1983), Easton *et al.* (1982) and Kanarek *et al.* (1982).

An important advancement in technology has been the innovation of the single bag method. In children weighing more that 15 kg, a bag containing a mixed solution of nutrients and minerals (but excluding lipids) can be infused. Using a laminar flow hood, a hospital pharmacist can 'tailor make' an appropriate mixture in non-vented plastic containers (Panter-Brick, 1983). However, some neonatologists use TPN solutions in bags which do contain all the nutrients as well as lipids (Rosbotham, 1986). Plastic bags must be protected by black outer covers to prevent photodegradation of light sensitive constituents. TPN is recommended in several conditions, including:

1. After extensive bowel resection (short bowel syndrome).
2. Protracted diarrhoea of infancy.
3. Extreme prematurity.

Total non-enteric nutrition necessitates considerable clinical and pharmaceutical expertise and laboratory support to minimize biochemical, bacteriological and surgical complications. Infusates must be prepared aseptically. Intensive nursing care must be present and the hospital laboratory should be able to use small aliquots of blood for microsampling. Where these facilities are lacking those requiring prolonged TPN should be referred to specialized centres.

Acidosis and/or dehydration must be corrected before TPN is commenced. The presence of liver disease or hyperlipidaemia may be a contraindication to the use of Intralipid infusions and such solutions must be used with great caution. There should be frequent biochemical monitoring and visual inspection of the serum to ensure it is not turbid as a result of persistent hyperlipidaemia.

Metabolic observations

Some basic daily clinical measurements are essential. The patient must be weighed, the total urine volume recorded and the quantity of any lost body fluids noted (e.g. via nasogastric or gastrostomy tubes). A state of positive nitrogen balance should be attained because the stools will be infrequent during TPN, therefore there is little loss of faecal nitrogen.

Composition of infusions

The infusate should contain the following:

Protein: fibrin hydrolysate, casein hydrolysate, crystalline amino acids.
Carbohydrate: glucose.
Fat: lipids.
Electrolytes: sodium, potassium, chloride, calcium, phosphate, magnesium.
Metals trace elements: zinc, copper, manganese, iodine, fluorine, chromium, selenium and iron.
Vitamins: A, C, D, E, K_1, B_1 (thiamine), B_2 (riboflavin), niacin, pantothenic acid, B_6 (pyridoxine), B_{12}, biotin, choline (cofactor for enzymatic reactions) and folic acid.

Amino acids

L-Amino acids are preferred to D-Amino acids because they are more effective in maintaining nitrogen balance and protein synthesis. There are a number of commercial preparations to choose from. At times of specific nutritional needs the non-essential amino acids may become essential or semi-essential (Harries, 1971a). Furthermore, quite apart from the eight amino acids known to be essential for adults, histidine, proline and alanine are required by the growing infant. Cystine and/or cysteine are also necessary for growth and so become 'semi-essential' or 'essential' as opposed to non-essential amino acids.

The infusion should be started at 0.5 g amino acids/kg per day and the maximum rate is 2.5 g/kg per day. Blood urea nitrogen, ammonia and pH should be monitored and quantitative assays of serum and urine amino acids are required.

Heird *et al.*(1988) have shown that the metabolic activity of low-birth-weight infants for parenterally administered amino acid mixture is not as limited as had been thought by other investigators. However, he has noted that the low-birth-weight infants

Table 3.4 Enteral feeding at different ages

Age	Weight (kg)	RDA[a] Fluid (ml)	Protein (g)	Energy (kcal) (MJ)		Feed
6 months	7.5	1120	15	790	3.30	SMA 'Gold Cap' 1120 ml Protein = 16.8 g; energy = 750 kcal (3.15 MJ)

9 months	9.0	1170	18	950	4.00	1. SMA 'Progress' 1170 ml
						    Protein = 33.9 g; energy = 760 kcal (3.20 MJ)
						2. SMA 'Progress' 1170 ml ⎫
						    Glucose polymer 25 g ⎬
						    Fat emulsion 25 ml ⎭
						    Protein = 33.9 g; energy = 972 kcal (4.08 MJ)

1 year	10.0	1200	20	1050	4.40	SMA 'Progress' 1200 ml ⎫ Glucose polymer 35 g ⎬ Fat emulsion 35 ml ⎭ Protein = 34.8 g; energy = 1077 kcal (4.52 MJ)
2 years	12.5	1250	22	1250	5.25	'Isocal' 1250 ml Protein = 42.5 g; energy = 1250 kcal (5.25 MJ)

[a] RDA for weight and age calculated from Appendices I.1 and I.2.
NB This regimen assumes continuous infusion. Volume of feed will be reduced if bolus feeding; extra water will be required to rinse tube after each feed.

Table 3.5 Composition of fat emulsion

Preparation	Composition (g/l)			
	Soybean oil	Safflower oil	Cottonseed oil	Phospholipid
Intralipid 10% and 20% (KabiVitrum, Sweden)	100/200			12
Lipofundin S 10% and 20% (Braun, Germany)	100/200			7.5–15
Travamulsion (Travenol Laboratories)	100			1.2
Intrafat (Daigo, Japan)	100			
Liposyn 20% (Abbott, USA)		200		1.2
Lipiphysan (Egic, France)			150	20

Adapted from JT Harries (1971a).

receiving TPN (Trophamine, Kendall McGaw Laboratories—plus L-cysteine-HCl) were not as able to use *N*-acetyl-L-tyrosine and cysteine-HCl as well as the term infants and older children.

Nitrogen balance studies allow the clinician to ensure that the protein intake is at a 'safe level'. The balance is the difference between nitrogen intake and nitrogen losses in the urine (as urinary urea), stools and sweat. Starvation and infections result in a negative balance and rapid growth in a positive balance.

Clinical nitrogen balance: urinary nitrogen excretion (in grams) is calculated from:

$$\frac{\text{mmol urea/24 h} \times 28}{1000} \times 6.5$$

1 mmol urea = 28 mg nitrogen; 6.5 is a constant to correct for urinary nitrogen, e.g. uric acid.

Lipids

Parenteral lipids provide a high energy yield as well as a source of essential fatty acids. Fat emulsion solutions are available as 10 or 20% preparations and are derived from soybean, safflower or cotton-seed oil with the fat mainly present as triglyceride (Table 3.5). Heparin has the desirable property of assisting the elimination of lipids by increasing lipoprotein lipase. Ultimate total daily dose of parenteral lipid emulsion should not exceed 4 g/kg per day (American Academy of Pediatrics Committee on Nutrition, 1983) and the infusion rate should be < 0.25 g/kg per hour (Table 3.6). One litre of 20% emulsion provides 2000 kcal (8.4 MJ) and is a rich source of the essential fatty acids linoleic and linolenic acids. The 20% emulsion has an osmolality of 330 mosmol/kg water and the 10% 280 mosmol/kg compared with a plasma value of approximately 290. Serum lipids must be monitored and infusion started only when the previous solution has been removed from the circulation. Visual inspection and nephelometry are imprecise. The light scattering index should be kept below 30 mg/dl.

Lipid emulsions are contraindicated: if serum bilirubin exceeds 100 mmol/l or if serum pH is less than 7.25.

Free fatty acids may displace bilirubin from albumin in the neonate with the risk of kernicterus. Lipids may also interfere with platelet function and should be withheld if the count is less than $50\,000 \times 10^9/l$.

A particular problem encountered when using fat emulsions is the leaching of plasticizers in the polyvinyl chloride (PVC) bag of the administration set. The leached quantity of di-2-ethylhexylphthalate (DEHP) in PVC relates to contact time and surface area of the plastic (Downie *et al.*, 1985).

Assiduous biochemical detection work has enabled the identification of an exogenous compound in the sera of premature babies receiving prolonged

Table 3.6 Use of intravenous fat

Age	Initial dose (g/kg per day)	Increase daily by (g/kg per day)	Maximum dose (g/kg per day)
Premature or growth retarded infant	0.5	0.25	3.0
Full term AGA[a] infant	1.0	0.5	4.0
Older children	1.0	0.5	2.0

[a] AGA = appropriate for gestational age.

intravenous therapy (Meek and Pettit, 1985). The rubber component of administration sets used for infusing parenteral solutions leaches out 2-(carboxymethylthio)benzothiazole (CMB). Theoretically the CMB could be hazardous, especially during jaundice, because it will compete for albumin-binding sites and is also known to be hepatotoxic in mice.

Infused intravenous lipid that is not hydrolysed by lipoprotein lipase, which is present in the endothelial cells of blood vessels, can be deposited in the lung and brain, especially in the growth-retarded baby. It is important to remember that nothing should be added to the lipid emulsions except fat-soluble sterile vitamin preparations. Both the growth-retarded and the premature baby are impeded in their ability to clear intravenous lipid particles, a process which is dependent on lipoprotein lipase activity. Moreover, those with growth retardation are less able to resolve the serum lipaemia than immature newborns, but with maturation this resolves.

Carbohydrate

Most centres use 10% glucose as the sole monosaccharide. A solution with a glucose concentration of 10% or more is too viscous for peripheral use. Glycerol present in Intralipid (Appendix II. 15) is another source of carbohydrate. High glucose loads in the range of 20–30 mg/kg per min may be hepatotoxic. Other sugars such as fructose, galactose and sorbitol have been suggested but fructose (via lactate and pyruvate) can cause a metabolic acidosis (Andersson *et al.*, 1969) and also hypoglycaemia (Sahebjami and Scalettar, 1971). In addition, sorbitol is metabolized to fructose. The recommended amount of glucose to be infused is 10–20 g/kg per day. Blood (venous or capillary) must be closely monitored for glucose levels. Although glucose is the preferred carbohydrate, a central and not peripheral catheter is indicated for a 20% solution. When using a peripheral vein the ratio of glucose to fat is 4:1, but this proportion can be higher when a central vessel is infused.

Vitamins

A multiple vitamin preparation, such as Multibionta Infusion (Merck) should be given daily (Appendix II. 13) This, given in dextrose saline at a rate of 0.15 ml/kg per day supplies all vitamin requirements.

During prolonged intravenous feeding the following should be given:

1. Folic acid — 0.1–0.5 mg/day.
2. Vitamin B_{12} — 100 µg/month.
3. Vitamin D — 7.5 µg/day.
4. Vitamin K — 3 mg twice a week.
5. Choline chloride — 150 mg/day.
6. Biotin — 0.5 mg/day.

Minerals

Weekly infusions of plasma (20 ml/kg) are not believed to provide adequate amounts of trace metals (Candy, 1980).

Alternatively iron can be administered as Imferon (Fisons Ltd) in intramuscular or intravenous injections. Daily intravenous needs of some essential trace elements are (Filer, 1981): zinc (100–300 µg/kg); copper (20 µg/kg); chromium (0.14–0.2 µg/kg) and manganese (2–10 µg/kg). Paediatric mineral supplements for addition to intravenous infusion are described on p. 232.

An American study into aluminium contamination of parenteral nutrition samples from 17 commercially available components demonstrated that calcium gluconate contributes more than 80% of the total aluminium load (Koo *et al.*, 1986). The investigators suggested lowering the aluminium content in calcium gluconate and recommended the use of other specific low-aluminium components to reduce the metal in parenteral solutions to less than 20 μg Al/l.

Technique of TPN

Because there is a considerable risk of septicaemia when using intravenous catheters, especially one which is centrally located, a peripheral or scalp vein should be used whenever possible. Bivins (1982) recommended a 0.22 μm filter when using intravenous fluids.

A fibreoptic light source can help in outlining subcutaneous vessels. Phlebitis and obstruction will necessitate frequent repositioning of the infusion site. Ultimately a catheter may need to be sited in a central vein under aseptic conditions.

Puntis (1987) has shown in a TPN study that percutaneously inserted fine Silastic central venous catheters (0.64 mm inner diameter or 0.94 mm outer diameter) performed as well as surgically

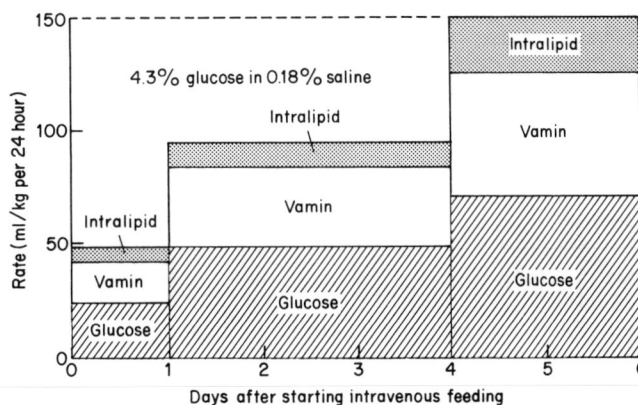

Fig. 3.1 Introduction of infusates for complete intravenous feeding. (Redrawn from Harries, 1971a.)

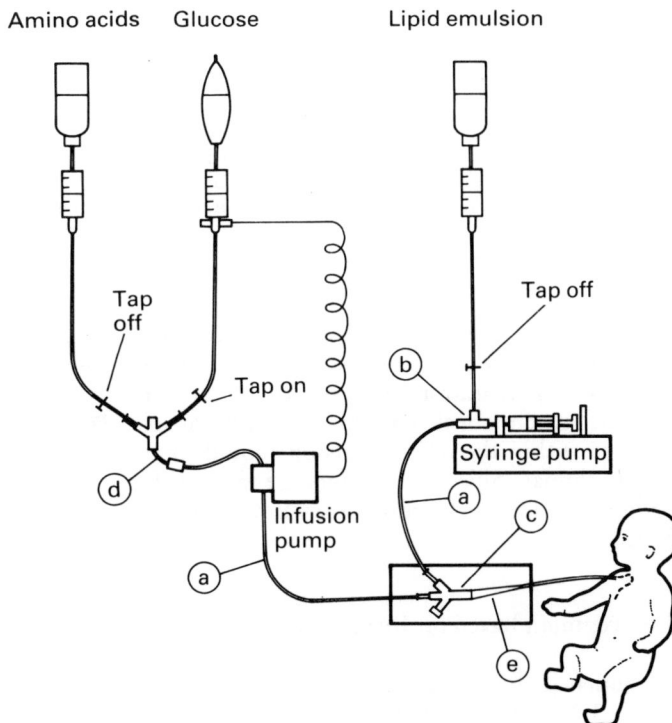

Fig. 3.2 Arrangement of infusion pumps, giving sets and infusate: (a) Extension set (S1028) (Avon Medicals Ltd); (b) three-way stopcock (4614-4) (Venflon, Viggo AB.); (c) dual injection site (V5600) (McGaw Laboratories); (d) L-S connector (409714/9) (B Braun, Melsungen AG); (e) Intravenous cannula (22-gauge, 8888-100107) (Argyle Medicut Sherwood Medical Industries). (Modified from Candy, 1980, with permission.)

Table 3.7 Infusion rates and additives for introduction parenteral nutrition and subsequent total parenteral nutrition in infants up to 10 kg body weight

	Duration (h/day)	Day 1	Infusion rates (ml/kg per h)		
			Days 2 and 3	Days 4 and 5	Day 6 and TPN
Intralipid 20% plus Vitlipid Infant[b]	20	0.3	0.6	0.8	1.0
Vamin Glucose plus Ped-El[c]	8[a]	2.5	4.0	5.0	6.0
Dextrose 10% (plus to each 500 ml: K_2HPO_4 17.42% : 4.0 ml NaCl 30% : 1.6 ml) plus Solivito[d]	16[a]	6.0	—	—	—
Dextrose 10% (plus to each 500 ml: K_2HPO_4 17.42% : 4.0 ml NaCl 30% : 1.0 ml) plus Solivito[d]	16[a]	—	5.5	—	—
Dextrose 15% (plus to each 500 ml: K_2HPO_4 17.42% : 3.5 ml NaCl 30% : 0.6 ml) plus Solivito[d]	16[a]	—	—	5.0	—
Dextrose 15% (plus to 500 ml: K_2HPO_4 17.42% : 3 ml) plus Solivito[d]	16[a]	—	—	—	5.0

[a] Order of infusion: Vamin → Glucose → Glucose → Vamin etc.
[b] Vitlipid Infant: 1 ml/kg, to a maximum of 4 ml, added to Intralipid syringe daily.
[c] Ped-El: 5 ml/kg to a maximum of 100 ml added to burette daily.
[d] Solivito: 1 ml/kg, to a maximum of 4 ml added to burette daily (contents of vial dissolved in 5 ml water for injection).
From *British Journal of Intravenous Therapy*, 1982, **3**: 35 by permission of I. W. Booth.
Intralipid, Vamin Glucose, Ped-El, Solivito, Vitlipid are all KabiVitrum Products.

placed Broviac catheters. Our preference too is for silicone catheters as they are less likely to cause thrombosis or perforation. The site of the tip of the longline must be checked radiologically because, if the tip is within the heart, infusions could produce arrhythmias. Silicone catheters are inert, soft and radio-opaque. Furthermore, they inhibit fibrin formation.

Feeding regimen based on Intralipid and Vamin

This regimen is demonstrated in Figs 3.1 and 3.2 and Table 3.7. The volume of the nutrient solutions should be increased slowly in the first 4 days as follows:

Day 1: One-third of total requirements (= 50 ml/kg) given as:

   20% Intralipid (or 10%).
   10–15% glucose.
   Vamin (or equivalent amino acid preparation).
   4.3% dextrose in 0.18% saline.

Days 2–4: Two-thirds of total requirements (= 100 ml/kg), therefore:

   Double volumes of Intralipid.

Table 3.8 Parameters and frequency of monitoring during TPN

Daily	Alternate days	Weekly
Na, K, Cl, Ca, Mg, P Glucose	Hb, WBC and differential counts Platelets	Total proteins, liver function tests, blood cultures (×2),[a] lipid electrophoresis
pH/bicarbonate status	Urea, creatinine Triglycerides	Urine culture
Nephelometry		Urine urea (for nitrogen balance *see* p. 32)
Urine osmolality ⎱ Urine Na, K ⎰ if indicated		

[a] For bacteria and *Candida*.
If a nasogastric or ostomy tube, of any description, is draining fluid measure volume and electrolyte content of the aspirate.
Phlebotomy — blood should be collected from veins remote from the intravenous sites.
Lipaemia will falsely lower estimated concentrations of water-soluble constituents and therefore venepuncture should be 12 hours after Intralipid has been administered (if possible).

Double volumes of glucose.
Double volumes of Vamin.
Double volumes of dextrose/saline.

Days 5 and 6: Give total requirements (= 150 ml/kg).

Precautions and complications

A meticulous aseptic technique is essential when handling the infusion apparatus, particularly upon injecting into the system. Septicaemia is more probable when central catheters are used; common sources of infection are *Staphylococcus aureus* and *albus*, *Candida* sp., *Pseudomonas* sp. and *Escherichia coli*. Sudden termination of TPN can cause hypoglycaemia. The sodium load in the amino acid preparation can provoke cardiac failure unless this particular source of salt is allowed for when calculating total daily needs (some antibiotics such as ampicillin and flucloxacillin contain sodium too). Cholestasis and rarely cirrhosis or liver failure are known hazards of TPN. There are data to suggest that intravenous amino acids mixtures play a role in the development of cholestasis in the very-low-birth-weight infant (Brown *et al.*, 1987). There is a clear association between the withdrawal of enteric

feeding and intestinal mucosal atrophy as well as pancreatic hyposecretion.

Non-enteral feeding causes a reduction in brush border enzyme activity, therefore a return to early normal feeding is important; alternatively, small volumes of oral nutrients should be used whenever possible. The development of gut hormones is dependent upon the presence of luminal food nutrients. Recently there has been much interest expressed on the topic of aluminium toxicity. Accumulation of this metal can result in anaemia, bone disease and encephalopathy. Solutions used in TPN might contain aluminium in concentrations up to 3400 µg/l (McGraw *et al.*, 1986), yet EEC provisional regulations set the maximum level in drinking water at 200 µg/l.

For details of monitoring during TPN *see Table 3.8.*

Regrading on to enteral nutrition

Oral feeds should be reintroduced very slowly with full TPN back-up. Feeds should be dilute and given in small frequent doses. A suggested protocol for changing from TPN to oral feeds is given in Appendix IV. 18.

4

Protein–Energy Malnutrition

Protein–energy malnutrition (PEM) includes marasmus, kwashiorkor and intermediate deficiencies. These disorders can be grouped together and some workers regard marasmus as successful adaptation to nutritional stress and kwashiorkor as representing the failure of an attempted adaptation. A comparison of marasmus and kwashiorkor is given in Table 4.1.

More than 15 million children die annually from malnutrition and associated infections (Editorial, 1982). Mortality can be very high except for those taken to specialized resuscitation centres where less than 5% die (Ashworth, 1979).

PEM is a spectrum of disease ranging from life-threatening kwashiorkor and marasmus to deficiencies of specific dietary constituents such as folate or vitamin A. Most children with severe PEM have parasitic infections commonly due to *Giardia lamblia*, *Strongyloides stercoralis* or *Ascaris lumbricoides*. These children have immunological deficit(s) and this, combined with their achlorhydria, accounts for intestinal colonization and subsequent diarrhoea.

PEM is not limited to non-industrialized countries. Fad and strict vegetarian diets and medically unsupervised elimination regimens all have the potential for causing PEM.

Definition/classification

Many classifications have been suggested to delineate the syndromes of PEM. The Wellcome Committee categorization, which is both simple and practical, is based on the presence of oedema and weight for age (Fig. 4.1) (Editorial, 1970; Waterlow, 1972). Alternatively, the severity of PEM can be determined by expressing the actual weight as a percentage of the expected weight of a healthy child of the same age using a standard.

Severity	Standard
First degree (mild)	89–75% of expected weight for age
Second degree (moderate)	74–60% of expected weight for age
Third degree (severe)	60% of expected weight for age

Characteristics

Conditions such as reduced gastrointestinal motility, prolonged transit time and potassium depletion are common in PEM and can exacerbate this syndrome (Fig. 4.2).

Bacterial overgrowth of the upper gastrointestinal tract can also occur.

Table 4.1 Comparison of marasmus and kwashiorkor

	Marasmus	Kwashiorkor
Weight	↓ ↓ ↓	↓ ↓
Oedema	– – –	+ + +
Depigmentation	– – –	↑ ↑ ↑
Hair changes	±	+ +
Vitamin levels	↓ ↓ ↓	↓ ↓
Small intestine — villous atrophy	+ +	+ + +
Lactase/sucrase/maltase	↓ ↓	↓ ↓ ↓
Pancreatic enzymes	↓	↓
Fatty liver	+	+

Modified from Gryboski and Walker, 1983, *Gastrointestinal Problems in the Infant*, 2nd edn, Philadelphia, W. B. Saunders. ↓ = slightly reduced; ↓ ↓ = moderately reduced; ↓ ↓ ↓ = markedly reduced.

Fig. 4.1 Wellcome Committee categorization of PEM. Standard weight = 50th percentile of weight for age (Harvard growth standards).

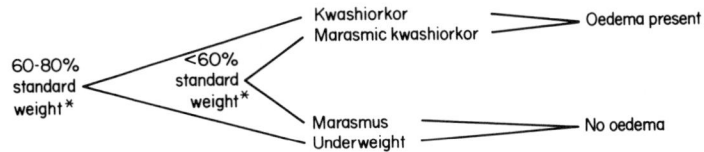

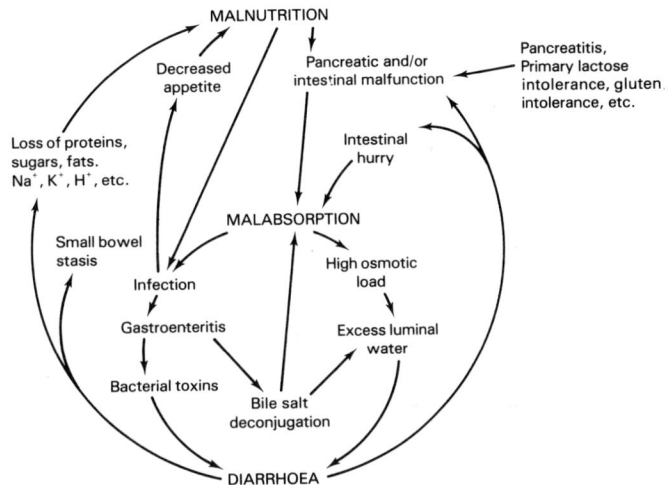

Fig. 4.2 The vicious cycle of diarrhoea and malnutrition. (Courtesy of WF Balistreri.)

Mechanisms of malnutrition during infections with intestinal parasites

1. Anorexia plays an important role in PEM. The loss of appetite can be the consequence of abdominal pain and distension secondary to parasitic infestations of the bowel.
2. Reduced calorie intake — children with protracted diarrhoea, due to parasites such as giardiasis, do not have an adequate food energy intake.
3. Mucosal atrophy is a dominant feature in PEM. The damage to the microvilli is more severe in protein-deficient children (kwashiorkor) than in those with energy deficiency (marasmus). In addition, the epithelial cells of the villi, bearing the brush-border disaccharidases become injured, thereby resulting in carbohydrate malabsorption.
4. Protein-losing enteropathy and iron deficiency. Iron deficiency, from intestinal bleeding, is well known, e.g. with hookworm infections (*Necator* sp. and *Ancylostoma* sp.). The loss of blood and mucus from the bowel causes hypoproteinaemia (e.g. *Entamoeba histolytica*) and this exacerbates PEM.
5. Hypercatabolism — systemic infections will

cause an increased rate of catabolism and if identified necessitate a high energy feeding regimen (200 kcal/kg per day or 840 kJ/kg per day). Because immunocompetence is compromised in malnutrition there is an increased susceptibility to infections. Tuberculosis and bronchopneumonia are important causes of secondary problems. A major viral complication of PEM is measles which has a high mortality in malnourished infants.

Some species of bacteria deconjugate bile acids and thus impair lipid- and fat-soluble vitamin absorption and *fat malabsorption* correlates with the degree of protein depletion. An altered *bile acid pool* is linked with a greater concentration of free bile acids and diminished conjugated bile acids. As a result micelle formation is lowered and fat uptake reduced. There is also an atrophy of the pancreas in kwashiorkor. Abnormalities of the liver are common in PEM and dietary toxins (e.g. aflatoxin) will increase hepatic deterioration. Indeed, it has been hypothesized that chronic aflatoxin poisoning could cause kwashiorkor (Hendrickse *et al.*, 1982). Infections and diarrhoea are responsible for a decline in nitrogen absorption. The *absorption of simple carbohydrates* by facilitated diffusion is impeded in severe PEM and hexose absorption (active transport) is often reduced. Immunity may be impaired. There is oedema of the gut and many nutrients are mal-absorbed (including vitamin B_{12}). Atrophy of the gastric mucosa and hypochlorhydria are also seen (Herbst *et al.*, 1969).

Treatment

Lack of nutritional knowledge and financial resources within a household, the community and society at large are responsible for the appalling global mobidity and mortality associated with PEM. The prevention of PEM ought to be regarded as the consequence of adverse social/economic conditions rather than primarily a medical problem. Simple measures such as the encouragement of breast feeding, personal hygiene, improved sanitation and the establishment of adequate and safe drinking water would do much to prevent many enteric infections in malnourished infants. Furthermore, the Thirty-first World Health Assembly in 1978 recommended 'regulating inappropriate sales promotion of infant foods that can be used to replace breast milk' (WHO, 1981).

The main principles in the management of PEM are:

1. Correct dehydration and electrolyte imbalance (by enteric or intravenous route) (*see* Chapter 2). In the presence of wasting it can be difficult to assess the severity of the dehydration. Mild dehydration can often be dealt with orally or by a nasogastric tube. Vomiting or persistent diarrhoea is an indication for the intravenous route (*see* p. 35).
2. Treat underlying infection(s) and/or parasitic infestations.
3. Treat other deficiencies and associated conditions, e.g.
   a. Iron deficiency;
   b. Folate deficiency;
   c. Vitamin A deficiency;
   d. Vitamin K deficiency;
   e. Magnesium deficiency;
   f. Hypoglycaemia;
   g. Candidiasis;
   h. Scabies.
4. Nutritional rehabilitation ('catch-up' growth). Anthropometric measurements and the use of appropriate reference charts or standards are essential for the proper assessment of growth (*see* Appendix I for standards). By the very simple act of measuring mid upper arm circumference (MUAC), community health workers in Bangladesh could predict the 56% of children who would die within a month (Briend *et al,*, 1987). MUAC is a better screening technique than other anthropometric indices at identifying those at high risk of death from invisible malnutrition in underprivileged communities. An MUAC of less than 110 mm denotes obvious malnutrition.

Oral rehydration

For details of oral rehydration *see* Chapter 2 but, while re-correcting dehydration, it is necessary to remember there is often failure to excrete sodium and excess water in PEM because of impaired cardiac and renal function.

Infection

Pneumonia and septicaemia (usually Gram-negative organisms) are the most common fatal infections. It has been suggested that anaerobic infections might also play a role (Ashworth, 1979). Some recommend antibiotics for severely malnourished infants even when the infection cannot be identified. The catabolic effect of infections increases nutrient requirements and worsens the effects of malnutrition.

Deficiencies

Vitamin A deficiency is one of the most common disorders seen in PEM. It has been estimated that 100 000 infants develop blindness from vitamin A deficiency and an equal number die from associated conditions. Even in the absence of xerophthalmia, vitamin A should be given to the following:

1. Infants under 12 months of age: vitamin A 15 mg by intramuscular injection (single dose) or vitamin A 30 mg orally once.
2. Children over 12 months of age:
   a. Vitamin A 30 mg by intramuscular injection (single dose) or vitamin A 60 mg orally for 2 days only;
   b. Then daily oral multivitamins to provide vitamin A 0.9–1.5 mg per day;
   c. Conclude treatment by giving 30 mg (<1 year) or 60 mg (>1 year).

3. Anaemia: Ashworth (1979) advised whole blood where haemoglobin was under 4 g/dl (maximum volume 10 ml/kg — over 3 hours).

Refeeding — acute phase

Once rehydration has been corrected small milk feeds should be given slowly every 2 hours. If the child is breast feeding every effort must be made to ensure this continues. It is preferable to use a cup and spoon for the non-breast-fed child, but naso-gastric feeding may be needed if insufficient feed is taken. A cautious and slow approach to refeeding is recommended (Walia, Rugmini and Khurana, 1982). Initially only half-strength feeds may be tolerated — a feeding schedule is shown in Table 4.2. Stabilization can be achieved on maintenance amounts of protein and energy (Harland, 1983); a suitable feed is given in Appendix III.7. Feeding in this way reduces the risks of cardiac and liver failure and lessens the probability of the child developing secondary lactose intolerance, hypo-glycaemia and hypothermia.

As weight falls due to loss of oedema and the appetite returns, full-strength feeds can be increased to 110 ml/kg giving 110 kcal/kg (462 kJ) and 2 g protein/kg. Providing the child is passing urine, potassium (4 mmol/kg per day), magnesium (2 mmol/kg per day) and a multivitamin preparation should be given.

Rehabilitation

Once full-strength feeds are tolerated intake can be stepped up to initiate weight gain. A high-energy feed providing approximately 150 ml/kg per day, 200 kcal/kg per day (840 MJ) and 4.5 g protein/kg per day given in 5—6 feeds provides

Table 4.2 Feeding schedule for a severely mal-nourished child based on 150 ml/kg body weight per day

Day	Strength of feed	Number of feeds per day
1	Half	12
2	Half	8
3, 4	Two-thirds	8
5 and onwards	Full	6

Adapted from Cameron and Hofvander (1983).

an opportunity for catch-up growth to take place over 4—6 weeks. If milk is both available and culturally acceptable, it can be fortified with sugar and oil to give a high-energy feed containing adequate protein (Appendix III.7). As fortification is needed to meet energy requirements, expensive protein preparations, e.g. Casilan (p. 265), are unnecessary (Ashworth, 1980). Realimentation formulae, designed to increase the rate of catch-up growth are marketed and their content is described (Appendix II.16). The staple cereal can form the basis of a feed but, owing to its bulky nature, this has a low energy density (Lindqvist, Mellander and Svanberg, 1981). It should be fortified, preferably using local produce.

Weight should be plotted against height weekly so that recurrent infection or inadequate intake can be identified. A record of food intake is valuable as it may explain a poor weight gain. Mild diarrhoea commonly persists. Unless the diarrhoea is serious the high-energy feed will not need diluting.

When solids are reintroduced the amounts initially need to be small, e.g. 150—200 ml (1—1.5 cups) for children of 1—3 years. In nutrition rehabilitation centres solids are introduced early in the recovery process and the emphasis is on parental education to avoid recurrence of PEM.

An introductory regimen for cereals has to be carefully planned. High-energy feeds can continue to be given until normal weight-for-height has been achieved. The child is then given the usual family diet. Many different mixes have been developed and choice varies according to local custom, availability and preference. A nutritionally adequate basic mix should contain a cereal, such as rice or maize, a protein source such as pulses, beans, milk, chicken, fish or eggs, a vitamin and mineral source, such as dark leafy vegetables, and fat or oil as an energy source. Fruit juice and fresh fruit should also be given at an early stage in the child's recovery.

Commercially processed weaning foods are widely available throughout the world but are too costly in less developed countries. Mothers need to be informed that their use is not essential and that a nutritionally adequate local mixture is satisfactory.

Hospitalized children with severe PEM should not be discharged until they have reached their target weight and can tolerate family food. This is of importance where facilities for monitoring progress are not available. The family diet may provide insufficient energy to maintain catch-up growth. The ability of children recovering from

PEM to achieve full catch-up growth is unclear, because children with PEM probably came from low socioeconomic groups and are likely to be shorter than those from more affluent families (Alvear *et al.*, 1986). An increased growth velocity can be maintained for many months provided an adequate energy intake is achieved.

Often home conditions and standards of hygiene are such that the mother may be unable to follow any complex hospital regimen. Junior hospital staff need to understand the importance of rehydration and the benefits of high-energy mixtures. Skills that have to be developed include a commitment to ensure that the dietary regimen is followed and, when resouces fail, initiative in seeking alternative solutions.

Prevention through education is of prime importance if the high global prevalence of PEM is to be reduced. Above all, education has to be appropriate to local economic/agricultural conditions and social circumstances. Clear and concise information must be conveyed by health workers.

Parents need to know how to mix rehydration fluids (*see* Chapter 2) in case diarrhoea and vomiting occur. Early intervention by parents can halt the development of PEM. Above all parents need to know how to use locally available foods to their optimal advantage. Quantities used must relate to local measures and household utensils, such as cups. Local cooking methods should be advocated as these have evolved in response to the prevailing conditions for the population.

5

Conditions Associated with Modified Dietary Requirements

Low- and very-low-birth-weight babies

Babies of low birth weight (LBW) are by definition less than 2.5 kg and those of very low birth weight (VLBW) less than 1.5 kg. Approximately one-third of LBW babies can be labelled as intrauterine growth retarded (IUGR) or small for gestational age (SGA). This contrasts with 'pre-term' which is the description applied to the baby who is immature and has a gestational age of 37 weeks or less. If the weight is appropriate for the gestational age (AGA) then the newborn is not growth retarded. The clinical problems and nutritional needs of the immature, as opposed to the neonate with IUGR, are dissimilar.

Oral feeding

Growth and energy

Many neonatologists feel that the growth rate in very pre-term infants should be close to that which is seen *in utero*. Table 5.1 shows some suggested nutrient intakes for LBW infants. Where nutrients have been omitted it must be assumed that the intake should be the same as for term infants until further data are available.

Because of the relatively high energy requirements of LBW infants a high caloric intake is desirable. However, if volumes above 150 ml/kg body weight daily are given either by oral or intravenous route, there is an increasing risk of patent ductus arteriosus. In contrast, if volumes are less than 120 ml/kg, the feed must have a high energy density in order to achieve an adequate energy intake. Hyperosmolar feeds may be linked to one of the causes of necrotizing enterocolitis and are also implicated in lactobezoar formation. The minimum energy requirement appears to be at least 120 kcal (500 kJ)/kg body weight per day and in practice this caloric intake is satisfactory for most LBW infants. This aspect of nutrition and the whole subject of the needs of low-birth-weight infants is well reviewed by the American Academy of Pediatrics (1985), and a committee of the European Society of Paediatric Gastroenterology (Wharton, 1987).

Table 5.1 Requirements which differ from those of term neonates

Nutrient	Suggested intake/kg body weight daily
Fluid	120−150 ml
Energy	120 kcal (500 kJ)
Protein	3.0 g
Sodium	<30 weeks gestation: up to 5.0 mmol 30−35 weeks gestation: up to 4 mmol
Calcium	5.5−6.25 mmol (220−250 mg)
Phosphorus	4.0 mmol (125 mg)
Iron	0.015−0.053 mmol (1−3.5 mg)
Copper	0.0095−0.0125 mmol (0.6−0.8 mg)

	Suggested total daily intake
Vitamin D	<34 weeks gestation: 0.025−0.05 mg >34 weeks gestation: 0.01−0.02 mg
Vitamin E	5.0 mg or 1 mg/g linoleic acid
Vitamin B_6	0.1 mg or 0.015 mg/g protein
Folic acid	0.1−0.2 mg
Vitamin K	1−1.5 mg at birth, repeated at 10 days if necessary

Protein and amino acid requirements

Less than 1.6 g protein/kg daily is insufficient for adequate growth and, furthermore, might result in hypoproteinaemia and subsequent oedema. Fortunately, the immature gut can conserve protein from week 29 of gestation (Sivan *et al.*, 1985). Protein intakes exceeding 4 g/kg daily can produce a raised blood urea nitrogen, hyperaminoaciduria and metabolic acidosis (which has an adverse effect on weight gain); 2.25 g/kg per day is recommended by the American Academy of Pediatrics (Committee on Nutrition, 1977), although this is considered low by some centres, who advocate > 3 g/kg per day (personal communication, W.C. Heird).

The quality of protein fed is as important as the quantity. Improved nitrogen retention takes place when the ratio of casein to whey is closer to mature human milk (70:30) than cows' milk (20:80) (DHSS, 1977; Brooke, 1982). The amino acid requirement of the LBW infant is different because of a deficiency of some key enzymes within the immature liver. For example, cystine is considered to be an essential amino acid for the LBW infant, and possibly glycine and taurine, as are cofactors such as carnitine — a fatty acid which is involved in fatty acid oxidation (Melegh *et al.*, 1987). Whey protein is richer in the specified amino acids than is casein. The elevated and harmful concentrations of some amino acids, such as phenylalanine and tyrosine found in casein-predominant formulae, may result in hyperaminoaciduria due to immature liver function; the suboptimal catabolism of these amino acids can lead to metabolic acidosis (Räihiä *et al.*, 1976).

At birth, the term infant's pancreatic activity for proteolysis is probably adequate. Pancreatic trypsin can be observed as early as 16 weeks of gestation and will then increase rapidly with advancing age. At term both trypsin and chymotrypsin secretion is only slightly lower than at 1 year of age and from 3 weeks to 12 months old serum trypsinogen values do not alter.

In general, infants fed on protein other than a high whey formula, such as casein protein or a soy-based formula, exhibit a slow weight gain and poor nitrogen retention. The Committee on Nutrition of the American Academy of Pediatrics (1983) advises that soy-based protein formulae should not be used for the routine feeding of pre-term and low-birth-weight infants. LBW infants require a greater protein:energy ratio than term infants who are not growth retarded. Provided that a suitable protein is used, 1 g protein per 35–40 kcal (145–165 kJ) should achieve a good weight gain with little risk of metabolic complications.

Lipids and bile salts

There is a reduced bile acid pool in the pre-term infant compared with the baby born at term. This digestive disadvantage might be aggravated by the decreased pool associated with poor weight-gaining infants. From gestational week 35, pancreatic lipase is present. Therefore, a very immature infant will have reduced lipolytic activity and be unable to utilize the ingested fats; but lingual lipase, which is present from gestational week 26, might complement lipolysis by pancreatic lipase. Milk triglycerides, the main source of human milk calories, are a poor substrate for pancreatic as opposed to lingual lipase in the immature. An advantage of untreated breast milk is its own lipase content which becomes functional in the duodenum having been activated by bile salts secreted with the bile.

However, pre-term serum lipase, although significantly lower than values which are obtained at term, will increase very markedly after 10 weeks of age. Moreover Cleghorn *et al.* (1988) have suggested that the rate of maturation of lipase is facilitated by the extrauterine environment. At 6 months of age, Cleghorn and his associates found premature infants had much higher serum lipase values than infants of the same age who were born at term. Even though pancreatic lipase increases by twofold by 1 month of age it still remains low at 1 year of age.

A number of investigators have shown that the use of medium-chain triglycerides (MCTs) will avoid the malabsorption of long-chain fatty acids present in human milk or standard formulae. However, Okamoto *et al.* (1982) and Whyte *et al.* (1986) demonstrated no improved growth or clinical benefit using MCTs. Because of the caution necessary for its introduction (p. 257), a feeding regimen including MCT takes longer to establish and, in the short term, may provide less energy than a conventional long-chain saturated fatty acid feed. Another reason for the failure of MCT to promote a higher growth rate may be its slightly lower energy content — 8.3 kcal (34 kJ)/g compared with 9 kcal (37 kJ)/g of long-chain fat.

Unabsorbed long-chain fatty acids in the small intestine interfere with calcium absorption (Andrews and Lorch, 1974), although improved calcium handling has not been demonstrated with MCT. A further advantage of high levels of MCT in the diet seems to be its greater influence on gluconeogenesis (glucose synthesis from a non-carbohydrate source) compared with long- and short-chain fats.

Current evidence suggests MCT in premature formulae might be advantageous. Yet in large quantities it may cause intestinal symptoms; it would seem that unsaturated vegetable fat should form the major fat source in such formulae.

Carbohydrates

Pre-term infants might malabsorb lactose because small bowel intestinal lactase activity does not develop fully until the last few weeks of a term gestation, although Weaver *et al.* (1986) using indirect techniques, involving urinary lactose and lactulose ratios, suggested that 98% of lactose is hydrolysed even in very pre-term infants. The substitution of glucose for lactose results in an unacceptably high osmolar load. Sucrose and maltose, although well utilized by LBW infants, are rarely used in infant formulae. A glucose polymer containing short-chain oligosaccharides (from two to ten monosaccharide units) used in this situation appears to be well tolerated (Raffles *et al.*, 1983).

Lactose assists in the absorption of intestinal calcium and in the promotion of normal gut flora. Neither of these effects can be seen with glucose polymers. The substitution of part of the disaccharide sugar lactose in a pre-term formula for another carbohydrate would seem to be beneficial.

Renal function and sodium

In infants of less than 34 weeks' gestation, the renal function is considerably reduced. The adaptive capacity of the kidney is low and sodium homeostasis must be carefully watched. Urinary sodium losses are highest in very immature babies and hyponatraemia can develop (Engelke *et al.*, 1978). Tubular function matures rapidly after birth and requirements will change. For the first 4 weeks in infants of less than 30 weeks' gestation, 5 mmol/kg daily is necessary. For infants of 30−35 weeks, 4 mmol/kg for the first 2−4 weeks; after 35 weeks of gestation 2.5−3.0 mmol/kg should be adequate in the first 2−4 weeks. Distal tubule maturation should be advanced sufficiently to warrant a normal sodium intake after this time.

Minerals

Iron

Iron stores in the pre-term infant are low and anaemia is likely to occur. However, early supplementation of iron has several disadvantages including the provocation of haemolytic anaemia which can be due to vitamin E deficiency. Yet one controlled trial in Canada of vitamin E supplementation showed it had no beneficial effect in preventing the anaemia of prematurity (Zipursky *et al.*, 1987). Iron supplements are believed to be unnecessary in the first month of life and they do antagonize the anti-infective properties of human milk. After this period the amount of iron given depends upon the birth weight of the infant: for a birth weight of less than 1000 g, the infant requires 0.07 mmol (4 mg) iron/kg body weight daily, of 1000−1500 g, 0.53 mmol (3 mg)/kg, of 1500−2500 g, 0.035 mmol (2 mg) iron/kg daily should be sufficient. Supplements may need to be continued to 12−15 months.

Copper

Copper deficiency can cause osteoporosis and metaphyseal abnormalities with radiological findings not dissimilar to those observed in rickets. Copper and zinc, in common with iron, accumulate in the fetal liver towards the end of gestation, and thus prematurity deprives the newborn of adequate stores. In addition the routine supplementation of iron in some milk formulae reduces the bioavailability of copper and zinc. Furthermore, the bioavailability of copper depends partly on the relative amounts of other metals, such as zinc and cadmium (*see* Appendix II.10). As yet the precise needs have to be determined, and deficiency states may arise (Yuen *et al.*, 1979; Aggett *et al.*, 1980; Editorial, 1987)

Selenium

Blood transfusion provides 0.5 mg selenium/kg per day. A mean intake of 1.73 µg/kg per day will result in a fall of selenium in prematures fed enterally (Friel *et al.*, 1984). Those on total parenteral nutrition require 3 µg/kg per day.

Calcium and phosphorus

Hypomineralization of bone leading to rachitic

changes is frequently seen in LBW infants. Those under 1500 g should be regularly monitored for evidence of rickets by studying the bone alkaline phosphatase (ideally but not essentially the isoenzyme) and confirming the diagnosis with an X-ray of the wrists. The absorption of calcium is inefficient in very small infants. The quantity and type of fat, the relative amounts of calcium and phophorus and vitamin D will all affect calcium absorption. Formulae designed to meet the requirements of LBW infants should have a higher calcium and phosphorus content than a normal formula. The use of phosphate and calcium supplements added to milk in response to blood monitoring are described by Whitelaw (1986).

Requirements for calcium and phosphorus are summarized in Table 5.1. The optimum calcium: phosphorus ratio has not been defined and the present recommendation is the same as for term infants in the range of 1.2−2.0. There is not adequate evidence for an increased magnesium requirement, although high retention rates of magnesium seem to need a higher intake than that supplied by breast milk or a normal infant formula.

Vitamins

Poor absorption, increased utilization and rapid tissue growth would suggest an increased need for all vitamins. Where infants are fed mature breast milk or the total intake is less than 300 kcal (1250 kJ) daily, a multivitamin supplement is required. However, it is recommended only from the age of one month. The routine use of a multivitamin preparation for LBW infants is less justifiable.

Vitamin D

Cholecalciferol (vitamin D_3) metabolism in preterm infants relates to the gestational age. Prior to 32 weeks there is inadequate absorption and hydroxylation of vitamin D and daily supplements of up to 0.05 mg should be given. After this age an intake of 0.01−0.02 mg appears adequate.

Vitamin E

The requirement for vitamin E is affected both by the amount of polyunsaturated fatty acids and by the level of iron in the feed; iron catalyses the generation of lipid peroxidases from unsaturated fats. A ratio of 1 mg α-tocopherol to each gram of linoleic acid is advisable with a minimum intake of 5 mg α-tocopherol if the feed is supplemented with iron.

Vitamin C

There is a theoretical extra requirement for ascorbic acid (vitamin C) because of the higher ingestion of protein by LBW infants, particularly if a casein-based feed is taken or hypertyrosinaemia and/or hyperphenylalaninaemia exist. It has been suggested that 50 mg vitamin C daily is adequate.

Vitamin B6

A high protein indicates an increased requirement for pyridoxine (vitamin B_6) and a minimum amount of 0.015 mg/g of protein, or a total of 0.1 mg daily appears to be adequate.

Vitamin K

There is decreased absorption of quinones (vitamin K) during the first few days of life because the gut flora is not yet established and the vitamin synthesis by bacteria has not commenced. A dose of 1−1.5 mg initially is advisable.

Folic acid

The need for extra folic acid is not universally accepted but 0.1−0.2 mg daily will prevent a deficiency state arising.

Enteral feeding

Feeding a LBW infant using the transpyloric route (jejunal or duodenal) is claimed to be beneficial because the problems of gastric distension are avoided. Also pulmonary aspiration is less of a risk when feeding is via the intrajejunal/intraduodenal system because milk is infused beyond the pyloric sphincter thus reducing episodes of regurgitation. However, the mere presence of such a tube can induce reflux into the stomach. Some have demonstrated no advantage in transpyloric feeding in terms of growth (Drew *et al.*, 1979; Laing *et al.*, 1986). Infusing milk of whatever source directly into the small bowel is clearly less physiological than infusions. Even using a soft rubberized Silastic tube within the jejunum might predispose to perforation or necrotizing enterocolitis. The infusion of hyperosmolar feeds can cause 'dumping' and fat malabsorption because lingual lipase is not utilized. The position of the tip of the tube should be checked radiologically because it is often impossible to aspirate from a soft small bore catheter to check for bile and an alkaline pH. In addition proteins, toxins and pathogens are a greater hazard if infused via a 'bypass system'. For these and other reasons many of us now advocate a return to intragastric feeding (Laing *et al.*, 1986). Transpyloric feeding, if practised, should be confined to units having the specialized nursing and medical expertise.

Constant infusion rather than intermittent bolus feeding is preferred, because it has been shown to result in greater weight gain than intermittent feeding (Toce, Keenan and Homan, 1987), although this requires vigilance on the part of the nursing staff to ensure that the tube remains in position. The calcium and phosphorus content of the feed may be altered because of settling and separation during the infusion period.

Nutritional options

There are a number of alternatives open to the mother and physician when deciding on the type of feed that is most suitable: the mother's own milk, pooled and pasteurized bank breast milk, enriched human milk, and baby milk formulae. Each has its advantages and disadvantages and factors such as the wishes of the parents, cultural concepts, the availability of a milk, the weight, the gestational and postconceptional age of the infant should be taken into account before a decision is made.

Mother's own milk

There is some evidence that an infant fed with his own mother's untreated milk has some, but not total, protection against necrotizing enterocolitis. This benefit is diminished if the milk is stored or preserved by pasteurization or freezing. Heating of the milk renders nutrients less available (Zoeren-Grobber *et al.*, 1987).

The nutrient content of milk from mothers who deliver pre-term is different to that from mothers who deliver at term. This is possibly due to immature mammary gland function or to a stress reaction resulting in a prolonged colostral phase. The protein, sodium, chloride, magnesium, zinc, copper and tocopherol content of the pre-term milk is higher than term milk, while phosphorus content is lower.

A major present day deterrant relating to the use of raw human milk, particularly if pooled, is the risk of transmitting the human immunodeficiency virus (HIV) to the immunocompromised newborn. Antenatal screening of all mothers would identify carriers and reduce, but not nullify, HIV infection in the neonate.

Infants fed on pre-term milk require calcium and phosphorus supplementation and at times sodium; if an iron supplement is given then additional zinc, copper and vitamin E will be required. Additional iron is needed to prevent late anaemia which develops because the storage *in utero* has been curtailed.

The energy content of pre-term and term milks is similar. A simple laboratory test ('creamatocrit') enables the paediatrician to assess the calories of sampled human milk when it is centrifuged in a haematocrit tube (Lucas *et al.*, 1978). This basic technique ought to be more widely practised to determine the energy value of breast milk in a non-thriving baby. The formula is:

Energy value = 290 + (66.8 x creamatocrit) kcal/l

For example, a tube of milk is found to have a creamatocrit of 5%. The calorific value is therefore:

290 + (66.8 x 5) = 624 kcal/l (or 2.62 MJ/l).

All studies examining human milks have demonstrated a very wide range of nutrient content between various mothers and in the same mother, when sampled at either breast and different phases of a feed and over a 24-hour period. This variation in composition can make management complex. In addition, mothers may experience greater difficulty in expressing milk or indeed breast feeding in a hospital setting, when compared to the non-clinical atmosphere of home. The regular use of an efficient electric breast pump in private and relaxed surroundings may improve lactation (Whitelaw, 1986).

Pooled human milk and 'lacto-engineering'

The nutrient content of pooled breast milk tends to be less variable than that from one mother. Despite this deficiency, particularly of protein and energy, there have been reports of infants fed pooled human milk achieving the desired intrauterine rate of growth, but in all case the infants have been fed volumes in excess of 180 ml/kg daily. A high volume intake is associated with an increased incidence of patent ductus arteriosus and necrotizing enterocolitis. If milk from a donor other than the infant's own mother is used without prior freezing to 4°C for 48 hours (Pittard and Bill, 1981) or pasteurization (Lucas and Roberts, 1979) there is a risk of bacterial contamination. Storage and processing of the milk alters both nutrient availability and protective function (Whitelaw, 1986). Many now advocate raw breast milk which can be safely stored at 4–6°C for 72 hours but the contentious and emotional topic of HIV has made such a policy controversial. Bacteriological quality control of pooled human milk is advisable. Some recommend that donor mothers discard the first few millilitres at the start of expression but others have disputed the need for this commonsense practice.

Because of the slow growth noted with pooled breast milk attempts have been made to enrich its content.

Human milk or modified human milk 'lacto-engineering' techniques. Lindblad *et al.* (1982) suggested that the protein intake of breast milk could be increased by adding a concentrated human milk isolate that doubled the protein load. This method did not cause the urea to rise. Furthermore, because it contained high secretory IgA (SIgA) activity against *E. coli* O-antigen the label 'hyperimmune breast milk' was suggested by the innovator. While the techniques of 'lacto-engineering' are interesting, widespread global application is a remote hope. Furthermore, one study has failed to show advantage in terms of growth (Schanler *et al.*, 1985a) and has demonstrated suboptimal retention of calcium and phosphorus (Schanler *et al.*, 1985b) in infants fed supplemented human milk.

Special LBW formulae. Special milk formulae have been designed to meet the increased requirements of the LBW infant. Appendix II.5 lists some formulae of this type. The energy density of formulae presently available is normally either 84 kcal (350 kJ)/100 ml which is equivalent to 24 kcal (100 kJ) per fluid ounce, or 95 kcal (395 kJ)/100 ml which is equivalent to 27 kcal (112 kJ) per fluid ounce. The use of feeds exceeding 84 kcal (350 kJ)/100 ml is associated with lactobezoar formation (aggregates of dense milk curds causing stomach outlet obstruction). The incidence of this phenomenon has increased in recent years and may be associated with LBW formulae. A formula which complies with these recommendations and which is not fed in excess of 150 ml/kg per day is unlikely to cause biochemical abnormalities. Studies have shown

that energy and nitrogen balances in very-low-birth-weight infants fed a low-birth-weight milk formula are greater compared with similar breast-fed infants (Brooke *et al.*, 1987; de Curtis and Brooke, 1987). Where such a formula is thought to be desirable, but is not available, a feed of similar composition can be prepared using a whey-based low-solute baby milk powder. The usual concentration of a feed of this type is 12% (12 g powder made up to a total volume of 100 ml). This can be concentrated to 20% dilution using 20 g powder made up to a final volume of 100 ml. Appendix II.9 shows the composition of a normal infant formula at 12% and 20% dilutions and of a premature milk formula. Sodium may still need to be supplemented with this regimen. Particular care must be taken in the preparation of a concentrated feed and infants should not be discharged home on anything but a standard dilution.

The Committee on Nutrition of the American Academy of Pediatrics (1983) advises that soy-protein formulae should not be used for the routine feeding of premature and low-birth-weight infants. It is difficult to generalize about an optimum feeding regimen because there are many conflicting data. The reasons for the low birth weight — whether due to prematurity and/or intrauterine malnutrition — influence such decisions. Infants who are growth retarded are better equipped to use an enriched milk formula than immature infants. For infants below 1200 g there are arguments for delaying oral feeding until after 2 weeks of age, but only if the expertise for parenteral nutrition and reliable biochemical monitoring is available. Certainly the use of high-energy feeds (84 kcal or 350 kJ/100 ml) during this period would appear to carry many risks. For infants above 1200 g the use of the mother's own breast milk alone seems to be the optimal regimen for the first 2 weeks. After this period, if growth velocity is impaired then the use of a premature formula either alone or in conjunction with the mother's own milk to achieve an intake of 120–150 ml fluid/kg daily should be adequate. The use of mineral, vitamin and trace element supplements must be calculated on an individual basis depending upon the infant's age, size and feed intake.

There are still many problems to be overcome in this field of nutrition. The first target must be to establish actual requirements of LBW infants.

Research is needed into formulae so that the bioavailability, balance and solubility of nutrients in feeds can be improved. Future developments

Table 5.2 Reasons for malnutrition in cancer

Cause	Effect	Result
Chemotherapy, e.g. vincristine	Physiological anorexia, nausea, alteration of taste perception, constipation	Poor food intake
Anxiety, depression, separation from family	Psychogenic anorexia, food refusal, food aversion	
Irradiation of head and pharynx, chemotherapy, e.g. methotrexate	Difficulty in eating and swallowing, stomatitis, oesophagitis, mouth ulcers	
Irradiation of abdomen and pelvis chemotherapy, e.g. cytosine arabinoside	Damage to mucosa of gastrointestinal tract, vomiting, poor digestion and absorption, diarrhoea	Poor nutrient retention
Surgery, infection	Hypermetabolic state, fever, catabolism	Increased nutrient requirements

Table 5.3 Staging the state of nutrition in cancer patients

Stage	Criteria
Nourished	Weight for height greater than or equal to the 5th percentile
	Weight less than the 5th percentile
	Albumin concentration greater than or equal to 3.2 g/dl
Malnourished	Weight for height less than 5th percentile
	Weight loss greater than or equal to 5%
	Serum albumin concentration less than 3.2 g/dl

must include formulae that are adapted to the needs and digestive capabilities of these very small infants. Ideally, we also seek a human milk substitute that is not an allergenic threat and bestows on the newborn some immunological benefit.

Cancer

The major nutritional complications of advanced cancer (Table 5.2) include anorexia, muscle wasting, both impaired protein synthesis and glucose intolerance, and a range of other metabolic abnormalities. One important aspect of satisfactory nutrition in malignancy is that it is associated with improved survival in localized disease (Donaldson *et al.*,

1981). It has been claimed that physicians have failed to recognize the importance and significance of malnutrition in neoplastic disorders (Rickard *et al.*, 1983). The incidence of malnutrition ranges from 6 to 50% depending upon the nature and severity of the malignancy.

Staging of the state of nutrition will enable objective changes to be assessed (Table 5.3). Anthropometric measurements, using skin-fold calipers to record subscapular thickness, are essential (Kibirige *et al.*, 1987). If the weight loss is equal to or exceeds 5% or the weight is less than the 5th percentile weight for height or the albumin concentration is under 3.2 g/dl, then the label of PEM has been applied (Rickard *et al.*, 1983). Transferrin may be an indicator of low energy intake and PEM.

Chemotherapy and radiotherapy

Chemotherapy and radiotherapy can induce an enteritis causing malabsorption. Bowel damage secondary to radiation has been observed in more than one-third of childhood malignancies. Radiation enteritis is determined by the total radiation dose and is common where therapy needs 50 grays. Chemotherapeutic agents, particularly actinomycin D and doxorubicin, can potentiate radiation enteritis. Also liver disease and even fibrosis may result from radiation. A number of anti-cancer drugs interfere with the proliferation of intestinal crypt cells and maturation of the intestinal mucosa. Cisplatin is nephrotoxic and can result in magnesium loss (Gonzalez and Villasanta, 1982). Malignant disease may be associated with reduced serum retinol and vitamin A which can adversely affect immunocompetence (Strauss, 1978). Furthermore, the use of high-calorie milk-containing solutions may precipitate or aggravate gastrointestinal symptoms arising from cancer therapy (Hyams *et al.*, 1982). Mucosal atrophy of the bowel secondary to radiation will produce decreased disaccharidases and subsequent diarrhoea when carbohydrates are ingested.

Protein metabolism in cancer

Muscle wasting is a not uncommon feature of malignant disease. It has been shown convincingly that there is a decreased rate of protein synthesis in skeletal muscle that is associated with a reduced RNA content. There is also an increased rate both of whole-body protein turnover and of specific protein synthesis in the liver.

Glucose metabolism in cancer

Carter *et al.* (1975) have shown a disturbed pattern of glucose metabolism and a decreased sensitivity and responsiveness to insulin in women with metastatic breast cancer. However, such changes could be secondary to anorexia and are seen in other abnormal states, e.g. starvation or infection, and the anomaly has not been detected in children. For a review *see* Lundholm *et al.* (1982).

The elevated free fatty acids noted in malignant conditions can interfere with glucose and pyruvate oxidation.

Obviously, cachexia is in part responsible for the morbidity and mortality in cancer.

Diet and cancer

One of the main objectives in dietary management is to increase the intake of energy and protein. For preference this should be achieved by the use of normal foods with the addition of high-energy, high-protein supplements as described in the section on enteral feeding. Appetite might be improved if parents are encouraged to bring foods prepared at home to the hospital and are then allowed to eat with the child. Meals should be small, appetizing and are offered frequently; timing of meals must be flexible enough to enable the child to eat when he or she wants. In hospital a range of favourite foods should be available at all times.

Specific problems should be dealt with. If diarrhoea is severe there may be disaccharide intolerance or fat malabsorption and the appropriate dietary treatments for these conditions should be instituted (pp. 82 and 74). The use of hyperosmolar high-energy supplements may precipitate or aggravate gastrointestinal symptoms arising from cancer therapy (Hyams *et al.*, 1982). The alteration in taste perception and the metallic mouth taste caused by some drugs often make red meats unacceptable and alternatives such as poultry, cheese or fish may be preferred. Cold foods are a better option if the child is nauseated. Constipation is best dealt with by using a pharmaceutical bulking agent and a high intake of fluid because a high-fibre diet is low in energy density.

Difficulty in eating and swallowing owing to soreness of the mouth and throat also requires an adequate fluid source. Soft low-acid food should be suggested; chilled foods and drinks cause less discomfort and, provided that the lesions are not on the tongue, a straw may be preferred to a cup. Sucking ice-cubes, ice-lollies or popsicles can be soothing and these can be fortified by freezing one of the mixtures given in Appendix III.5.

If an adequate intake of fluid and nutrients cannot be achieved orally then a nasogastric feed may need to be used as described Appendix III.1. A fine-bore nasogastric tube can enable a continuous infusion to take place overnight while the child is asleep, the tube being removed in the morning. In the presence of severe bowel disease associated with aggressive anti-cancer treatment, intestinal surgery and radiotherapy, total parental nutrition (TPN) might be the preferred option. Survival might not be influenced by TPN although short-term benefits can be achieved, such as a feeling of well-being; this is dealt with in Chapter 18. There is a greater risk of sepsis in the malnourished immunologically compromised child but this risk is decreased if TPN is started early and continued for as long as possible. Rickard *et al.* (1983) suggest that the recommended dietary allowance (RDA) for all nutrients should be infused for a period of 21−28 days.

Poor nutrition may adversely affect the outcome of chemotherapy, e.g. doxorubicin has been shown to have a greater cardiotoxic effect in poorly nourished patients. Mood changes in children with protein−energy malnutrition are well documented and in sick children poor nutrition can contribute to depression. The provision of nutritional support forms a part of the total programme of treatment.

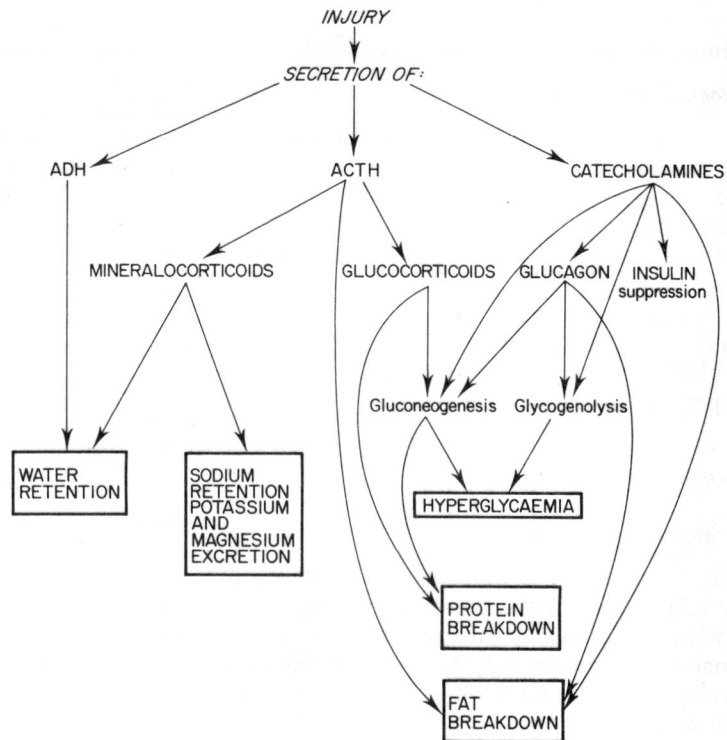

Fig. 5.1 The metabolic effect of injury.

Burns and trauma

In the USA, 100 000 patients are hospitalized annually for burn injuries and almost 8000 of these die: more than one-third of these cases are under the age of 15 years. Severe burns can cause a cascade of metabolic and nutritional changes (Fig. 5.1). The sequelae of serious thermal injury or trauma are such that a multidisciplinary approach is recommended (Stern and Davey, 1985). This support group should include a trained counsellor or even a child/family psychiatrist after the acute medical/surgical phase of management. The guilt felt by adults as a result of the incident may be underestimated, but is such that prolonged family psychotherapy may be essential if disharmony is to be avoided and parents should be encouraged to join the multidisciplinary team.

Initial assessment involves the recognition of shock and the maintenance of an airway in the acute situation. The approximate total surface area of the burn is evaluated by applying 'Wallace's Rule of Nines':

1. Each upper limb represents 9% of the surface area.
2. Each lower limb represents 18% of the surface area.
3. Head and face represent 9% of the surface area.
4. Front or back trunk represents 18% of the surface area.

Complications

Immediately after the burns, the physician must ensure that there are adequate fluids, electrolytes and protein replacements.

Respiratory complications (from carbon monoxide)

These are common where burns have arisen from an accident in a confined space. They include:

1. Inhalation of toxic gases.
2. *Shock lung* which should be suspected when respiratory problems develop 18–36 hours after the onset of severe hypotension as a result of shock from burns, haemorrhage or septicaemia.
3. Central venous pressure monitoring is essential if extensive limb burns prevent conventional blood pressure taking (Novak *et al.*, 1983).
4. Pneumonia.

5. Hyperventilation.
6. Pulmonary oedema with fluid overload.

Neurological complications

1. Confusion due to hypoxia from hypotension and shock.
2. Convulsions — the consequence of cerebral oedema from water intoxication.
3. Antidiuretic hormone (ADH) production, the product of a painful burn and water/electrolyte overload may all have a role.
4. Fluid restriction is indicated if burns exceed 10–15% of total body surface area.
5. Hyperpyrexia can cause a seizure.

Other complications

These include:

1. Septicaemia — this is unusual before the third day and is seen in the presence of deep burns or when a site has an impaired blood supply.
2. Renal — myoglobinuria, the result of damaged muscle, and haemoglobinuria can be associated with oliguria.
3. Gastrointestinal haemorrhage may be the result of an acute ulcer at almost any site in the intestinal tract.
4. Skeletal — the prevention of contractures by physiotherapists in the acute period is of major importance.

Basal metabolic rate

Burns or skeletal injury increase the basal metabolic rate (BMR). This metabolic change correlates with additional evaporative water loss from the site of the burn. Furthermore, an elevated rate of gluconeogenesis from amino acids may contribute to the raised metabolic rate.

The aims of treatment are (Davies *et al.*, 1981):

1. The relief of pain.
2. Management of hypovolaemic shock.
3. Prevention of burn wound infection.
4. Dressing control of the damaged skin area.
5. Early detection and treatment of burn wound infection. Impaired host resistance is often unidentified in burn injuries. Infection is a leading cause of death in burn injuries. Serum transferrin and skin antigen testing for cellular immune response can identify those at high risk of infectious complications (Jensen *et al.*, 1985).
6. Early autografting of deep–partial and full-thickness skin loss.
7. Nutritional support (Table 5.4). Malnourished post-operative and post-trauma patients are at increased risk of sepsis and mortality.
8. Prevention of contractures and hypertrophic scars.
9. Psychological support.
10. Rehabilitation.

For a concise overview of treatment, *see* Herndon *et al.* (1985).

Fluid requirements

Fluid requirements are high in burned and injured patients and early replacement is vital. Since much of the fluid loss results from exudation it may be preferable to base estimations on surface area (Herndon *et al.*, 1985). However, because surface area relates to height (Appendix I.19), accurate measurement may be difficult, so Herndon estimates fluid requirements, after the initial early shock period, to be 1500 ml/m^2 total surface area plus 3750 ml/m^2 burned surface area daily. Novak *et al.* (1983) suggested that in addition to the normal physiological requirements for age and size an additional (2 x percentage burned area x weight in kg) be given. Whichever formula is selected, intake should be sufficient to maintain a urine output of about 25 ml/kg per day.

Nutrient metabolism and requirements

Energy metabolism

It is acknowledged that the provision of an adequate energy intake is important in determining the survival of a burned or injured child (Solomon, 1981). Some experts suggest intakes of 200–300% of the RDA for age, while others state that requirements may not be greatly in excess of those for a well-nourished child of the same age. Although BMR is elevated this may be counterbalanced by the enforced inactivity of the child. A summary of methods of calculating energy and protein requirements is given in Table 5.4. Estimations of individual energy needs are always imprecise and careful monitoring of

Table 5.4 Summary of nutrient requirements in burns

Reference	Age/size	Energy (kcal/day)[c]	Protein (g/day)
Sutherland, 1955	Children	1.3 × normal requirement[a]	1.5 × normal requirement[a]
Curreri *et al.*, 1974	Adults	25 kcal/kg + 40 kcal × percentage burn	—
Solomon, 1981	Infants 0–9 kg	Normal requirement[a] + 15 kcal × percentage burn	Normal requirement[a] + 0.75 g × percentage burn
	1–3 years 10–13 kg	Normal requirement[a] + 20 kcal × percentage burn	Normal requirement[a] + 1.0 g × percentage burn
	3+ years	Normal requirement[a] + 30 kcal × percentage burn	Normal requirement[a] + 1.5 g × percentage burn
Hildreth and Carvajal, 1982	Children	1800 kcal/m² body surface area[b] + 2200 kcal/m² burned surface area	—
Bell *et al.*, 1984	Children	kcal = 2 × BMR (calculated from ideal body weight)	—

[a] Normal requirements — *see* Appendix I.2.
[b] Body surface area and BMR — *see* Appendix I.19.
[c] 1 kcal = 4.184 kJ.

weight to obtain a weight gain commensurate with age is the only method of ensuring an adequate intake.

The provision of a suitable protein/energy ratio is important to allow rapid regeneration of damaged tissue. This usually means that protein should contribute 25% of the energy intake during the early stages of recovery, decreasing to 16% as healing proceeds and catabolism lessens. Solomon (1981) recommends a nitrogen/calorie ratio of 1:130–150.

Protein metabolism

Wound exudate and hypercatabolism coupled with gluconeogenesis causes large amounts of amino acids and nitrogen to be lost. In addition, there appears to be a diminished ability to synthesize new protein by damaged tissues and organs.

There are some indications that protein requirements can be increased to 400–600% of the RDA, although others have demonstrated adequate nitrogen balance in children receiving an intake only slightly in excess of the RDA (Sutherland, 1955). Because dietary and parenteral protein and amino acids increase the renal solute load, it is essential that excess protein is not given and blood creatinine and urea monitored. An intake of up to 300% of

the RDA for weight (Appendix II.2) is usually tolerated provided adequate fluid is also given. The creatinine/height index can be used to assess skeletal muscle protein mass when both arms are burned and anthropometric measurements cannot be made. This ratio reflects skeletal muscle catabolism (Jensen *et al.*, 1985).

Carbohydrate metabolism

Hyperglycaemia, glycosuria and a diabetic type of glucose tolerance test are common in burns and severe trauma. This is due in part to glycogenolysis, increased gluconeogenesis and high levels of catecholamines causing both insulin suppression and peripheral insulin resistance. Administration of exogenous insulin does not significantly alter this picture; the inclusion of oral or parenteral glucose will diminish but not abolish the high rate of gluconeogenesis which contributes to the negative nitrogen balance. Blood glucose levels should be monitored to ensure that the carbohydrate intake does not exceed the body's capacity for metabolism. Once the energy and protein requirement has been determined, the energy in the diet that does not come from protein should ideally be equally divided between carbohydrate and fat. High intakes of lactose

in the diet after burns or trauma may be contraindicated in young children because a temporary lactose
intolerance is sometimes seen.

Fat metabolism

Large quantities of fat are catabolized to meet the
increased energy requirements, particularly of
gluconeogenesis. As fat is a concentrated energy
source and a relative intolerance to carbohydrate
exists, its use is not contraindicated and it should
supply 35–40% of the energy intake (*see above*)
despite the fact that serum free fatty acid levels are
raised in trauma and infection; this increase is
probably due to the effects of catecholamines and
glucagon on the adipose tissue.

Minerals and vitamins

Sodium retention in the early post-injury period
necessitates a restriction of sodium intake to the
minimum RDA for weight. Potassium and other
intracellular ions are released during protein breakdown and excretion is increased; supplements may
be needed to maintain adequate body levels. Adult
studies have indicated that both zinc and iron
should be supplemented to twice the normal
RDA; in addition, B vitamin requirements may be
500% RDA, fat-soluble vitamins 200% and vitamin
C needs increased by up to 1000%

Feeding in burns and trauma

The form which nutritional support of trauma-
tized children takes depends upon the extent and
type of the injury and the age and cooperation of
the child. In the early stages, when nutrient requirements are highest and gut function may be depressed, it is suggested that a mixture of enteral

and parenteral feeding is offered. Oral diet is indicated as it reduces the incidence of stress ulcers,
but it is unlikely that the regular ward diet will be
able to provide sufficient protein and energy to
meet requirements (Herndon *et al.*, 1985). Children
are likely to have poor appetites and the anorexia is
worsened by anxiety and stress caused by painful
procedures. To overcome this, parents and care
staff need to be very flexible and include in the
ward freezer popular items such as burgers, chipped
potatoes and ice cream which allows freedom of
choice and timing of meals. In addition, care should
be taken in planning procedures, including baths
and dressing changes, so that meal-times are avoided
whenever possible.

Despite these measures the use of high-energy,
high-protein supplements as described in Appendix
III.3 is recommended for drinks in between meals
and as a meal replacement if food is refused. Feeding
nightly via a nasogastric tube, in addition to meals,
may be necessary if voluntary intake is inadequate.
Because of the particular requirements of protein,
carbohydrate and energy, it may be advantageous to
use modular feeding preparations, as described in
Appendix IV.11 to achieve a suitable individual
regimen (Bell *et al.*, 1984).

Where burns or trauma to the face and/or
oesophagus are present, the high-energy, high-
protein diet will need to be in a liquid form. This
presents a particular challenge because many of the
proprietary liquid diets are fairly unpalatable. Careful selection of natural foods which can be homogenized and supplemented with dried milk powder,
cream and glucose polymer may be more acceptable, especially if the child can select foods and
watch them being prepared.

Because adequate nutrient requirement is crucial
and poor nutritional status is associated with complications of trauma (Jensen *et al.*, 1985), surveillance
of dietary compliance is necessary (McLaurin *et
al.*, 1983; Bell *et al.*, 1984). The quantities of consumed nutrients should be calculated daily and
efforts made to minimize and correct any shortfalls.

Section 2

GASTROINTESTINAL AND HEPATIC DISORDERS

6

Gastro-oesophageal Reflux

'...the infant, mewling and puking in the nurse's arms.'
As You Like It − Act II, Scene VII
Shakespeare

Gastro-oesophageal reflux (GOR) is a very common occurrence in the early months of life which invariably resolves with the passage of time. As the infant matures, the subdiaphragmatic segment of the oesophagus containing the distal sphincter elongates (Fig. 6.1); this is one of the major reasons for the resolution of the problem. Few babies do not vomit; indeed posseting — the regurgitation of small mounts of milk — may occur after every feed.

The term 'hiatal hernia' implies that the gastro-oesophageal junction is within the chest, i.e. there is herniation of the stomach through a hiatus in the diaphragm (Fig. 6.2). Sometimes the term 'partial thoracic stomach' and not 'hiatal hernia' is used. GOR and hiatal hernia are not interchangeable terms. Furthermore, it is necessary to distinguish between reflux and lower oseophageal incompetence. The latter suggests a failure of the anti-reflux mechanisms to function as opposed to an abnormal lower oesophageal sphincter. The reflux of small amounts of barium during radiological examination is not equivalent to gastro-oesophageal incompetence (GOI).

For an understanding of the precise anatomy of a paradoxically complex region refer to Carré (1979) and for an overall review *see* Gellis (1979).

Physiology of the oesophagus

The lower oesophagus functions as a sphincter and is able to prevent reflux of the stomach contents upward into the distal oesophagus. Although termed a 'sphincter' it does not have the usual configuration associated with such a structure. There is an area of increased intraluminal pressure in the distal oesophagus and on swallowing there is relaxation of the oesophagus and food enters the stomach.

Several characteristics of the lower oesophagus and stomach summate to create a valvular-like mechanism and, in addition, the gut peptide gastrin influences lower oesophageal sphincter pressure. Normally the oesophagus enters the stomach at an angle. Also part of the lower oesophageal sphincter (LOS) is in the abdomen (Fig. 6.2) and an increase in the abdominal pressure helps to bring the sidewalls of the oesophagus into apposition thus preventing reflux. Where there is a hiatal hernia the negative intrathoracic pressure acting on the LOS promotes reflux. Furthermore, the phreno-oesophageal ligament helps to maintain the integrity of the LOS (Fig. 6.2) as does the crura of the diaphragm and other neighbouring ligaments. Yet it is probably too simplistic to view the problem of reflux in solely anatomical terms (Balistreri and Farrell, 1983).

Clinical features

The major features are regurgitation and/or vomiting and sometimes pulmonary complications. Additional manifestations include oesophagitis,

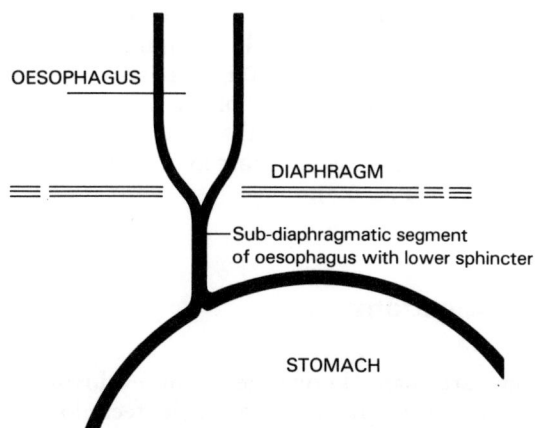

Fig. 6.1 Anatomical representation of gastro-oesophageal closure.

a

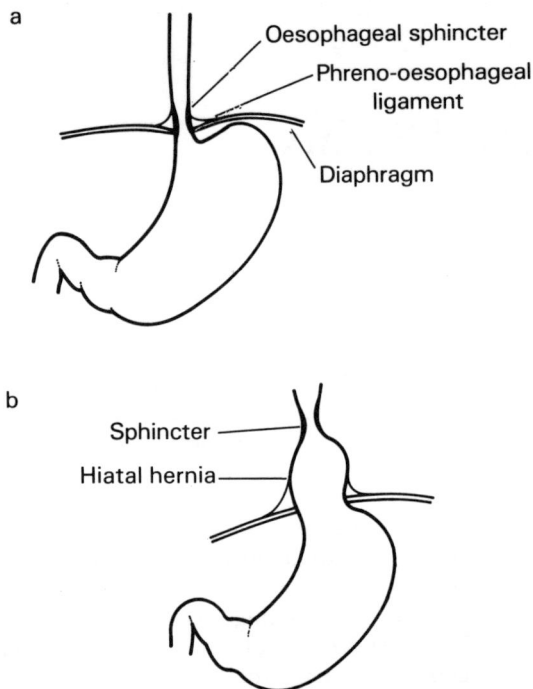

Oesophageal sphincter

Phreno-oesophageal ligament

Diaphragm

b

Sphincter

Hiatal hernia

Fig. 6.2 (a) The normal position of the lower oesophageal sphincter — part in the abdomen, part in the thorax. (b) The position of the lower oesophageal sphincter in hiatus hernia. (From Herbst, 1981.)

oesophageal stricture, haematemesis, iron deficiency anaemia and failure to thrive. Some experts (Leape *et al.*,1977; Herbst *et al.*, 1978; Ariagno *et al.*, 1982) have linked reflux and the sudden infant death syndrome or acute life-threatening events (Dr M. Brueton, personal communication). The incidence of reflux is 1:500 infants and symptoms usually present by 6 weeks of age. About 60% are symptom-free by 18 months, but 30% have persistent troubles. Death occurs in 5% and strictures also in 5% (Fig. 6.3).

Investigations

There are many known tests for evaluating the severity of reflux, but no single technique can consistently and infallibly detect abnormalities at the gastro-oesophageal junction. Suggested tests are given below.

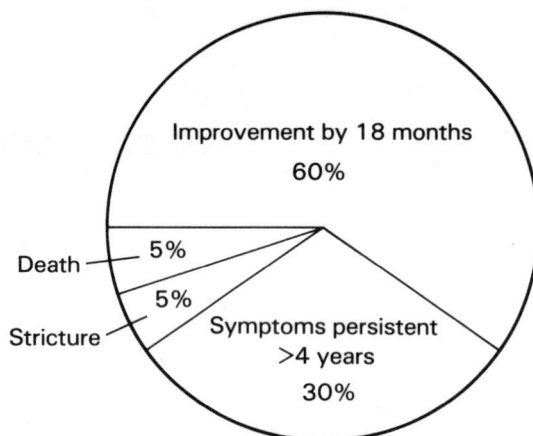

Improvement by 18 months 60%

Death 5%

Stricture 5%

Symptoms persistent >4 years 30%

Fig. 6.3 Natural history of gastro-oesophageal reflux. (Adapted from the data of Carré, 1959, *Archives of Disease in Childhood*, vol. 34, p. 344 — cited in Herbst, 1981.)

Barium swallow with fluoroscopy. The usual major failing is insufficient barium to obtain a good image. A single episode of reflux is not diagnostic. The height and amount of the refluxed material must be noted.

Oesophageal pH monitoring. Tiny intraoesophageal pH microelectrodes have been designed with diameters less than 2 mm (e.g. Microelectrodes Inc., New Hamsphire). Such a probe is positioned approximately 3 cm above the distal oesophageal sphincter and coupled with a recorder; 12–24 hours of monitoring is carried out. A pH of less than 4.0 for more than 15 minutes is abnormal (Tables 6.1 and 6.2).

Tuttle test of acid reflux. Hydrochloric acid (0.1 N) or unsweetened apple juice is ingested and the oesophageal pH is monitored for 30 minutes. A drop in pH below 4 in two or more episodes is considered abnormal.

Oesophagoscopy Modern fibreoptic equipment enables evidence of oesophagitis or stricture to be observed. The presence of oesophagitis in the absence of corrosive poisoning confirms significant reflux. In addition to visualizing the lower oesophagus, a biopsy may be taken which allows a diagnosis of monilial or herpetic disease to be made and for the severity of inflammation to be determined.

Radioisotopic scanning. A feed containing the isotope technetium is ingested and the oesophagus is then scanned. The volume of refluxed fluid can be calculated. Aspirated technetium in the lungs can be noted and will explain chronic lung disease in

Table 6.1 Oesophageal pH monitoring

Duration 24 hours	Normal infants ±1 s.d.
Episodes below pH 4	10.6 ± 8.2
Episodes >5 min	1.7 ± 2.1
Longest episode (min)	8.1 ± 7.2
Percentage time below pH 4	1.9 ± 1.6

From Boix-Ochoa *et al.* (1980).

Table 6.2 Continuous 24-hour oesophageal pH monitoring in 200 asymptomatic infants from 0 to 15 months of age

Age (months)	Percentage time below pH 4
Newborn	1.16
1	1.78
2	2.53
6	3.22
8	3.85
15	2.55

At 4 months differences are significant ($P < 0.01$) = 4.21%. From Vandenplas and Sacré (1986).

appropriate cases. Oesophageal motility can be studied during swallowing, preferably using [81m]Kr or ^{99m}Tc colloid. The ^{99m}Tc colloid milk scan has been used for many years (Gordon, 1986).

Other methods include oesophageal manometry and the methylene blue string test (Euler and Ament, 1977; Christi, 1978).

Management

Most infants respond to simple and conservative measures such as being held upright after feeds. This is usually only needed for a short time postprandially but in severe cases the child will need to be retained upright (30–45°) for much of the day and night (Fig. 6.4). Positioning in the prone position with the head elevated to 30° is recommended by Meyers and Herbst (1982). However, in one small series the 'chalasia chair' was found to be detrimental (Orenstein *et al.* 1983).

Feeding

Small volumes of milk should be offered frequently as opposed to larger amounts infrequently. Occasionally, constant intragastric infusion of milk will result in alleviation of the symptom. Vomiting may be reduced upon increasing the density of the feed by the use of special preparations (e.g. Carobel,

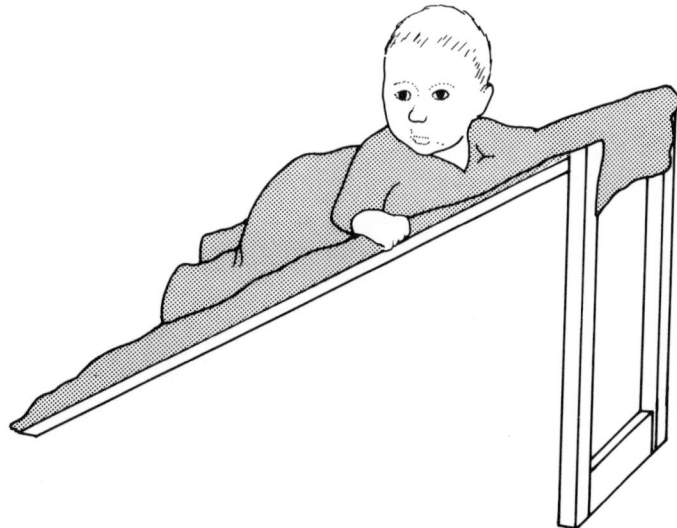

Fig. 6.4 The 'saddle'. The child is elevated to a prone 30° position to help alleviate gastro-oesophageal reflux. (From Meyers and Herbst, 1982.)

Nestargel, Appendix II.14). Alternatively, the addition of 2−5 g of an infant-type baby cereal such as rice, groats or gruel to each 100 ml feed often relieves the symptoms, but it can lead to occult gastrointestinal reflex episodes, possibly increasing the risk of oesophagitis and respiratory dysfunction, (Vandenplas and Sacré, 1987). Since this type of starch is pregelatinized it requires no further cooking.

A starch gel can be formed by the addition of 2−4 g cornflour (maize starch) or arrowroot to each 100 ml feed. Starch should be added to the cool milk then the whole feed stirred over a rapid heat for a few minutes until thickening has occurred. Mothers need to be advised to increase the size of the hole in the teat when giving a thickened feed.

For breast-fed infants a thick gel can be prepared by any of the above methods and fed by spoon prior to breast feeding. For those on a weaning diet, it is often beneficial to increase the amount of solid food and reduce the intake of fluids; toddlers and young children should be discouraged from drinking excessively. Gastric emptying is delayed by fat and the substitution with a semi-skimmed milk may be of value provided that an adequate energy intake can be achieved (*see* p. 000). Parents can find the persistence of the odour from vomiting unpleasant and indeed socially embarrassing; the smell arises from fatty acids, e.g. butyric acid. This can be remedied by replacing a butterfat-based baby milk with one containing vegetable oils. Where it is thought that regurgitation or rumination is a behavioural problem, an improvement can often be achieved if the carer stays with the child and distracts his/her attention for 20−30 minutes after each feed.

Medication

Bethanechol 8.7 mg/m^2 per day divided into three doses lowers the lower oeophageal sphincter pressure (Moroz *et al.*, 1976). However, it can cause agitation and is contraindicated where there is oesophageal stricture or restrictive airways disease. Other drugs such as alginic acid influence reflux but serious complications can arise such as the formation of bezoars (Keipert, 1979). Metoclopramide > 0.5 mg/kg per day can result in extrapyramidal side-effects and domperidone, a dopamine receptor antagonist, 0.6−1.2 mg/kg per day given orally in three divided doses is preferable. Cisapride facilitates acetylcholine release from myenteric nerves and may have a role in the pharmacological management of reflux.

Surgery

There is an operative mortality of 0.6% (Herbst, 1981). However, some with recurrent apnoea and others who fail to respond to conservative therapy may eventually require surgery.

Because gastro-oesophageal reflux diminishes with age, surgery should be reserved but not exclusively so for the older child. Several techniques are available; these include the Nissen and Belsey fundoplication in which the fundus of the stomach is wrapped around the lower oesophagus. Other surgeons prefer gastropexy. Carré (1985), in his excellent review of management, recommends the Belsey Mark IV type of fundoplication.

7

Malabsorption Syndromes

His stomack is the kitchin, where the meat
Is often but half sod, for want of heat.
Francis Quarles (1592–1644)

Coeliac disease (gluten-sensitive enteropathy)

Coeliac disease is one of the major chronic disorders of the small intestine and is due to a permanent intolerance to gluten, the germ protein of wheat and some other cereals. Just as cows' milk protein intolerance can be an associated complication of enteritis, so similarly a temporary gluten intolerance might occasionally arise as a secondary phenomenon (Visakorpi and Immone, 1967; Walker-Smith, 1970). The incidence of coeliac disease ranges from 1:3000 (England and America) to a peak of 1:300 in the Galway region of western Ireland. The decreasing incidence of coeliac disease has been linked to increased breast feeding, a decrease in protein and osmolality of infant milk and later introduction of weaning in Western countries (Stevens *et al.*, 1987).

Coeliac disease was originally described in the first century AD by Aretaeus of Cappadocia. Almost 100 years ago a vivid and classic clinical description of this alimentary tract disease was written by Samuel Gee in the *St Bartholomew's Hospital Report* of 1888 'Faeces, being loose, ... bulky, ... pale, ... stinking'. In more contemporary times Dicke in Holland (1950) noted the link between wheat and steatorrhoea.

Clinical features

Commonly, coeliac disease presents before the age of 2 years and usually within 6 months of starting cereals but may only be diagnosed in late childhood or even adulthood. Frequently, these children are referred to paediatricians because of irritability, apathy, a delay or regression of motor development, hypotonia, malaise, anorexia, failure to thrive, the passage of foul, bulky stools and vomiting.

The gastrointestinal symptoms can be subtle as the infant's main feature might be small stature. Following the introduction of a strict gluten-free diet an impressive growth spurt is seen; however, it might take 2–3 years before the peak velocity of growth height is achieved (Fig. 7.1). Muscle wasting is a useful sign. Usually it is most evident around the shoulders, hips and/or buttocks. Abdominal distension is often seen (Fig. 7.2) and constipation is not uncommon. Oedema may arise secondary to a protein-losing enteropathy that has caused hypoproteinaemia. The infant should be examined for digital clubbing and clinical evidence of anaemia.

There is a highly significant increase in the incidence of histocompatability antigens HLA-B8, -DR3 and -DR7 when compared with controls. The former antigen has a very high frequency within the Galway population mentioned above. Furthermore, a lymphocyte antigen independent of the HLA system has been identified in many cases of coeliac disease (Mann *et al.*, 1976).

The precise mechanism of the toxic effect of gluten is unknown. Gluten is a large complex molecule which consists of gliadin, glutenin and globulins. Electrophoresis shows gliadin to be composed of about 40 different compounds — the α-gliadin fraction is the most toxic (Kendall *et al.*, 1972).

On histology there is a diffuse lesion of the proximal small intestine with atrophy of villi (Figs. 7.3 and 7.4), lymphocyte infiltration and deepening of the crypts of Lieberkühn. However, these findings are not pathognomonic of coeliac disease or of a transient gluten intolerance. In addition to loss of villi and crypt hyperplasia there is inflammatory cell inflammation of the lamina propria and an increase in the intraepithelial lymphocytes. Severe villous atrophy is likely to be accompanied by a deficiency of the brush border disaccharidases — lactase and/or sucrase. This information is useful in determining the need for a temporary limitation

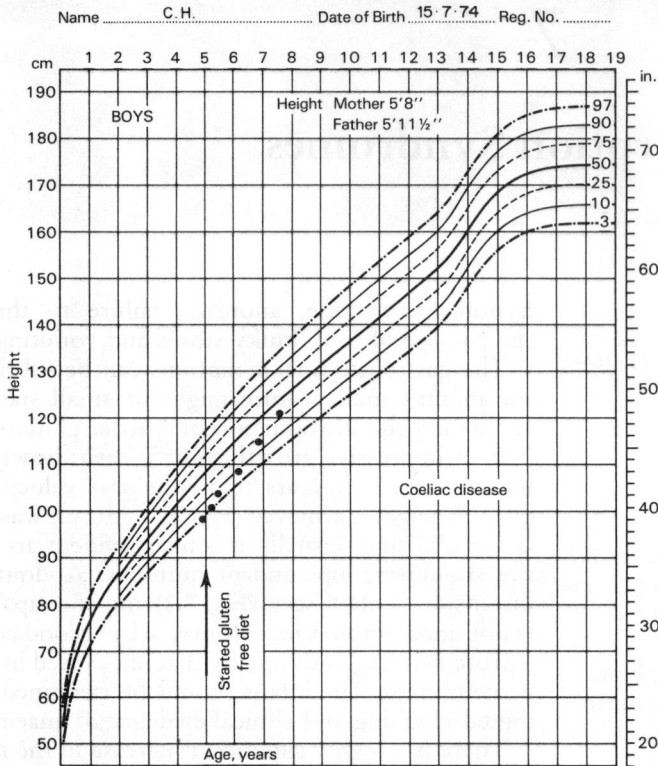

Fig. 7.1 Growth chart of child with coeliac disease showing improvement following gluten-free diet.

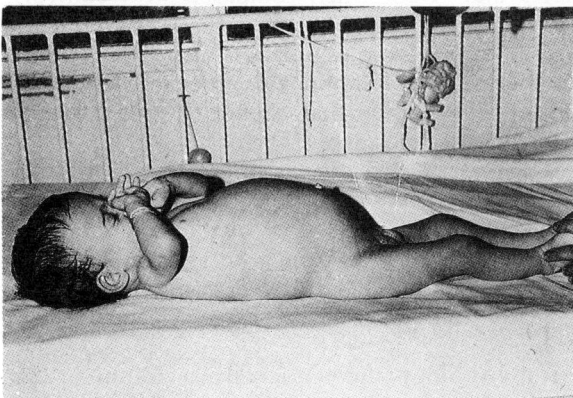

Fig. 7.2 Abdominal distension in a child with coeliac disease.

of lactose and/or sucrose if enzyme activity is subnormal.

Diagnosis

Diagnosis is made histologically from a small bowel biopsy at the ligament of Treitz (duodenojejunal flexure). Formerly, damage to the villi (subtotal or total villous atrophy) was considered diagnostic of coeliac disease, but now such findings are not thought to be conclusive evidence of a gluten sensitivity. There are many other causes of such pathology within the small bowel, e.g. gastroenteritis, cows' milk protein intolerance and giardiasis. To justify a diagnosis of coeliac disease three small bowel biopsies are suggested over an unspecified period of time:

1. Initial biopsy revealing damaged or flattened villi.
2. Normal biopsy findings on a gluten-free diet.
3. Histological relapse following a gluten-containing diet — or challenge with 20 g daily of gluten powder.

These so-called 'Interlaken' criteria were agreed upon at a meeting of the European Society for Paediatric Gastroenterology (Meeuwisse, 1970).

There may be difficulties in distinguishing coeliac disease from a transient gluten intolerance. If challenge with gluten causes no histological and/or clinical deterioration and if gluten were responsible originally then, following a normal biopsy, the

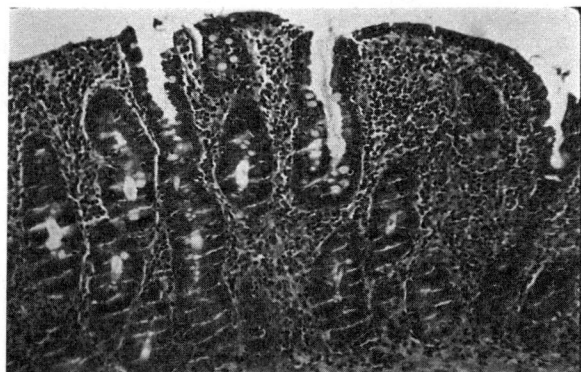

(a)

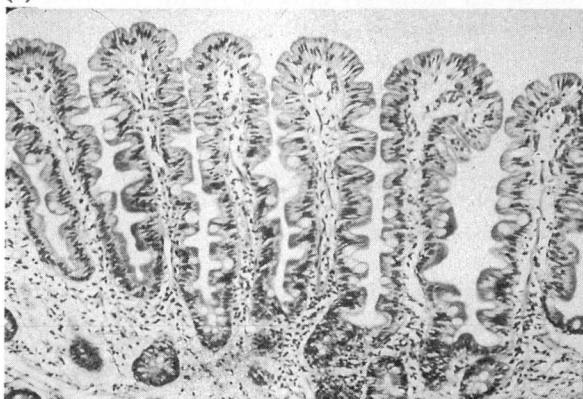

(b)

Fig. 7.3 (a) Histological appearance showing flattened villi of the proximal small intestine in coeliac disease. (b) Normal appearance for comparison — tall fingerlike villi.

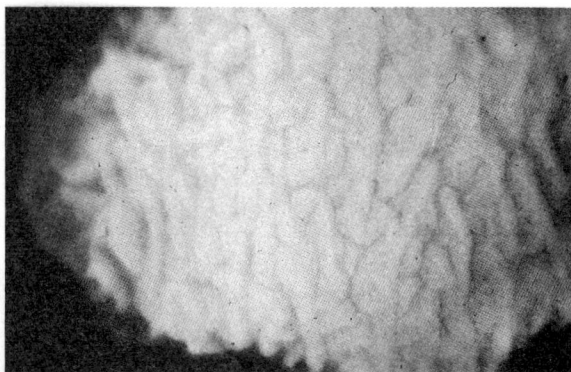

(a)

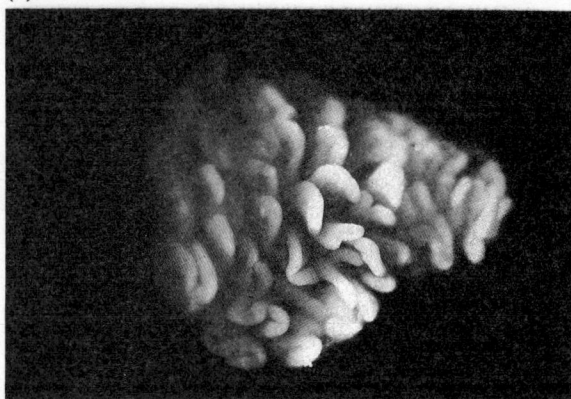

(b)

Fig. 7.4 Dissecting microscope views showing (a) the flat mucosa seen in coeliac disease; (b) normal mucosa for comparison.

problem is a temporary and not a permanent intolerance.

Gluten challenge

Various methods of gluten administration and times of post-challenge biopsy have been proposed. Some paediatricians favour the use of up to 20 g/day of commercially prepared gluten powder; this has the disadvantage that the gluten ingested is not in the same form as cooked gluten in food, and its toxicity may be altered. If natural foods are used it is important to ensure that an adequate amount is taken: 10 g wheat protein daily (equivalent to 130 g bread or 90 g flour) for a period of 3–4 months appears to be sufficient in many but not in all with coeliac disease. In a few, even the so-called 'two-year rule' is insufficient time to induce a relapse (Walker-Smith, 1986).

Investigations

The following investigations are available, although some are only used in a research setting.

Faecal fat excretion is monitored over 3 days using carmine markers to time the collection together with calculation of the total fat intake during the study. In 80% of cases of coeliac disease, there is steatorrhoea but this may only be evident later in the disease and, indeed, in some infants there is no increase in the stool fat content.

Stool smear for fat globules is less reliable than faecal fat excretion but a quick simple screen; > 100 globules per high-power field is abnormal (Drummey *et al.*,1961). However, this investigation is rarely positive in coeliac disease:

1. An abnormal fat collection result is > 10% excretion.

2. Fat excretion exceeding 3.5 g/24 hours in infants is only abnormal in some cases.
3. Fat excretion exceeding 4.5 g/24 hours in children, is only abnormal in some cases.

Xylose absorption (Rolles *et al.*, 1975) — there is a high degree of correlation between an abnormal biopsy and a low 1-hour blood xylose after a load of 5 g (14.2 g/m²) as a 10% solution. (D-Xylose is a pentose sugar absorbed in the proximal small intestine.)

Blood test for detection of antibodies to gliadin (Unsworth *et al.*, 1981) — although Cacciari *et al.* (1985) found close correlation between anti-gliadin antibody and coeliac disease using immuno-fluorescence in prepubertal coeliacs, this test may be non-specific for coeliac disease.

Presence of serum and IgA class reticulin antibodies (Seah *et al.*, 1973; Mäki *et al.*, 1984).

Organ culture in vitro of small intestinal tissue using alkaline phosphatase as a brush border enzyme marker (Katz and Falchuk, 1978). This is a sophisticated research model.

Leucocyte migration inhibition factor (LIF) test using subfractions of gluten. Blood lymphocytes from most cases of coeliac disease respond to stimulation by producing increased LIF (Ashkenazi *et al.*, 1978).

Skin testing — positive reactions with intradermal injection of a peptic/tryptic digest of gluten have been reported in 52% of 23 untreated coeliac patients (Baker, 1975; Anand and Truelove, 1977).

Anaemia — the commonest type of anaemia in coeliac disease is due to iron deficiency; megaloblastic anaemia is rare in coeliac disease. Serum iron, serum folate and red cell folate are all usually reduced in those more than 1 year old.

Gut hormones — there is a characteristic gut hormone profile (Besterman *et al.*, 1978).

Differential diagnosis

1. Cystic fibrosis.
2. Cows' milk protein intolerance (Visakorpi and Immonen 1967; Young and Pringle, 1971).
3. Soy protein intolerance.
4. Tropical sprue.
5. Giardiasis.
6. Lymphoma of small intestine.
7. Immune deficiency.
8. Bacterial overgrowth of bowel.

Dietary management of coeliac disease

The treatment for coeliac disease and gluten-induced enteropathies is a gluten-free diet (*see* Appendix IV.29). Whether the enteropathy is thought to be true coeliac disease — requiring life-long adherence to the diet — or a transient gluten intolerance, the principles of management are the same.

There is general agreement that wheat and rye should be completely excluded from the diet. The position is less clear when oats and barley are considered (Baker, 1975), although there is clinical evidence that they are toxic. In England it has been demonstrated that 12% of children with coeliac disease are adversely affected by the inclusion of oats in their diet. In most centres in the UK, oats and barley are allowed in the diets of treated coeliacs unless they appear to cause problems. All four cereals, along with beer and malt, are generally excluded by North American gastroenterologists and paediatricians.

Compliance with this restrictive diet is likely to be poor, particulary among adolescents. Failure to comply with the diet during childhood is associated with short stature and depressed brush border enzyme activity, particularly lactase (Colaco *et al.*, 1987).

Foods allowed and forbidden

All wheat, rye, barley and oats, and products derived from them, should be excluded from the regimen.

Processed foods

With the enormous variety of manufactured food products available in Western countries, it is impossible to give comprehensive instructions for the avoidance of gluten in processed foods (see Appendix IV.28). Unless the ingredients are included on the packaging it is wise to omit them. Carefully scrutiny of labels each time a food is purchased is important as the composition of complex products can change. In the UK, owing to the efforts of the Coeliac Society of Great Britain, manufacturers whose products are guaranteed free of wheat products put a gluten-free symbol on their packaging. The Coeliac Society also publishes a list, regularly updated, of British foodstuffs which are gluten-free. In all countries where stringent food regulations exist and information is available, dieticians should be able to compile a list of gluten-free manufactured products.

Special gluten-free foods

In countries where wheat is the staple cereal, it is advantageous to include the use of specially prepared gluten-free equivalents of bread, biscuits, cookies and pasta. Without these products the diet can prove to be expensive unless substantial amounts of pulses, lentils and nuts are taken, as animal protein foods will be needed in large quantities to provide an adequate energy intake for a growing child. Special foods are generally prepared from purified wheat starch and this has given rise to some controversy recently as to whether the small portion of residual cereal protein left over after treatment of wheat starch is harmful. There is no evidence to suggest that this small residue causes adverse effects in coeliac disease and biopsies demonstrate that the mucosa returns to normal when these products are included in the diet. There are standards laid down for gluten-free foods by the Committee on Foods for Special Dietary Use of the Codex Alimentarius Commission of the World Health Organisation. These standards state that a residual cereal nitrogen content of 0.05% is acceptable, providing that the residual material contains no gliadin.

In the UK, there are a number of proprietary breads, bread mixes, biscuits, flours and pasta available for purchase or on prescription for use in coeliac disease. A full list of these foods is available from dieticians and from the Coeliac Society of Great Britain.

Research has been carried out recently on the use of strains of wheat thought to be naturally lacking in a fraction of the gliadin molecule, but so far they have not proved to be of any practical use.

Vitamin and mineral supplements

Various deficiency states have been described in coeliacs prior to treatment. Because of the generalized malabsorption, it is advisable to give a multivitamin supplement, including a water-miscible form of the fat-soluble vitamins (*see* Appendix II.13). If there is a prolonged prothrombin time, parenteral vitamin K is indicated initially, especially prior to any small bowel biopsy. A trace element preparation, administered either orally or parenterally, may be useful in children with long-standing malabsorption or failure to thrive (*see* Appendix II.13).

Supplements should not be considered a permanent part of a gluten-free regimen; a varied diet will provide an adequate intake and vitamins and minerals are absorbed normally after the improvement of the small bowel histology and may thus be discontinued when the child has shown a good response to diet.

Complications

Failure to thrive

Where diagnosis has been delayed infants or children may present with severe failure to thrive resembling frank protein—energy malnutrition (PEM). These children will achieve catch-up growth and show an earlier response to dietary treatment if they are given a generous protein and energy intake as well as supplemental vitamins, minerals and trace elements. Steatorrhoea is the consequence of defects in absorption, lipolysis, micelle formation and the enterohepatic circulation as well as suspected exocrine pancreatic insufficiency (Branski and Lebenthal, 1981) Because fat is malabsorbed a medium-chain triglyceride milk may be better tolerated than one containing long-chain fatty acids. Precautions should be taken to ensure that this is not introduced too rapidly (Appendix IV.7). Alternatively, a high-protein, high-energy milk based on skimmed milk can be used (Appendix III.10).

Coeliac crisis. This is a rare life-threatening complication in which dehydration provoked by diarrhoea accompanies malabsorption. Although this was not an uncommon mode of presentation in Western countries some years ago, it is rarely seen now, probably owing to increased awareness and earlier referral. However, children in less developed countries may still present in this dramatic manner, particularly where a hot climate or intercurrent infection exacerbates dehydration. Acidosis, hypokalaemia and hypoglycaemia, along with low serum levels of calcium and magnesium, may be encountered. Correction of the fluid, electrolyte and mineral status is of first importance. When the infant is able to take oral feeds he should be treated with a multiple malabsorption regimen, excluding not only gluten but milk and soy protein and disaccharides, until the diagnosis has been established.

Lactose intolerance and food allergy

A secondary deficiency of small bowel disaccharidases is an almost invariable finding when biopsy material is assayed for intestinal enzyme activity. However, this secondary deficiency may not be important in the majority of infants and children. In a small infant with severe symptoms or in coeliac crisis the initial diet should be free of lactose. In children who do not fall into these categories, a low lactose diet should not be instituted unless there is good evidence that the child is not thriving on a gluten-free diet alone.

Various food allergies have been described in children with coeliac disease: most commonly milk, egg and soy proteins seem to be involved. However, a diagnosis of food intolerance alone or transient gluten intolerance should be suspected if a coexisting food allergy is found. There is no reason to routinely exclude milk or other foods in the initial stages, unless the child is severely ill: — malignancy of the small bowel (particularly lymphoma and reticulum-cell sarcoma) — suspected but unproven in confirmed childhood coeliacs; miscellaneous—rickets and osteoporosis (due to malabsorption of vitamin D), stunted growth and developmental retardation, peripheral neuropathy, anaemia (usually hypochromic and microcytic), hypoproteinaemia and hypoprothrombinaemia (due to malabsorption of vitamin K) — have all been described.

Problems arising from a gluten-free diet

Dental problems

There is no evidence to suggest that a gluten-free diet has a deleterious effect on tooth development and the incidence of caries appears not to be increased in coeliac children. Parents should be warned, however, that caries will result if they ply children with sweets in order to compensate for dietary restrictions. Delay in diagnosis and subsequent poor nutrition can lead to enamel hypoplasia, which may be severe.

Constipation

A gluten-free diet is necessarily low in cereal fibre, the main source of this in Western diets being wholemeal wheat products. Constipation can be a problem in those children who do not care for

vegetables and fruit. Even when reasonable quantities of these items are eaten difficulty can still be encountered. The inclusion of pulses, beans (including gluten-free varieties of baked beans), nuts and lentils should be encouraged as they can be helpful. A recent innovation in the UK has been the introduction of gluten-free bread enriched with soy bran (Appendix IV.30). This compares favourably with wheat bran in its properties and should prove useful where constipation is a problem.

Intestinal resection (short bowel syndrome)

This term is used where, following surgery, there is a residual small bowel length of less than 75 cm from the duodenojejunal junction to the caecum. In a term newborn, the length of the jejunum and ileum is 250–300 cm measured along the anti-mesenteric border, but it is shorter in the pre-term baby (Benson, 1955). Apart from atresia of the small gut the most common reasons in the newborn for small bowel resection are: volvulus, necrotizing enterocolitis, meconium ileus and inflammatory bowel disease (IBD).

For large bowel resection, Hirschprung's disease as well as IBD are the most common reasons.

The severity of symptoms and the prevalence of short- and long-term complications relate to the site and the extent of the bowel removed, residual surface area and gut motility. Removal of mid-small bowel gives rise to fewer problems than proximal or distal small bowel resection. Also the presence of the ileocaecal valve is extremely important and influences the outcome. The experience of Wilmore *et al.* (1971) suggests a minimal length of 15 cm of small bowel where the ileocaecal valve is present, if the neonate is to survive. However, in the absence of this 'valve' the least length needed is 40 cm. Yet Holt *et al.* (1982) described an infant with a small bowel length of only 12 cm who had survived beyond 2 years.

Symptoms

The severity of symptoms relates directly to the surface area of small bowel villi remaining after surgery. Diarrhoea is the chief symptom, with or without the following:

1. Short transit time.

2. Monosaccharide intolerance.
3. Disaccharide intolerance.
4. Bile salt malabsorption.
5. Bacterial overgrowth.
6. Depressed salt/water transport.

Rapid transit time, sugar intolerance, unabsorbed bile salts and bacterial overgrowth are just some of the reasons for the problem of persistent and sometimes intractable diarrhoea. With resection of short bowel segments, the malabsorption is mild but with massive resection bile salt depletion becomes profound and steatorrhoea predominates. The malabsorbed dietary fat is converted to hydroxy fatty acids by bacteria and these exacerbate the diarrhoea. Hepatic synthesis of bile salts from cholesterol to replace faecal losses is controlled by a negative feedback mechanism. Bile salts facilitate the absorption of fatty acids and monoglycerides which are derived from dietary triglycerides following lipolysis by lipase.

Bile salts form aggregates called micelles (*see* Fig. 13.8) which solubilize insoluble lipids and provide a mechanism for transport to the intestinal mucosa. If extensive resection occurs, the liver cannot compensate by synthesizing adequate amounts of bile.

Adaptation and pathophysiology

Flint (1912) originally demonstrated the phenomenon in dogs of compensatory enlargement of the small gut surface area following resection. This was attained by dilatation. In addition, Flint observed lengthening of the villi and deepening of the crypts of Lieberkühn. Yet, using piglets as a model, Rickham (1967) was unable to show consistent histological changes of compensation. Resections of the proximal small bowel are associated with greater compensatory changes than those seen when surgery is to the distal small bowel. Removal of the distal small gut is linked to serious and chronic sequelae because of the relative inability of the jejunum to compensate, in contrast to the ileum. A jejunal remnant of 11 cm has attained a length of 1 metre after 4 years (Kurz and Sauer, 1983). For a concise and comprehensive review of the regulatory mechanisms of the small bowel *see* Dowling (1982).

Enteral nutrition results in the release of enteroglucagon from ileal endocrine cells (Milla, 1986). This is the major trophic hormone involved in adaptation secondary to intestinal resection (Sagor *et al.*, 1982). Luminal nutrients, especially fat, are essential for adaptation. The specific activity of some mucosal enzymes($Na^+-K^+ATPase$, enterokinase etc.) increase, although brush border disaccharidases are decreased secondary to reduced surface area.

Investigations

Short transit times are demonstrated with carmine markers. For bacterial overgrowth, an aerobic/anaerobic culture of small bowel contents with a colony count is grown to see if bacteria are more than 10^7/ml.

Specific malabsorption studies are carried out to show impaired uptake of nutrients, e.g. carbohydrates: use 1-hour blood xylose technique (p. 68) or hydrogen breath test (p. 71) as a screen or sugar tolerance tests for specific substrates. Stools are tested for pH, and the presence of reducing sugars with the Clinitest reaction and by stool sugar chromatography.

Enzyme assay of small bowel tissue or enteric fluid is performed for assay of lactase, sucrase, enterokinase and peptide hydrolases (Richards *et al.*, 1971; McCarthy and Kim, 1973).

1. Balance studies — fat/proteins to assist nutritional management.
2. Vitamin B_{12} malabsorption test (Schilling test, *see* p. 11).
3. Faeces — bile acid estimation, Sudan III stain stool test and electrolyte content.
4. Urine — measure urinary oxalate excretion and electrolytes (increased in most infants who have had an extensive resection).
5. Breath tests to calculate breath excretion of either radioactive carbon dioxide ($[^{14}C]$glycocholic acid) or hydrogen to support a diagnosis of bacterial overgrowth or $[^{14}C]$xylose breath test or ^{13}C-labelled bile acid breath test (p. 106).

Management

Specific non-nutritional problems

1. Diarrhoea — cholestyramine is useful where a large bile acid loss causes watery stools, but it impairs the absorption of several nutrients

including the fat-soluble vitamins, folate, iron and calcium.

2. Antibiotics for aerobic/anaerobic bacterial overgrowth.
3. Water and electrolyte imbalance following colonic resection particularly in the immediate postsurgical period.
4. A high fluid intake is needed, especially in hot environments.

Parenteral nutrition

Severe malabsorption and diarrhoea will sometimes necessitate non-enteric feeding. However, even though not well absorbed, introduce some nutrients into the bowel early on to help maintain normal mucosa (trophic effect) and gut hormones.

Oral nutrition

Although long-term parenteral nutrition may be necessary for a minority of children and has been successfully carried out at home (Dorney *et al.*, 1985; Lin *et al.*, 1987), oral nutrition should be commenced as soon as possible. The secretion of enterogastrone requires the presence of nutrients in the gut lumen and this in turn will hasten adaptive mucosal changes. Human milk contains a factor which stimulates mucosal hyperplasia and this increases the brush border enzymes so there are advantages in using the mother's own milk. Heat treatment or freezing destroys this factor. However, in practice, there are often low levels of lactase in the small intestine, particularly after resection of the proximal small bowel and lactose intolerance is common. It is possible to add a lactose-splitting enzyme to milk (e.g. Lactase, Kremers Urban, Wisconsin) but the usefulness of this has not been fully evaluated. Milks with a reduced lactose content are described in Appendix IV.1. Whichever regimen is selected, it is important that small volumes of a hypo-osmolar feed are used. Although adaptation to a high osmolar load does occur, episodes of abdominal distension, vomiting and diarrhoea may indicate a failure to tolerate a hyperosmolar feed rather than suggest intolerance to a specific nutrient (Cashel *et al.*, 1978).

A modular feeding regimen is suggested initially, because this offers flexibility of concentration and nutrient content and permits an individual regimen

to be devised and allows for any dietary intolerances. This module should be a dilute carbohydrate preparation such as Caloreen; if fat malabsorption is suspected, include medium-chain triglycerides (MCTs) because they do not require solubilization by bile salts. However, because of their small particle size they do have a high osmolality and must be introduced very slowly. The inclusion of some long-chain triglycerides (LCTs) is advisable to provide essential fatty acids and because LCT is a potent stimulator of enterogastrone. The use of milk-based protein modules is contraindicated in temporary milk protein intolerance secondary to surgery (Postuma *et al.*, 1983). Furthermore, soy protein may not be tolerated and the use of protein hydrolysates as the module will increase the feed osmolality. It is most important that increases in feed volume and concentration take place slowly and that the volume and strength are not raised simultaneously. A suggested regimen for an infant on a modular regimen is illustrated in Appendices IV.17 and IV.18.

Elemental formulae have been used with success in short bowel syndrome, as the constituents do not require intestinal enzymes or bile salts for their digestion (Christie and Ament, 1975). However, most preparations currently available have been designed for adults and care must be taken to ensure that the nutrient requirements of the infant and young child have been met. A further potential problem is that elemental products have a very high osmolality so must be introduced cautiously. This type of product is described in Appendix IV.10. Predigested formulae such as Pregestimil (Appendix IV.5) are useful in the management of bowel resection but also have the disadvantage of a high osmolality.

The fluid requirements of infants who have undergone gut surgery are high and may be increased by 25—50%. It is difficult to achieve such an intake unless the feed is given by constant infusion. Bolus feeding might give rise to adverse reactions. Electrolyte losses can be high where the colon has been resected and requirements for sodium and potassium may be increased by as much as five times above normal. The addition of sodium and potassium salts to the feed will greatly increase the osmolality and, in the immediate post-surgical period, most of the electrolyte requirement should be met intravenously until the gut has become accustomed to the hyperosmolar feed. Calcium, magnesium, zinc and iron may well need supplementation because long-term deficiencies of these elements have been described. A full supplement of water- and fat-soluble vitamins and trace elements should be given to compensate for the malabsorption.

Sequelae

Malnutrition during a critical period of brain growth can cause mental retardation and permanent small stature. End-stage liver failure, associated with total parenteral nutrition, is the principal cause of death where there has been massive small bowel resection (Cooper *et al.*, 1984).

Complications

The major deficiencies caused by gut surgery are summarized in Fig. 7.5 and these can be minimized by correct choice of feeding regimen and the addition of dietary supplements where necessary.

Gastric hypersecretion is sometimes seen after resection of the proximal and distal small bowel, but is relatively uncommon in infants. Where present it impairs pancreatic enzymes as a result of lowered duodenal pH. Gastric acid is an irritant to the small bowel mucosa and is a factor contributing to a rapid gut transit time and subsequent diarrhoea.

Bacterial overgrowth of resected sections of bowel should be considered and investigated if steatorrhoea continues despite dietary manipulation. Renal stones may arise from the enhanced absorption of oxalate from the colon after ileal resection. A high fluid intake should be maintained. In addition, the diet should contain adequate amounts of magnesium as this is necessary to keep the oxalate in solution. Foods which are high in oxalate should be avoided by older children. A list of such foods is given in Table 7.1.

Other sequelae include osteoporosis (Kurz and Sauer, 1983). There needs to be a prospective awareness of rickets arising months or even years after surgery (Touloukian and Gertner, 1981).

Abetalipoproteinaemia (Bassen— Kornzweig syndrome)

This is a rare disorder of lipid metabolism inherited in an autosomal recessive manner and characterized by the following: failure to thrive and steatorrhoea

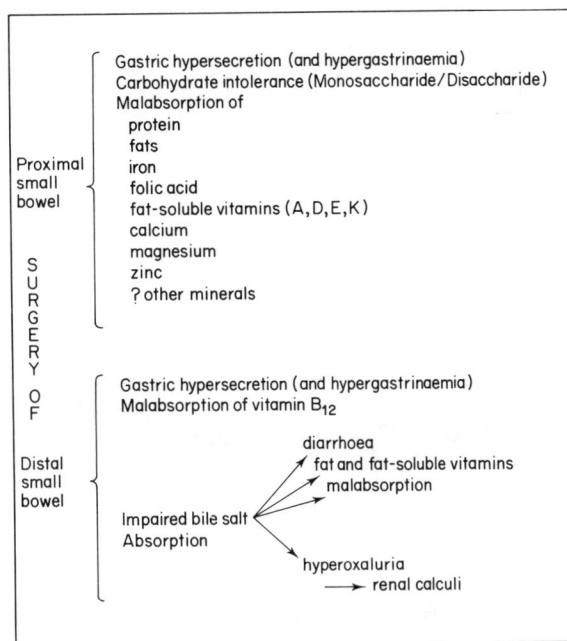

Fig. 7.5 Major deficiencies caused by gut surgery.

Table 7.1 Foods high in oxalate

Rhubarb	Cocoa, chocolate
Spinach	Wheatgerm
Beetroot	Beans
Parsley	Nuts

early in infancy and progressive ataxia (degeneration of spinocerebellar tracts) and retinitis pigmentosa later in childhood. Although acanthocytes (thorny red cells) in the peripheral blood smear are pathognomonic it can be difficult to distinguish these malformed erythrocytes from burr cells.

The primary defect is the deficiency of apoprotein B and low-density lipoprotein (LDL) β-lipoprotein. LDL is needed to form chylomicrons and in its absence dietary fat accumulates within the engorged enterocyte as it cannot be transported away. β-Lipoproteins transport more than 50% of the cholesterol of human plasma and their deficiency leads to abnormally low levels of lipids in the plasma. Dietary triglycerides are normally re-esterified in the intestinal mucosa and then transported through the lymphatic system as chylomicrons. However, without β-lipoproteins, chylomicrons cannot be formed. Coagulation abnormalities in patients presenting with haemorrhages have been described in

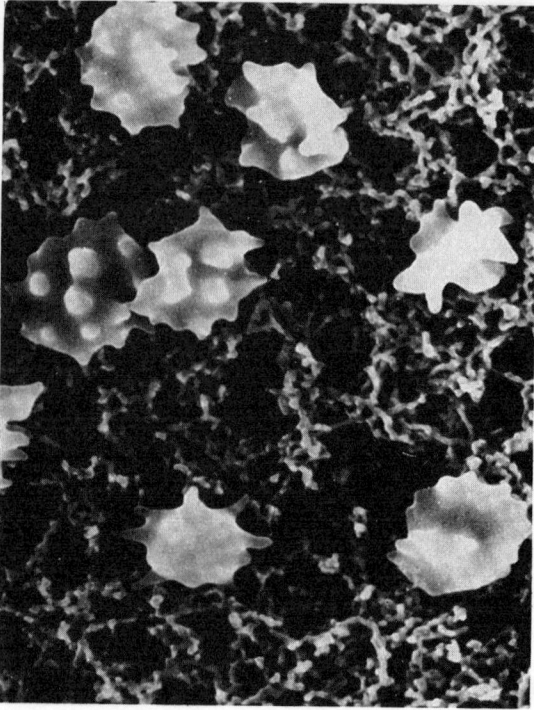

Fig. 7.6 Scanning electron micrograph of an acantho-cyte in abetalipoproteinaemia. (From Gryboski J and Walker WA (1983) *Gastrointestinal Problems in the Infant*, p. 624, WB Saunders, Philadelphia.)

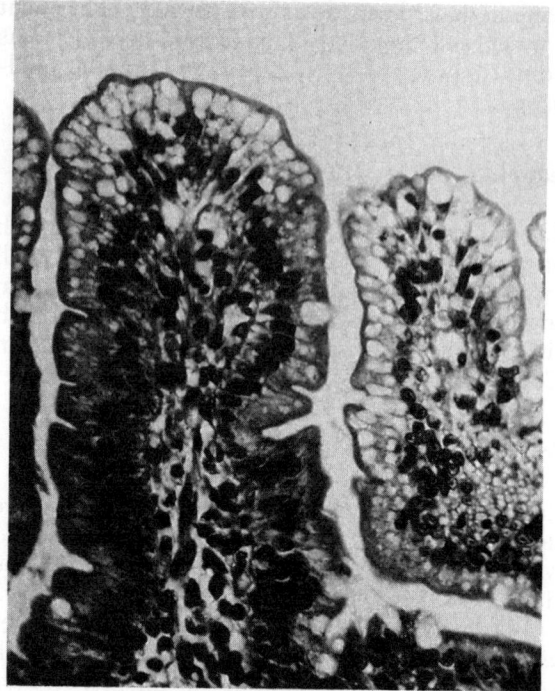

Fig. 7.7 Small bowel biopsy in abetalipoproteinaemia. Note the epithelial cells are vacuolated by lipids which cannot be transported.

abetalipoproteinaemia. A jejunal biopsy will show distended small intestinal epithelial cells full of triglyceride (*see* Fig. 7.7).

Investigations

1. Blood film — shows acanthocytosis of erythro-cytes (crenated red cells with spiny/thorny excrescences; Fig. 7.6).
2. Plasma cholesterol low (<2.0 mmol/1).
3. Plasma triglyceride low (<0.25 mmol/l).
4. Lipid electrophoresis — only HDL band present (high-density lipoprotein = α-lipoprotein).
5. Jejunal biopsy shows normal villi morphologi-cally but distended with lipid drops (Fig. 7.7).

Management

Early treatment in infancy prevents retinal and neurological complications (West and Shaw, 1981).

Dietary treatment

Some of the clinical manifestations of abetalipo-proteinaemia resemble those of deficiencies of the fat-soluble vitamins A, D, E and K, and it is essential that these are given in a water-miscible form as soon as the diagnosis is made. If an oral supplement such as Ketovite liquid (Appendix IV.13) is not absorbed, then it may be necessary to use a parenteral source of these vitamins. Initially, a minimal fat regimen as described on p. 76 for intestinal lymphangiectasia is recommended. The gradual introduction of MCTs can be tried to improve the energy content of the diet but fat absorption should be monitored during this process, because in some variants of this condition the transport of MCTs is defective. If MCTs are in-deed malabsorbed, the energy content of the diet may be inadequate for normal growth. After weaning the fat content of the diet should remain as low as is practical.

8

Protein-losing Enteropathies

There are many disorders which cause protein loss from the mucosal surface of the gastrointestinal tract. Altered gut permeability may be seen in ulcerative colitis, enteritis, coelic disease, kwashiorkor, cystic fibrosis and nephrosis. Protein loss will also occur if there is lymphatic stasis as in primary intestinal lymphangiectasia, congestive heart failure, constrictive pericarditis and lymphoma. A small protein loss can be a problem in the presence of malnutrition and/or malabsorption. The basis of therapy is to treat the primary cause and to reduce the dietary fat to lower mesenteric chyle flow and the intestinal leak of protein. Medium chain triglycerides (MCTs) which travel by the portal vein do not increase lymph flow and provide an important source of energy.

Pathogenesis

Serum albumin will fall if hepatic synthesis cannot compensate for the enteric loss of protein (Table 8.1). Proteins that have the longest half-life (albumins and γ-globulin) are more depressed than proteins with a short half-life (e.g. fibrinogen).

Quantitation of the enteric protein loss

Using albumin labelled with $^{51}CrCl_3$, quantitative losses can be determined. A 4-day stool collection is made after intravenous $^{51}CrCl_3$-labelled albumin. As chromium salts are neither excreted nor absorbed from the bowel, this metallic marker is ideal. The protein loss from the gastrointestinal tract is calculated from a plasma decay curve of radioactivity and stool isotopic counting. Other labelling methods include ^{67}Cu-labelled ceruloplasmin.

A much simpler and non-invasive alternative is to measure α_1-antitrypsin in a random faecal sample α_1-Antirypsin is a glycoprotein protease inhibitor which is resistant to degradation in the gut. This method has the advantage of being non-isotopic and is readily carried out. Furthermore, α_1-antitrypsin in the stool enables the response to therapy in inflammatory bowel disease to be monitored (Crossley and Elliott, 1977; Keaney and Kelleher, 1980; Hill et al., 1981)

Dietary treatment

In addition to a high-protein source of nutrition the composition of the long-chain triglycerides (LCTs) in the diet may need to be modified. However, where protein loss is due to altered gut permeability there is no need to restrict fat unless there is steatorrhoea. A low-LCT, high-protein diet for infants and children is described in the section on lymphangiectasia on p. 76. Where fat does not need to be restricted then a high-protein, high-energy regimen as described in the section on enteral feeding (p. 34) can be followed. It is important to monitor vitamin, mineral and trace element status in all cases of enteropathy causing malabsorption and supplement accordingly.

Intestinal lymphangiectasis

This disease was first described by Waldmann (1966) and is characterized by congenital abnormalities of the small bowel lymphatic system. Hypoplasia of the lymphatic channels may be seen in the limbs too. Obstruction to the lymphatic drainage of the intestine results in rupture of the lacteals with leakage of lymph into the lumen of the bowel. There is marked protein loss from the bowel mucosa and there may also be fat loss. Chronic loss of lymphocytes and immunoglobulins from the gastrointestinal tract increases susceptibility to infection. An acquired form of the disease is caused by constrictive pericarditis, congestive heart failure or obstruction of other lymphatics.

Table 8.1 Normal albumin data

Subjects	Serum albumin level (g/100 ml)	Albumin synthesis (mg/kg per 24 hours)	Albumin degradation (percentage plasma albumin pool/ 24 hours)	Exchangeable albumin pool (g/kg)	Intravascular albumin (%)
13 days– 14 months	3.3–4.3	180–300	10–11	6.0–8.0	33–43
3–8 years	4.2–5.0	130–170	6–9	3.0–4.0	46–51

From Rothschild *et al.* (1972).

Clinical features

The disorder may present with failure to thrive, steatorrhoea, oedematous limbs, repeated infections and tetany. Chylous effusions may develop. The gastrointestinal symptoms include diarrhoea, abdominal distension and pain.

Pathology

The lymphatics of the lamina propria and/or submucosa and/or serosa and mesentery are dilated and macrophages may be present. Enterocytes at the tip of the villi contain lipid droplets (Fig. 8.1).

Investigations

The following findings are characteristic of intestinal lymphangiectasis:

1. Low total protein (3.4–5.5 g/100 ml; Vardy *et al.*, 1975).
2. Low serum albumin (1.1–2.7 g/100 ml; Vardy *et al.*, 1975)
3. Low immunoglobulins.
4. Lymphopenia.
5. ± Anaemia (low serum iron and folate).
6. Hypocalcaemia.
7. Abnormal xylose tolerance test (*see* p. 68).
8. Stool fat increased.
9. Increased stool protein loss (^{51}Cr-labelled albumin or iodine-125).
10. Stool smear for lymphocytes — many seen.
11. α_1-Antitrypsin clearance studies.
12. Small bowel biopsy — dilated lacteals.
13. Barium studies of small bowel: increased intestinal and mucosal folds, spiculation, jejunization of ileum, dilatation of lumen.
14. Lymphangiography to demonstrate obstruction.

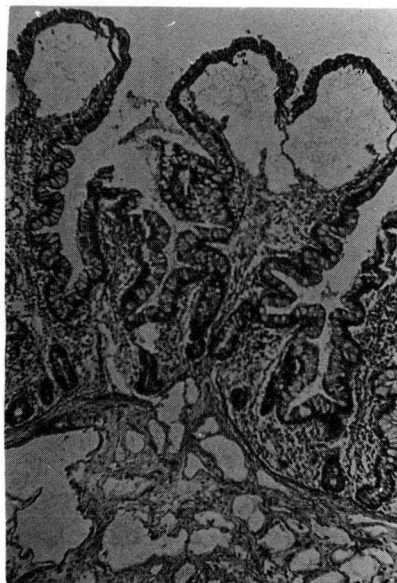

Fig. 8.1 Small bowel biopsy showing dilated lymphatics and presence of lipids in intestinal lymphangiectasis.

Treatment

Localized disease might be remedied with resection at site of obstruction or the creation of an anastomosis. Complete remissions have been described. The aim of dietary treatment, in essence, must be to provide nutrients in a form in which they can be readily absorbed. The presence of long-chain fats increases the intralymphatic pressure which may result in the rupture of the channels leading to an increased loss of lymphocytes and protein from the lacteals (Vardy *et al.*, 1975).

The early removal of most of the long-chain

triglycerides (LCTs) is essential. MCTs are absorbed directly into the portal venous system, bypassing the lymphatics (p. 127) and can be used to replace the energy which is normally derived from dietary LCT. It is important to introduce MCTs very slowly so initially a low-fat feed based on skimmed milk powder can be used. This feed can also be used in situations where MCT formulae are not available. It is important that approximately 1.0 g LCT/100 ml feed or per 60–70 kcal (250–290 kJ) is included in order to prevent deficiency of essential fatty acids. Once the infant is tolerating this then the energy intake can be improved by gradual introduction of either an MCT formula such as Portagen (Appencix IV.7) or an MCT emulsion, e.g. Liquigen (Appendix IV.14).

The protein intake in intestinal lymphangiectasia depends upon the quantity being lost from the gut. This loss should decrease once the LCT content of the feed is reduced. Generally the requirement is 5–10 g protein/kg actual weight daily, although serum protein and blood urea levels should be monitored to ensure that the correct intake has been achieved. Infant formulae incorporating MCT will not provide sufficient protein unless large quantities are consumed, and a modular regimen might be needed. Alternatively, a protein module (Appendix IV.12) can be used to supplement an MCT formula.

Fat-soluble vitamins are poorly absorbed and up to twice the recommended dosage in a water-miscible form such as Ketovite is suggested. If the feed is based on skimmed milk or a specially designed modular regimen, then water-soluble vitamins may also be indicated. Since anaemia is a feature of this condition, iron will be required at least until intestinal protein losses are minimal.

When weaning foods are introduced they should contain no LCT; foods such as potato, rice, fruit and vegetables must form the basis of the diet. In older children, the LCT ought to be less than 10 g daily and only foods with a very low fat content (Appendix IV.25) should be included. Additional energy in the form of glucose polymer and MCT will be necessary to achieve sufficient energy for normal growth and a high-protein, high-energy, low-fat drink could be a useful source of nutrients as described in Appendix III.10. Additionally MCT can be used in cooking as described in Appendix IV.27.

9

Disorders of Carbohydrate Digestion and Absorption

Carbohydrates and malabsorption

Impaired carbohydrate digestion and absorption is not uncommon in infants. The problem may arise because of an inherited enzyme deficiency or, more commonly, be the consequence of damage to the small bowel mucosa as the result of an infection, enteropathy or surgery.

The main carbohydrate ingested in man is starch and, to a lesser extent, the disaccharides lactose and sucrose as well as the monosaccharides glucose and fructose. In babies and infants lactose from breast or cows' milk is the principal sugar. This disaccharide facilitates the presence of the organism *Lactobacillus acidophilus* which enhances calcium and phosphate absorption.

Basic chemistry of sugars

D-Glucose is an important carbohydrate. It is a hexose sugar, i.e. it contains six carbon atoms, the carbon atoms being numbered from the aldehyde on C-1 (Fig. 9.1).

Glucose molecules can be linked to form a disaccharide or a polysaccharide such as starch which is made up mainly of amylopectin and, to a lesser extent, amylose (Figs 9.2 and 9.3). Amylose is formed by a straight chain of 200—2000 glucose units linked via α-1,4 oxygen bonds (the α designation means the OH at C-1 is below the plane of the ring). Salivary and pancreatic α-amylases can attack the interior α-1,4 junctions but not the outermost links — therefore maltose (2 glucose units) + maltotriose (3 glucose units) are the final products.

Amylopectin is highly branched containing 250—5000 glucose units. The main linkage is α-1,4 but at the branch site a third unit of glucose is joined in the 6 position. Salivary and pancreatic α-amylases attack the interior α-1,4 glucose—glucose links, but cannot hydrolyse the exterior bonds or those at the branching points. Therefore the end products

of starch digestion are maltose, maltotriose and α-dextrins. α-Dextrins are hydrolysed to glucose by mucosal α-dextrinase (isomaltase).

The major catalytic enzymes responsible for carbohydrate hydrolysis are: maltase (maltose and maltotriose to glucose); lactase (lactose to glucose and galactose); sucrase (sucrose to glucose and fructose).

Lactase activity is at its peak level in the term newborn which explains the lactose malabsorption seen in very immature babies.

The epithelial cells in the proximal jejunum have the highest concentration of the brush-border enzymes. There is least activity in the terminal ileum. A summary of carbohydrate digestion is given in Table 9.1.

Monosaccharides

Glucose—galactose malabsorption

Glucose—galactose malabsorption is an autosomal recessive defect leading to impaired absorption of

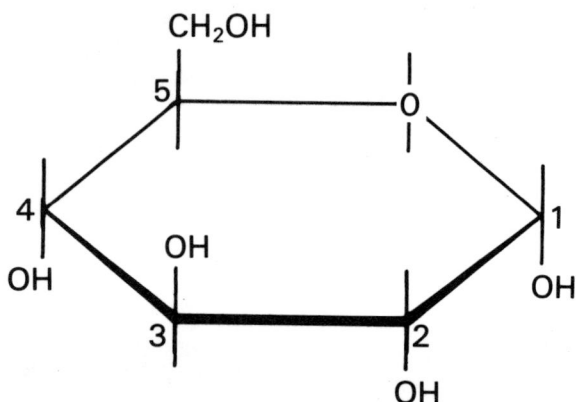

Fig. 9.1 Haworth projection formula of sugars (1929). For clarity, all carbon atoms have been omitted except the sixth.

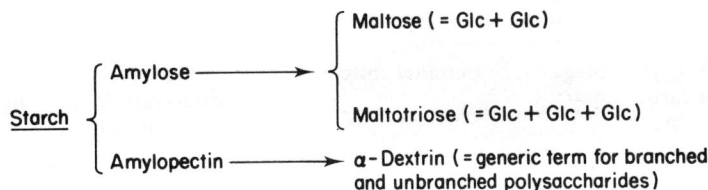

Fig. 9.2 The composition of starch. Glc = glucose.

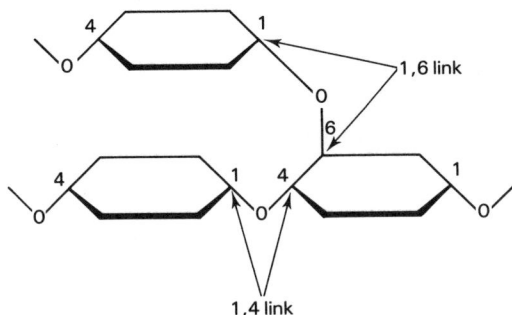

Fig. 9.3 The structure of amylopectin showing 1,4- and 1,6-links between glucose molecules.

the two separate monosaccharides transported by a common mechanism (Lindquist *et al.*, 1962). In most infants the condition becomes less severe by the age of 7 months. It is important that the clinician distinguishes glucose—galactose malabsorption from the unrelated disorder of galactosaemia.

Glucose, galactose and fructose are the monosaccharides derived from the hydrolysis of disaccharides by the brush-border enzymes of the small bowel villi. Walker-Smith (1979) draws a clear distinction between sugar intolerances causing a clinical syndrome and sugar malabsorption where there is laboratory evidence of disordered sugar absorption. Transient monosaccharide secondary intolerance (or malabsorption) arising from an infective enteritis or small bowel enteropathies is not uncommon and probably is underdiagnosed, e.g. glucose intolerance in rotavirus infection.

Presentation

Diarrhoea is seen when the baby is given a glucose solution such as an electrolyte preparation or a lactose-containing feed, be it breast milk or normal formula. The stools are explosive and watery. Presenting features are similar to those seen in disaccharidase deficiencies (*see below*).

Diagnosis

Diagnosis is based on the following:

1. pH of stool supernatant is <5.5 (pH is both less helpful and reliable than Clinitest).
2. Presence of stool reducing substances. Clinitest (Ames & Co.) reaction strongly positive (Kerry and Anderson, 1964). In neonates oligosaccharides may be present and give a positive Clinitest result. Various drugs, too, can give a false-positive Clinitest reaction, e.g. cephalexin and nalidixic acid. Sucrose is a non-reducing sugar and so the Clinitest will produce false negative findings in those malabsorbing this carbohydrate.
3. Test for presence of glucose in stools (glucose oxidase methods, e.g. Clinistix, Labstix, Tes-tape, Hema-combistix).
4. Hydrogen breath test (*see* p. 83).
5. Stool chromatography for sugar (the most commendable of the laboratory diagnostic techniques, *see* p. 83).
6. Glucose tolerance test: flat response + symptoms. Fast 4—6 hours. Obtain fasting serum glucose. Give glucose 1 g/kg and galactose 1 g/kg. Measure serum glucose at 15, 30, 60 and 120 minutes. Results: glucose will not rise above 1.1 mmol/l (20 mg/100 ml) if glucose—galactose malabsorption is present.
7. Lactose tolerance test: flat response + symptoms. Fast 4—6 hours. Obtain fasting serum glucose. Give lactose 2 g/kg as a 10% solution. Measure serum glucose at 15, 30, 60 and 120 minutes. Results: *see above*. Also test stools during the study or immediately afterwards for the Clinitest reaction.
8. Jejunal biopsy: normal small bowel architecture is found in congenital glucose—galactose malabsorption. If the villi are damaged then this disorder is a secondary as opposed to a primary phenomenon. In such a situation, the activity of the disaccharidases lactase and sucrase will be reduced and they can be assayed.

Table 9.1 Carbohydrate digestion

Diet (percentage of carbohydrate intake)	Luminal enzymes		Oligosaccharides and disaccharides presented to mucosa	Mucosal enzymes	End products
Starch (60%)			Maltose Maltotriose (α-1,4 linkage)	Maltase ⟶	Glucose
	Amylopectin	Salivary and ⟶ pancreatic α-amylases	α-Dextrins (α-1,6 linkage)	α-Dextrinase (isomaltase) ⟶	Glucose
	Amylose	Salivary and ⟶ pancreatic α-amylases	Maltose Maltotriose (α-1,4 linkage)	Maltase ⟶	Glucose
Sucrose (30%)		⟶	Sucrose	Sucrase ⟶	Glucose and Sucrose
Lactose (10%)		⟶	Lactose	Lactase ⟶	Glucose and galactose

Modified from Gray G M, *Gastroenterology* **58**, 100, 1970.

Management

Glucose, galactose and lactose must all be excluded from the diet. The alternative milk substitutes include a low lactose preparation containing fructose such as fructose formula Galactomin (Appendix IV.1) or a feeding regimen using a protein module that is free of lactose, such as Comminuted Chicken (Appendix IV.12). The fat module selected can be based on long- or medium-chain fats, though MCTs should be avoided where possible because they will increase the osmolality.

The carbohydrate module must be fructose or laevulose. The use of fructose as the sole carbohydrate carries with it some potential danger. The osmolality will be high because fructose has a small particle size compared with a disaccharide or a polymer. In addition, because fructose is initially metabolized to lactic acid via glycolysis, it is likely to worsen acidosis in acidotic states (e.g. hypoxia); therefore, it should be introduced very slowly into the feed, while blood glucose levels are maintained by a parenteral dextrose infusion. The protein and fat modules can be introduced fairly rapidly (unless MCT is used) to give an adequate energy intake.

The initial oral feed should not contain more than 2% fructose nor exceed a total of 5 g fructose in the first 24 hours. The quantity of fructose can be increased to full strength (7–8% fructose) over a period of 5–6 days. Small infants may develop diarrhoea at concentrations of greater than 6% fructose and should this arise then additional energy in the form of extra protein and fat can be given.

Where the malabsorption is a secondary, therefore temporary, phenomenon, glucose can be introduced cautiously after symptoms have disappeared and the infant is gaining weight. Introduction of glucose to replace fructose in the feed should take place gradually over about 5 days. Once the infant appears to tolerate glucose then lactose can be reintroduced in a similar manner.

In the case of the primary enzyme defect or where a secondary intolerance persists then the infant may require a weaning diet that is free of glucose, galactose and lactose. Such a diet is extremely limited and a list of suitable foods is shown in Appendix IV.21. As the infant gets older glucose is better tolerated. Later, starchy foods, such as cereal or potato, may be accepted in small amounts.

Transient/secondary intolerance to fructose

Fructose, a ketohexose released from the hydrolysis of sucrose, is absorbed by a process called facilitated diffusion. It has a specific entry mechanism as it moves across the enterocyte. Damage to the villi can cause malabsorption of this monosaccharide. The clinical features are not dissimilar to those seen in other sugar intolerances.

Diagnosis

Diagnosis is based on the following:

1. Jejunal biopsy will exclude villous atrophy and brush-border disaccharidases should be assayed. The presence of damaged villi accompanied by low enzyme activity will explain any carbo-hydrate malabsorption.
2. Hydrogen breath test (*see* p. 83).
3. Stool chromatography for sugars (*see* p. 83).

Hereditary fructose intolerance

The condition (HFI, Fig. 9.4b) was first described by Chambers and Pratt (1956). It is characterized by nausea, vomiting, hypoglycaemia, hepatomegaly, jaundice and aminoaciduria following the ingestion of fructose or sucrose. Symptoms do not appear until fruit juices or sucrose (present in some milk formulae) appear in the diet. An aversion to sweets can be a useful diagnostic clue. Fructosaemia and fructosuria develop when fructose or sucrose are consumed. This is a rare autosomal recessive disease in which there is reduced activity of fructose, 1-phosphate aldolase. Dietary fructose is converted

to glucose by this enzyme in the liver and in its absence there is an associated inhibition of fructose, 1,6-diphosphate aldolase and glycogen phos-phorylase probably due to shortage of phosphate as fructose 1-phosphate.

Diagnosis

Diagnosis is made by the fructose loading test — fructose 0.25 mg/kg i.v. will result in hypoglycaemia and hypophosphataemia and lactic acidosis. It is a very dangerous test in a sick child. If the patient is stable the test is best done with intravenous fructose and a glucose drip must be on hand. Oral fructose can cause intestinal symptoms.

A clinical diagnosis can be made by noting the improvement on withdrawal of fructose.

Liver biopsy for assay will show reduced activity of the enzyme fructose, 1-phosphate aldolase. In advanced cases there will be histopathological features of cirrhosis.

Essential fructosuria

This entity has been called an anomaly rather than a disease (Froesch, 1972). Essential fructosuria which is of no clinical signifiance is seen mainly in Jewish families and is due to absence of the enzyme fructokinase causing a high blood fructose level, and fructosuria after fructose or sucrose ingestion.

Management

Sucrose and fructose should be removed from the diet. Some infant formulae contain sucrose and such preparations should be avoided. Instead a

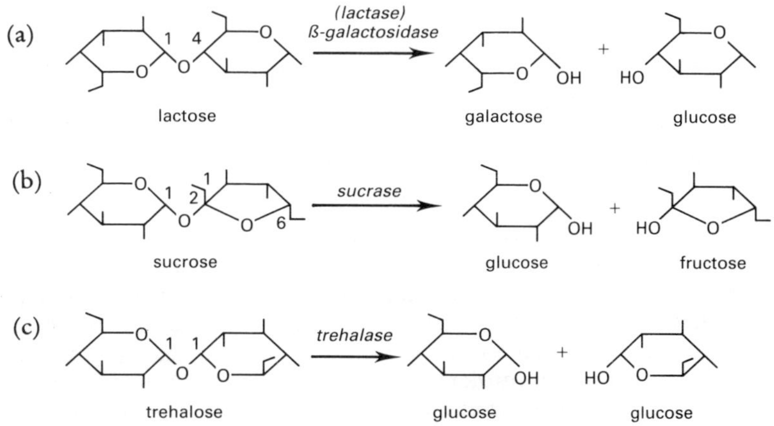

Fig. 9.4 The action of brush-border enzymes β-galactosidase (lactase) (a); sucrase (b); trehalase (c).

normal milk formula which contains only lactose or hydrolysed cornstarch as the carbohydrate is used. Unless an intolerance to other sugars, such as lactose, is suspected, there is no reason to use a specialized formula. Solids should be free of sucrose and fructose and a list of such foods is given in Appendices IV.22 and IV.23.

Glucose or glucose polymer can be used where necessary to sweeten foods. Care should be taken to see that medicines are not made up in a sucrose-containing syrup. In HFI a tolerance to fructose develops and foods containing small or moderate amounts of sucrose can be gradually introduced.

Disaccharides

Disorders of lactose absorption

The subject of lactose malabsorption (Fig. 9.4a) is a complex one and there is much disagreement about the classification of this entity. In global terms there are more lactose malabsorbers than those with normal absorption patterns. Malabsorbers are found in eastern Asia and in the Pacific and include the Chinese, Japanese, Koreans, Thais, Fijians, Philippinos, Australian Aborigines, Africans (Ibo, Yoruba, Hausa) and the American Negroes. Some Europeans and those from the Middle East may also malabsorb lactose; however, there is generally a low incidence within northern Europe and Scandinavia. For an interesting and comprehensive review of the biology and anthropological appraisal of lactose malabsorption *see* Johnson *et al.* (1974).

Secondary lactase deficiency

This transient phenomenon is by far the commonest variety of disaccharide malabsorption. Whenever neutral lactase, which is the membrane-bound brush-border enzyme involved in lactose hydrolysis, is diminished by mucosal injury malabsorption occurs. The following conditions are an example of some that may be associated with sugar intolerance:

1. Enteritis (viral, bacterial, fungal).
2. Parasitic infestation (e.g. *Giardia lamblia*).
3. Coeliac disease.
4. Cystic fibrosis (in 25%).
5. Cows' milk protein intolerance.
6. Protein—energy malnutrition.

7. Drugs (e.g. neomycin, methotrexate).
8. Small bowel resection.
9. Inflammatory bowel disease — rarely a problem.

Is the lower incidence of secondary lactose intolerance, which has now been seen for a decade in north European infants with gastroenteritis, a result of the switch from high-solute to low-solute milks? It has been suggested that carbohydrate malabsorption following enteritis was formerly more common because non-adapted formulae existed and they were more antigenic than present-day preparations. Perhaps sensitization to the particular milk being used in the early phase of an acute bowel infection, when there is increased macromolecular permeability, would predispose to cows' milk protein intolerance and reduced brush, border disaccharidase activity (Anon, 1987).

Congenital lactase deficiency

Holzel *et al.* (1959) originally described the very rare congenital disorder of lactose malabsorption, yet some authorities dispute the existence of this disease (Lebenthal and Rossi, 1981). Symptoms arise immediately after birth when breast milk or a formula is offered. Unlike the other intestinal disaccharidases, lactase develops early in the fetus from the third month of gestation to reach a peak of activity at the time of normal gestation (Auricchio *et al.*, 1965). Thus it is not unusual for an immature newborn to demonstrate a transient developmental intolerance to lactose. This phenomenon was described as 'ontogenetic' lactose malabsorption by Johnson *et al.* (1974) and is seen in the perinatal period or beyond 3—5 years of age in children of certain ethnic origins. It is characterized by reduced lactase activity. There is no convincing evidence that offering a baby the substrate lactose induces enzyme activity. Most observers accept as valid the conclusions of Plimmer (1906), although carried out on animals, that there is no lactase adaptation in man. Furthermore, intestinal lactase activity decreases at the time of weaning in most mammals.

Presentation

Diarrhoea is the major feature seen in malabsorption of lactose irrespective of the basic pathology. Explosive diarrhoea and the presence of watery acid stools becomes evident after milk ingestion. Non-hydrolysed disaccharides cause considerable movement of electrolytes and water into the gut

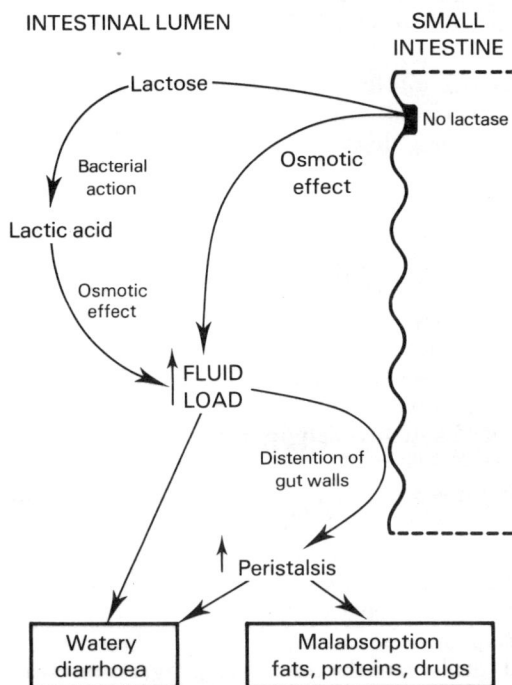

Fig. 9.5 The mechanism of congenital lactase deficiency. (Courtesy of WF Balistreri.)

lumen and this provokes osmotic diarrhoea (Fig. 9.5). Excoriation of the perianal area is common because of the acid stools. Lactose which is passed from the small bowel to the colon is fermented by bacteria to lactic acid. Abdominal distension with or without vomiting may appear and the baby will not thrive. In some situations blood (macro- or microscopic) will be in the stool and even mucus if there is an infective agent present in the colon (e.g. *Salmonella* sp. or, uncommonly, the rotavirus may be present in the small and large bowel). Cows' milk protein can produce an enteropathy in the upper gastrointestinal tract with lactose malabsorption and a colitis in the large bowel.

Diagnosis

Diagnosis is based on the following:

Clinitest reaction (Fig. 9.6) — test for reducing substances in the fluid portion of the stool — *not* Clinistix. Place a small volume of liquid stool in test tube, add twice its volume of water. To 15 drops of suspension add one Clinitest tablet.

Results:

0.25% or less = negative

0.25−0.5% = suspect
0.5%+ = abnormal

Stool pH — if < 5.5 sugar present (only valid if lactose is still being ingested - a test that is rarely helpful).

Stool chromatography for sugar

Hydrogen breath test: fast, then give lactose load of 1−2 g/kg. If the expired hydrogen in the breath exceeds 20 p.p.m. above the baseline sugar malabsorption is present (Metz *et al.*, 1976). Sample the room air and baseline expired breath before the test. Then measure hydrogen at 15, 30, 60, 90 and 120 minutes, taking duplicate samples at all times.

Lactose tolerance test (LTT): fast (4−6 hours in toddlers or infants, less in the neonate − particularly if immature or growth retarded). Normally there should be a rise in capillary blood glucose of 1.1 mmol/l = 20 mg/100 ml. Take blood samples at 0, 15, 30, 60 and 120 minutes. The sample at 15 minutes is important since some children peak then.

Jejunal biopsy: if the patient is not hypoproteinaemic or experiencing a disorder of the clotting mechanisms a small bowel biopsy is important if disaccharide malabsorption secondary to an enteropathy is to be excluded. Management is facilitated if enzymes are assayed (lactase, isosucrase/maltase) in addition to routine histophathology of the specimen.

Management

The dietary treatment of adverse reactions to lactose relates to the severity of the symptoms. Weight loss in a small infant necessitates the removal of virtually all lactose from the diet, while a less intense reaction may indicate a temporary reduction in lactose intake. A minimal lactose regimen means that no milk from any species can be used because lactose is the carbohydrate in human, cow, goat and sheep milk. A milk with a reduced lactose content should be used (Appendix IV.1). Because it is sometimes difficult to differentiate between adverse reactions to lactose and to other components of cows' milk, particularly protein, it may be prudent to use a preparation that does not include intact cows' milk protein. This type of formula (Appendices IV.3 and IV.4) is always free of lactose. Most pill-type medicines contain lactose as a filler. It is often not necessary to remove lactose entirely from the diet of an infant or young child; a reduction in the lactose concentration of the diet may be sufficient to alleviate symptoms. In situations where secondary intolerance to lactose is predictable, such as following gut surgery — particularly extensive small bowel resection — or persistent gastroenteritis, it may be appropriate to use a feed with a reduced lactose content as a routine measure. A normal infant formula which has been supplemented with glucose or maltodextrin rather than lactose would be the most suitable; milks with this type of composition are discussed in the section on normal milks (Appendix II.4). For older children who are receiving unmodified cows' milk, preparations of the enzyme lactase can be added to the milk to remove approximately 70% of the lactose (Biller *et al.*, 1987). No advantage in terms of growth or improved nutrient retentions has been shown in children with primary lactose intolerance from whom milk is withheld.

Small infants who are taking solid foods and who have shown a severe reaction to lactose should be offered a lactose-free weaning diet (Appendix IV. 19). The duration of a diet is a matter of clinical judgement. It is important that the infant should be tolerating the feed and gaining weight before any attempt is made to reintroduce lactose. Although lactase levels are not influenced by substrate concentrations, the reintroduction of this sugar into the diet should be done slowly to prevent the reappearance of symptoms. Approximately 10% of the low lactose formula should be replaced by a normal infant formula or breast milk for the first 24 hours. This 10% should not be given in one feed but should be divided and given with the low lactose formula. The quantity of lactose-containing milk can be increased over a period of 4−5 days until the low-lactose formula has been entirely replaced. If the low-lactose milk is also free of milk protein then additional precautions, as described on p. 94, should be followed.

Lactose and sucrose intolerance — management

Where there is severe trauma to the small bowel mucosa, both lactase and sucrase/isomaltase enzymes may be depleted leading to malabsorption of all dissacharides and starch (*see* Table 9.1). Digestion of glucose polymer, hydrolysed cornstarch or dextrins may also be affected because the hydrolysis of short-chain oligosacchahrides requires α-glucosidase which is a brush-border enzyme. For the young infant, treatment is identical to that of lactose intolerance alone with the proviso that the low lactose formula selected contains only glucose or glucose with fructose as the carbohydrate.

If symptoms persist then solids free of lactose and sucrose should be given. Care should be taken when introducing starch and only small quantities may be tolerated. Until normal gut function returns, it is possibly desirable to omit gluten from the diet because there may be a transient and secondary gluten intolerance. A list of suitable foods is shown in Appendix IV.29. When reintroducing disaccharides sucrase activity is likely to return before lactase.

Because the former is a substrate-dependent enzyme there will be little activity from a biopsy assay while the infant remains on a low sucrose diet. A small amount of sucrose (initially 1 g/100 ml feed) can replace glucose in the feed; this can subsequently be increased to 2 g/100 ml. Once this level is tolerated the infant can progress on to a low lactose diet already described.

Complete carbohydrate intolerance — management

In addition to reduced disaccharidase activity where there is severe damage to the mucosa of the small intestine, the absorptive mechanism for monosaccharides may also fail. Small infants, particularly those who are malnourished, do not have large glycogen stores and are inefficient converters of glucogenic amino acids to glucose by gluconeogenesis. It is vital therefore that a parenteral source of glucose is given. If total parenteral nutrition is not possible then, providing glucose is given parenterally, a carbohydrate-free oral feed may be tolerated. Examples of preparations containing protein and fat, either singly or in conjuction with each other, are described in the section on modular feeding in Appendices IV.11−IV.17. If it is felt necessary to give solid foods then only the protein foods — meat, poultry, fish and egg — are free of carbohydrate.

When the infant appears to be tolerating a carbohydrate-free regimen and is maintaining weight (weight gain is unlikely), then small quantities of a monosaccharide can be introduced. A mixture of glucose and fructose is likely to be better tolerated than a higher concentration of one sugar alone.

Initially a concentration of 1 g glucose/100 ml feed can be added in the first 24 hours. If the sugar does not appear in the stool and stool frequency does not increase, then 1 g fructose/100 ml can also be added. When a total of 6 g mixed carbohydrate per 100 ml feed is tolerated then the procedure and feeding regimen is as for lactose/sucrose intolerance.

Sucrase/isomaltase deficiency

Isolated deficiency of the brush-border enzyme complex sucrase/isomaltase (=sucrase/α-dextrinase) may be the result of an inherited autosomal recessive disorder (*see* Fig. 9.4b). The incidence in most populations is 1:500–1:30 000 (Gray *et al.*, 1976) but in the Eskimos of Greenland it is as high as 10% (McNair *et al.*, 1972).

Rarely, secondary deficiency of isomaltase/sucrase will be seen as a result of mucosal destruction (e.g. postenteritis, postintestinal resection, malnutrition). In this situation the disaccharidase lactase may also be decreased. The combined defect of the two enzymes, sucrase and isomaltase, always coexists. Isomaltase activity (measured as palatinase) concerns the α-1,6-glucosidic linkage.

Presentation

Clinical manifestations of sucrose intolerance arise from incomplete hydrolysis of this disaccharide and starch from the subsequent bacterial fermentation of the unabsorbed carbohydrate. Sucrose in the jejunum will increase the osmotic load of the intraluminal contents thus causing watery diarrhoea. Abdominal distension and cramp will arise when the carbohydrate load is excessive.

Diagnosis

Diagnosis is based on the following tests

Clinitest reaction (Fig. 9.6) because sucrose is a non-reducing sugar add 2 volumes of 1 N hydrochloric acid to 1 volume of liquid stool, then boil for 30 seconds before carrying out the Clinitest reaction (*see* p. 79).

pH: if < 5.5 sugar present.

Stool chromatography for sugar: where chromatography is available it is crucial that the stool is fresh and must be deep frozen from the time it is passed until sugar analysis is determined. Enzyme activity of stool bacteria will remove any disaccharides.

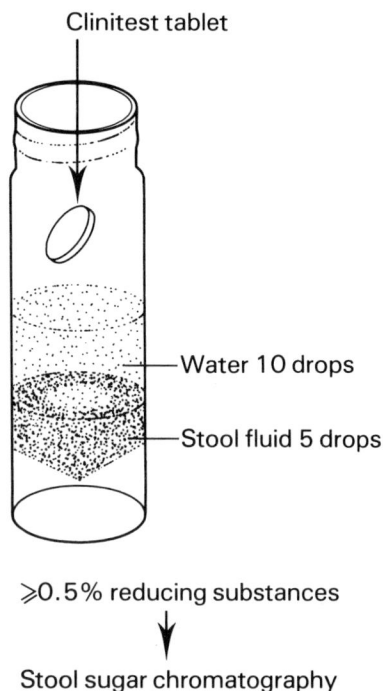

Fig. 9.6 The Clinitest reaction; *see* text for details.

Hydrogen breath test: fast 4–6 hours then give a sucrose load of 2 g/kg in a 10% solution and maltose 1 g/kg. If the expired breath hydrogen exceeds 20 p.p.m. above the baseline level sugar malabsorption is present (Metz *et al.*, 1976) (*see* p. 83).

Sucrose tolerance test: fast 4–6 hours then give a sucrose load of 2 g/kg in a 10% solution — for maltose use 1 g/kg. Introduce the solution by nasogastric tube in the baby or infant. The oral route can be used in the older child.

Fasting glucose: take a fasting capillary glucose then sample at 15, 30, 60 and 120 minutes. The rise of glucose should be > 1.1 mmol/l (=20 mg/100 ml). Note the number and nature of the stools as well as symptoms during the tolerance test. Also determine stool pH and Clinitest reaction during the study and for 6–8 hours after it is completed. A 'flat' test supports a diagnosis of enzyme(s) deficiency.

Jejunal biopsy: a small bowel biopsy at the ligament of Treitz should be obtained to exclude a secondary enzyme defect from mucosal damage. An enzyme assay is the definitive diagnostic but invasive procedure. Normal jejunal villi and absent or reduced levels of sucrase and isomaltase (palatinase) and subnormal total maltase activity would confirm a diagnosis of primary sucrase/isomaltase deficiency.

Management

Removal of concentrated sources of sucrose from the diet is the most important aspect of management. In infants this means ensuring that the normal milk formula used is sucrose free. In the primary condition where there is an isolated enzyme deficiency the ability to hydrolyse glucose polymers, hydrolysed cornstarch and dextrins should be normal. Sweetened fruit drink and syrups should be eliminated from the diet and care needs to be taken to ensure that any medicines do not have a sucrose base. When infant solid foods are introduced they should be free of sucrose and starch. A list of suitable items is given in Appendix IV.23.

In the older child without severe symptoms, the diet need not be so restrictive. Although the 1, 6-linkage of starch cannot be hydrolysed owing to lack of the isomaltase, these 'α-limit' dextrins constitute only about 30% of the hydrolysed starch molecule, and do not impose a high osmotic load in the gut lumen. In practice, foods containing starch can be given in limited quantities. Tolerance to starch improves with age, to sucrose to a lesser extent. Foods such as fruit containing natural sucrose complexed with fibre tend to be better tolerated than processed foods containing added sucrose. Parents and children tend to construct a diet which suits the individual, perhaps limiting their intake to one normal sized serving of starch-containing foods and one small serving of natural sucrose per meal. Soy flour can be used in place of wheat flour where the child wishes to eat more baked goods than can be tolerated. Soy flour has a relatively low starch content (15 g/100 g; wheat flour 80 g/100 g). Because it does not contain gluten it will not 'rise' and give a light, aerated product, Where only small amounts of fruit and potato are tolerated and green vegetables are not taken, a supplement of ascorbic acid and folate should be given.

Trehalase deficiency

This is a rare disorder due to the absence (or deficiency) of the intestinal enzyme trehalase (Fig. 9.4c). The major source of trehalose, a non-reducing sugar, is the young mushroom; it is converted to glucose in the older mushroom. This sugar intolerance is characterized by watery diarrhoea soon after young mushrooms are ingested. Treat by eliminating the offending source of the carbohydrate from the diet.

10

Food Intolerance and Aversion

There are few subjects that are so enigmatic, confusing and clouded with anecdotal clutter as that of food adversion (intolerance) and aversion (psychological intolerance or avoidance). Because of a paucity of prospective double-blind investigations, clinicians who ascribed to a belief in food intolerance, especially allergy, were in the recent past scientifically suspect. Definitions as yet have not been universally accepted; however, Lessof *et al.* (1980) suggested the term 'allergy' be applied only to those with immediate allergic responses to food and with the presence of specific IgE antibodies. Mast cells, basophils, eosinophils, macrophages and platelets can all be activated by IgE antibodies causing the release of preformed or instant mediators.

Clinical manifestations of food intolerance may include diarrhoea, abdominal pain, failure to thrive, urticaria, eczema, migraine, behavioural disturbances and inflammatory bowel disease (Cant, 1986).

Food intolerances

Food intolerance is an adverse and reproducible reaction which can be caused by:

1. *Allergic* reactions, which implies an unpleasant and immediate response to food(s) and the mechanisms may be via IgE antibody formation, a T-cell-mediated reaction, or the systemic formation of antigen—antibody complexes (Table 10.1).
2. *Pharmacological*, e.g. tyramine. There is a high concentration of tyramine in fermented cheese and this can elevate the blood pressure and produce symptoms. Caffeine in coffee and tea can, in the hypersensitive, cause symptoms such as anxiety and tachycardia.
3. *Toxic* effect, e.g. mycotoxins from storage of foods contaminated with moulds.

4. *Enzyme deficiency*, e.g. lactose intolerance due to alactasia (*see* p. 82). It has been suggested that a deficiency of the enzyme phenol sulphotransferase may have a role in food-induced migraine (Littlewood *et al.*, 1982).
5. *Food fermentation*: bacteria in the colon, particularly *Proteus morganii*, can produce decarboxylase, an enzyme that will convert dietary histidine to histamine. However, as histamine does not cause an immunological reaction its effect is pseudoallergic. In addition, this particular amine does not readily penetrate the gut mucosal barrier.
6. *Other intolerances*:
   a. Tartrazine is a common colouring substance contained in many foods, soft drinks and pharmaceutical products. Its mechanism of action may be mediated by IgD antibodies. Benzoates or sulphur dioxide preservatives and butylated hydroxyanisole or butylated hydroxytoluene antioxidants may have similar effects. Manifestations of symptoms due to food additives include urticaria, asthma, migraine, rhinitis. For the so-called hyperactivity syndrome and the Feingold diet *see* p. 97.
   b. Acetylsalicylic acid (ASA), present in vegetables and fruits, can cause a range of symptoms in sensitive patients including asthma, urticaria and rhinitis. Synthetic salicylates are found as flavouring products (*see* Appendix IV.35).

Food aversion

Food aversion, in contrast to adversion, is the result of either psychological intolerance or food avoidance. For a comprehensive and balanced account of this topic *see* Royal College of Physicians/British Nutrition Foundation (1984).

Table 10.1 Classification of hypersensitivity reactions according to Gell and Coombs (1963)

Type	Immunoglobulins	Effectors	Clinical
I Anaphylactic	IgE	Histamine SRS-A, ECF-A	Urticaria, angioedema, bronchospasm, anaphylaxis
II Cytotoxic	IgG, IgM	Complement	Cytotoxicity (e.g. haemolysis)
III Immune complexes	IgG, IgM	Complement	Immune complex (e.g. serum sickness)
IV Cell-mediated	None	T-lymphocyte, monocyte, macrophage	Delayed hypersensitivity

ECF-A = eosinophil chemotactic factor of anaphylaxis.
SRS-A = slow-reacting substance of anaphylaxis.

Investigations

Skin tests ('immediate') and the radioallergosorbent test (RAST) produce false-positives as well as negatives but fail to identify problems not due to IgE, that is reactions that occur after some hours. Small bowel biopsy will show damage to the mucosa which can occur in intolerances to cows' milk proteins, soy, chicken, rice, fish and egg.

There are also a number of unproven clinical and laboratory tests which some claim help in the diagnosis of food intolerance (David, 1987). These include:

1. The 'pulse test' (Coca, 1943) in which it is alleged the pulse rate will rise following the ingestion of a food that the patient cannot tolerate.
2. The 'sublingual food test' which necessitates dropping dilute solutions of different food allergens beneath the tongue to provoke symptoms but is of unproven value (Lehman, 1980a).
3. The 'cytotoxic food test', which unfortunately to date has no validity, involves exposing the patient's white blood cells to different foods and demonstrating a change in the leucocytes; again the findings are too inconsistent to be of value (Lehman, 1980b).
4. Using monoclonal antibodies, Walker-Smith (1984) has suggested that gastrointestinal food allergies are due to a relative lack of T-suppressor lymphocytes in the small gut epithelium.

Pathogenesis

The permeability of the gastrointestinal tract mucosa to food allergens is believed to be a major factor in the pathogenesis of antigenic food reactions. It is known that intestinal permeability is increased following an acute gastroenteritis. Noone *et al.* (1986) have demonstrated temporary changes in the gut after rotavirus enteritis by studying the differential permeation of the sugars lactose, lactulose and rhamnose. Studies using the inert probe, polythylene glycol, have shown increased intestinal permeability in allergic children which has been impeded by disodium cromoglycate (Fälth-Magnusson *et al.*, 1984). Moreover, using a radio-immunological method for measuring serum concentrations of human α-lactalbumin, pre-term infants have an increased absorption of macro-molecules than that seen at term (Axelsson and Jakobsson, 1986). Excessive uptake of such antigens might be associated with subsequent allergy. Changes in intestinal permeability can be provoked in an animal model by causing jejunal inflammation. Using the probe ^{31}Cr-EDTA, to study renal clearance, rats were infected with a nematode parasite, *Nippostrongylus brasiliensis*, and isolated loop studies demonstrated that permeability changes were localized to the site of inflammation and also reversible after healing (Ramage *et al.*, 1988). The integrity of the bowel mucosa is maintained in part by secretory IgA and the glycocalyx (a glycoprotein secretion coating the bowel enterocytes) as well as the mucosa-associated lymph tissues (MALTs). Alteration to this protective barrier will enable the uptake of undigested macromolecules and the risk of a subsequent allergic reaction (Tomasi, 1972; Walker and Hong, 1973). Brostoff *et al.* (1983) suggest that following food challenge there is the deposition of immune complexes in different target organs and sites which can result in migraine, arthralgia or eczema. Antigen-specific protection is related to oral or parenteral immunization as well as the secretory immunoglubulins IgA and IgM. The absorbed antigens are presented to the gut-associated lymphoid tissue (GALT) of the lamina propria. GALT is an important component of the immune system and it gathers information from an antigen-filled tube, the gut. It is comprised of nodular lymphoid tissues (Peyer's patches and mesenteric lymph nodes), the mucosal phagocytes and lymphoid cells as well as lymph nodes.

Treatment

Often treatment is unsatisfactory because of difficulties in identifying and then removing the offending allergen(s). Disodium cromoglycate has been of some help (Freier and Berger, 1973) and perhaps the next generation of so-called mast cell membrane stabilizers or food hyposensitization techniques might be more effective than those presently used.

Dietary management of adverse reactions to foods

Almost every food consumed by man has been cited as an allergen in the literature. Many food dyes which have a low molecular weight and are not allergens in themselves act as haptens and become allergenic if linked to a larger protein molecule. Some substances may undergo transformation to allergens only after they have been through the digestive process. Cooking or food processing can also affect allergenicity: a hard boiled egg is less allergenic than a raw one. Certain combinations of food may be allergenic while failing to give rise to symptoms when eaten separately. Allergy to one food is likely to produce cross-reactions with biologically related compounds: if eggs are not tolerated then chicken should be suspected until proved otherwise; likewise beef and veal in milk protein allergy and broad beans, peas and lentils where peanuts are known to be allergenic. The allergenicity of some items may be dose related: one strawberry may be tolerated while a plateful will produce urticaria.

However, from this morass of facts it is usually possible to select items which are likely offenders. Certain foods are linked with particular symptoms

Table 10.2 Allergic symptoms related to foods

Disease spectrum	Most common foods
Migraine	Chocolate, cheese and dairy products, citrus fruits, alcohol, tea and coffee, pork, fish and shellfish, wheat, vegetables (especially onions), fatty fried food
Urticaria and angioedema	Nuts, eggs, fish and shellfish, yeasts, salicylates, azo dyes, antioxidants, preservatives and flavourings, pork, chocolate, banana, berry fruits, particularly strawberries
Asthma and eczema	Milk, cheese and dairy products, egg, chocolate, nuts, fish and shellfish, chicken and beef, beans, yeast, azo dyes
Gastrointestinal	Milk and dairy products, egg, chicken, wheat, rice, soy, pork, fish and shellfish
Hyperkinesis	Salicylates, food colourings, flavouring, emulsifiers and stabilizers

and this may be of help when deciding which foods should be avoided (Table 10.2).

It can be seen that the most common food allergens reported are milk, cheese and dairy products, egg, fish and shellfish, chocolate, citrus fruits, meat (particularly pork), nuts and wheat. For dietary management of food intolerances, *see* Fig. 10.1.

Elimination diets

A careful diet history in relation to clinical features is most important: if symptoms are continuous then the culprit is likely to be something that is taken daily; occasionaly a reaction occurs within hours of eating a food, and the cause is readily identified. Those with intermittent symptoms should keep a food diary including every item eaten or drunk with brand names of processed food where applicable. A careful scrutiny of foods ingested 48 hours prior to the development of symptoms, preferably on at least two occasions, should result in a 'short list' of offenders. These foods, and those biologically related to them, are then removed from the diet for a period of 4–6

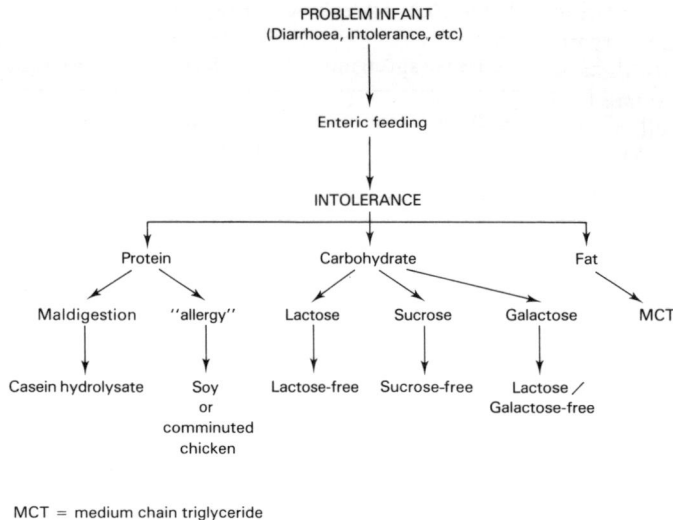

Fig. 10.1 Dietary management of food intolerances. (Courtesy of WF Balistreri.)

MCT = medium chain triglyceride

weeks with the intake/symptom record being continued. After this time the offending item(s) should be given, ideally in a disguised form, to see if symptoms reappear. Failure to test in this objective way may result in many foods being wrongly branded as allergens and the child being condemned to a more restricted diet than is necessary. If a full diet history fails to give any clues it is worth while excluding the most common allergens, according to symptoms, for 4–6 weeks before embarking on a full elimination diet (Hathaway and Warner, 1983). It is important that all traces of allergens are removed so manufactured products, which may contain hidden ingredients, should be completely avoided.

A full elimination diet should only be proposed as a last resort, because this is a major undertaking for all concerned (Cant, 1986). It requires patience, meticulous attention to detail and record keeping, and careful supervision of the child. The duration of the earlier more restricted stages of the diet should be kept as short as possible. Prolongation may result in nutritional deficiencies, particularly of vitamins, minerals and trace elements, as well as inflicting psychological trauma on the child and his family.

An essential prerequisite to an elimination regimen is a diet record of all foods consumed over a 4- to 6-week period when symptoms are apparent. Using this record it is possible to design an elimination diet suited to the child. A list of foods or food types is drawn up with a logical sequence of reintroduction in the shortest possible time using only foods that are normally consumed.

The first stage in the regimen is to find an acceptable substance or substances that will maintain a reasonable nutrient intake during the reintroduction period and which do not give rise to symptoms. This may be a small number of ordinary foods with low reported allergenicity, possibly combined with the use of a hypoallergic chemically defined elemental diet. This should be maintained until the child has been symptom free for at least one week — or longer in the case of intermittent symptoms. If symptoms still persist, it may be necessary to remove all natural foods from the diet and rely entirely on an elemental diet to maintain nutrition. Preparations which have been used as a basal elimination regimen include Flexical and Vivonex (Appendix IV.9). A suggested protocol for an elimination diet is given in Appendix IV.34.

Cows' milk protein intolerance

Cows' milk protein intolerance/(CMPI; cows' milk protein sensitive enteropathy/cows' milk allergy), presents itself differently in the primary and secondary forms of this disease. As a primary disorder there is often a history of atopy in the family and the protein intolerance commonly arises within weeks, but sometimes days, of starting cows' milk. Also eczema and/or asthma may develop.

Secondary intolerance is usually the result of an acute enteritis (Firer *et al.*, 1988) or coeliac disease and presents with gastrointestinal symptoms, e.g. vomiting, loose mucosy stools containing macro- or microscopic blood and failure to thrive. Furthermore, hypoproteinaemia may arise as a result of a protein-losing enteropathy (Lebenthal *et al.*, 1970). Some babies with CMPI are said to manifest with rhinitis and urticaria with or without iron deficiency. This poorly understood condition is overdiagnosed by many and too infrequently by others (7–0.3%). To further complicate this saga, cows' milk antigen may be transmitted through human milk. CMPI can be the scapegoat for those seeking a diagnostic label to explain vague symptoms and/or signs ('colic', irritability, rhinitis etc.). There are more than 20 protein fractions in cows' milk: β-lactoglobulin (not present in human milk) is the commonest culprit but α-lactalbumin, casein and bovine serum albumin can cause this enteropathy (Strobel, 1986). Some of the milk antigens can cross-react with those found in goats' milk, but this non-bovine source of nutrition, which is not without risks will be of some help. The gastrointestinal mucosa has a vast surface area and is exposed to the many proteins found in cows' milk which can enter the epithelial cell ('enterocyte'). In the absence of adequate secretory IgA (SIgA) or in the presence of a diseased or an immature mucosal surface that has not undergone maturation ('closure'), proteins may enter the lamina propria. CMPI can be triggered following enteritis (Harrison *et al.*, 1976) or presumably in other instances of small bowel disorders such as coeliac disease. In this situation, damage to the villi has impaired the integrity of the mucosal barrier and allowed the absorption of protein antigens.

A useful clue to the diagnosis is the not infrequent presence of occult or gross blood and/or mucus in the stools in an infant previously thriving on breast milk.

Diagnosis

At present there is no widespread agreement concerning the criteria for diagnosing CMPI. Over the decades the means of diagnosis has moved away from clinical observations and directed towards sophisticated immunocytological techniques.

Goldman's criteria (Goldman *et al.*, 1963) — symptoms must subside following dietary elimination of milk and become exacerbated within 48 hours of its reintroduction (three challenges in all). Extreme caution is needed upon challenging an

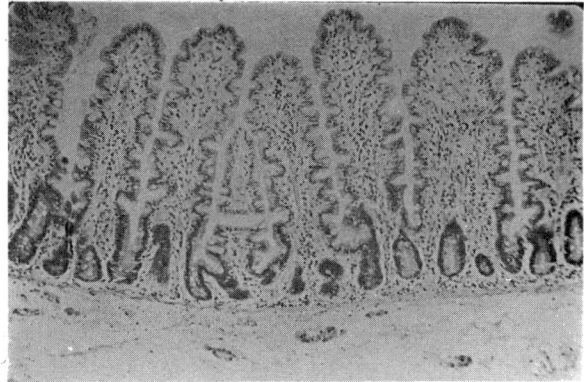

(a)

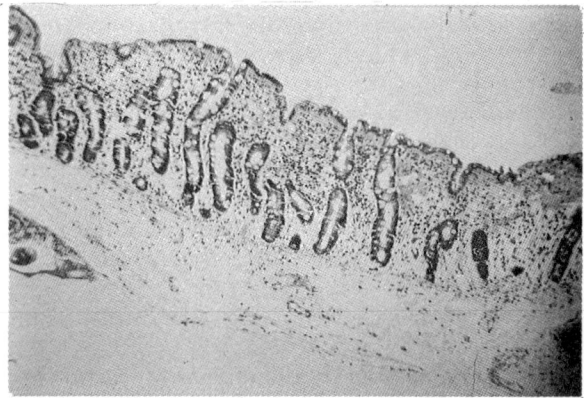

(b)

Fig. 10.2 Jejunal biopsy specimens. (a) Normal — note finger-like villi. (b) Cows' milk protein intolerance showing partial villous atrophy. (Courtesy of Dr M Brueton.)

infant because an anaphylactic type reaction may occur. Shock and rarely death has followed milk ingestion in this situation.

Serial jejunal biopsies will show abnormal mucosal structures (Fig. 10.2). The extent of the damage is patchy, variable and non-specific. The histopathology can resemble coeliac disease. Also the lamina propria may be infiltrated with eosinophils and/or have an increase in IgE plasma cells (Kilby *et al.*, 1975; Shiner *et al.*, 1975). The mucosa improves when milk proteins are removed.

Proctoscopy/sigmoidoscopy — if a paediatric proctoscope is not available use an otoscope. The mucosa may be friable, haemorrhagic and similar to that seen in colitis (Gryboski, 1967). Other investigative and research aids that might support the diagnosis include:

1. Iron deficiency (hypochromic and microcytic anaemia) with a reduced haemoglobin and serum iron.
2. Eosinophilia (>450 × 10/dl).
3. Positive skin testing to milk proteins.
4. Total IgE increased.
5. RAST positive to cows' milk proteins.
6. Serum IgA reduced (Walker, 1975).
7. Cows' milk precipitins in serum.
8. Stools:
   a. Presence of Charcot—Leyden crystals (eosinophils);
   b. Precipitating antibodies against cows' milk; look in supernatant of a freshly spun stool.
9. One-hour blood xylose reduced by 50% (comparing pre- and postchallenge blood xylose levels; Morin *et al.*, 1979).
10. Complement activation (decreased complement C3 post-milk challenge; Matthews and Soothill, 1970).
11. Duodenal juice: presence of precipitating antibodies to cows' milk (Kuzemko and Simpson, 1975).
12. Antigen-induced lymphoblast transformation (Endre and Osvath, 1975).
13. Production of a lymphokine (*in vitro*) by β-lactoglobulin (Ashkenazi *et al.*, 1980).
14. Measure ^{51}Cr-labelled autologous erythrocytes in the stool following a challenge with cows' milk proteins (Bjarnason *et al.*, 1983).

Differential diagnosis

The following conditions need to be excluded:

1. Lactose malabsorption.
2. Coeliac disease.
3. Irritable colon syndrome (toddler's diarrhoea).
4. Enteritis.
5. Enteropathy (giardiasis, chicken, fish, rice or egg intolerance etc.).
6. Intractable diarrhoea of infancy.
7. Intestinal lymphangiectasis.
8. Intestinal malrotation.
9. Immune deficiency syndrome.

The difficulty is that lactose malabsorption can coexist with CMPI as can gluten intolerance (Visakorpi, 1970). Once the intestinal mucosa heals, lactose will be tolerated and later milk proteins.

Dietary management of cows' milk protein intolerance

Efforts have been made to identify infants at risk from developing cows' milk intolerance (i.e. those with a family history of atopy) in order that they are not exposed to antigens at an early age. Exclusive breast feeding was not found to be protective against the development of atopy or respiratory tract infections (Savilahti *et al.*, 1987).

The nutritional requirements of children with cows' milk allergy are usually normal. However, if there has been prolonged failure to thrive prior to diagnosis an increased energy intake may be necessary. This can be achieved by adding extra carbohydrate in the form of a glucose polymer to the feed chosen for treatment. Details are described in the section dealing with high-energy feeds in Appendix III.3.

Formulae alternative to whole cows' milk protein

Alternatives to cows' milk fall into three broad categories: cows' milk-based feeds which have been appropriately treated to reduce allergenicity; milk of another species, such as human, goats' or sheep's milk; protein from another source, which can be either animal, vegetable or synthetic.

Cows' milk-based feeds

Heat-treated cows' milk. Heat treatment of cows' milk alters the proteins to make them less allergenic (McLaughlin *et al.*, 1981). There are other reports which indicate that heat treatment increases the allergenicity of milk by creating new antigens (Bleumink and Young, 1968). Heat-treated cows' milk feeds may be tried for mild cases, or in situations where special formulae are not available. However, many infants react to more than one class of milk protein and this type of formula is only likely to be tolerated by a small proportion of milk-intolerant infants. Heat-treated milks retain their full lactose content and will not be tolerated by infants with coexisting alactasia.

Some examples of heat-treated milks are:

1. Canned evaporated whole milk (Appendix II.7).
2. SMA (Ready-to-feed) (Appendix II.4).

Milk protein hydrolysates. Cows' milk protein products which have undergone enzymatic hydrolysis into their constituent peptides and amino acids are frequently used in the treatment of cows' milk protein intolerance. These milks are generally lactose free with glucose added as the carbohydrate. A small proportion of infants have been reported to react to these products. Care must be taken to ensure that the product used is suitable for infant use and contains adequate vitamin and mineral supplementation.

Hydrolysed products designed for use as an infant formula and which contain adequate vitamin and mineral supplementation include:

1. Nutramigen (Appendix IV.5.)
2. Alfare.
3. Pepdite.

Milk of another species

Human milk. Where lactation in the mother has not entirely ceased, continuation of breast feeding can be encouraged. Pasteurized and banked human milk has been used for very sick infants in hospital as a temporary measure. A supplement of iron and vitamins A, B, C and D should be given with breast milk. This regimen would not be suitable for infants who are suspected of being lactose intolerant. In addition, unless the mother excludes cows' milk protein from the diet, allergies can be transmitted via breast milk (Van Asperen *et al.*, 1983).

Goats' milk. This is sometimes tolerated by infants allergic to cows' milk protein. However, a number of the proteins of cows' and goats' milk do cross-react and many infants show symptoms when challenged with goats' milk. Furthermore, folate deficiency is a potential cause of megaloblastic anaemia because goats' milk contains only 6.5 µg/l of folate compared with 42 µg/l in cows' milk. Goats' milk may also be deficient in vitamins B_{12}, C and D. Boiling of goats' milk is thought to alter the protein in such a way as to reduce allergenicity; goats' milk should always be pasteurized or boiled before it is offered to infants because of the risks of tuberculosis and brucellosis. However, spray dried goats' milk powder is less likely to carry any risk of infection. Neither undiluted nor diluted goats' milk is to be recommended for babies less than 6 months of age (Taitz and Armitage, 1984). Until raw goats' milk or even the pasteurized version is radically modified in terms of its high solute load, vitamin depletion and low energy content, it cannot be regarded as an acceptable substitute for conventional milks.

Sheep's milk. Although there is immunological cross-reaction between bovine and sheep β-lactoglobulin, fortunately there is said to be no evidence of clinical studies showing cross-allergenicity (Bahna and Heiner, 1980).

Protein from other sources

Homogenized animal protein. Animal protein which has been homogenized to a fine enough consistency to pass through an infant feeder can be used. These preparations require careful supplementation to ensure an adequate intake of all nutrients. A 'home-made' preparation can be used where no special formulae are available. Well-cooked chicken breast can be finely homogenized with boiled water in the ratio 25 g cooked chicken to 75 ml water. The instructions given for administration of comminuted chicken meat (p. 000) can be followed. It is unlikely that a fine enough consistency will be achieved for the feed to be given via a feeding bottle and a cup and spoon may be used instead.

Preparations suitable for infant feeding include:

1. Comminuted Chicken Meat (Appendix IV.12).
2. Albumaid Complete.
3. Meat Base Formula.

Vegetable proteins. The most common vegetable-based milk substitutes contain soya which has a high biological value and a bland taste. These preparations are free of lactose and would therefore be suitable for lactose-intolerant infants. Some adverse reactions have been noted in milk intolerant infants fed with soy formulae (Strobel, 1986). However, these have mainly been products based on soy flour; most infant formula marketed now contain a soy protein isolate which is less likely to give rise to problems.

Care must be taken to use a product specifically designed for paediatric use. Products designed for adult vegans in general are not nutritionally adequate; methionine content is low and vitamins and minerals may not be added.

Soy protein isolates which are suitable for infants include:

1. Formula S (Appendix IV.3).
2. Wysoy.
3. Nursoy.

Chemically defined diets

Chemically defined diets are based on synthetic amino acid mixtures with a source of fat and carbohydrate, and are theoretically the least likely product to cause allergy. They have several disadvantages, such as low palatability and high osmolality which are more fully discussed in the section in Appendix IV.9. Suitable feeds of this type are:

1. Neocate.
2. Flexical.

Reintroduction of cows' milk. Where milk protein is to be reintroduced after a period on a milk-free diet care should be taken to minimize the risk of an anaphylactic reaction developing. This acute reaction has been seen in infants who only exhibited fairly minor symptoms while receiving cows' milk on previous occasions. Ideally, prior to a cows' milk challenge a small bowel biopsy should show a normal healed mucosa. Also lactose tolerance should be proven by either a lactose tolerance test (*see* p. 79) or a hydrogen breath test (*see* p. 83) or stool Clinitest reaction and sugar chromatography (*see* p. 83) following a lactose load of 2 g/kg. If the mucosa still reveals features of CMPI, postpone the challenge. However, a normal mucosal pattern does not exempt the child from the risk of an adverse reaction to a cows' milk challenge. In addition milk should then be applied topically to the skin.

A severe cutaneous reaction would suggest persistence of milk intolerance, but the absence of a skin response does not nullify the risk of anaphylaxis. An intravenous drip should be *in situ* and observations maintained for about 12 hours following the provocation. The patient must have immediate access to resuscitation facilities. Without the presence of on-site experienced and capable medical staff we would not expose the patient to this potentially hazardous procedure.

The first oral introduction of milk should be carried out under medical supervision and should only consist of 5 ml or 1 teaspoon of milk on the first occasion. If this does not provoke an acute reaction it can be considered safe to progress more rapidly. In the next feed, 30 ml cows' milk formula can replace 30 ml milk substitute; in the following feed the cows' milk can be increased to 60 ml with a corresponding decrease in the milk substitute. This stepwise introduction can continue until all the milk substitute is replaced by a cows' milk formula — usually over a 24–48 hour period.

It should be remembered that, if a normal cows' milk formula is used, then lactose is also being introduced at the same time. If doubt exists about a possible lactose intolerance a lactose-free formula should be introduced initially, followed by a normal cows' milk-based feed. Many children with quite severe reactions to foods outgrow their allergy by the age of 2 years (Bock, 1985).

Cows' milk protein-free diet for older infants and children. In children over the age of one year, milk or a milk substitute is not an essential ingredient in the diet. Provided that an adequate intake of protein, energy and calcium is achieved, the fluid intake can consist of non-milk-containing beverages.

Very small amounts of cows' milk protein can provoke an allergic response and, for the diet to prove effective, all traces of bovine protein must be eliminated. Dairy products such as cheese, yoghurt, ice cream, cream and butter are obvious sources of milk protein, but in fact almost all manufactured foodstuffs may contain one or more types of milk protein.

In countries where food legislation demands that the ingredients be shown on the packaging of processed foods, parents can be instructed to read the labels and omit any items which contain milk, casein or whey products. Where such information is not available, all processed food should be avoided.

Soy protein intolerance

Features

Intolerance to soy protein is said to be uncommon because it is not readily identified and so is underdiagnosed. Whenever cows' milk protein intolerance is suspected and a switch is made to soy milk there is the possibility of allergic reactions recurring (Eastham *et al.*, 1982). This non-bovine protein can cause bloody diarrhoea, fever, vomiting, anaemia, weight loss and at times mild eosinophilia. Ament and Rubin (1972) described an intolerance to soy protein which caused flattening of the small bowel villi that was morphologically indistinguishable from coeliac disease. Moreover, the villi became atrophied as early as 24 hours after soy challenge. The lesion was reversible within 4 days following removal of the offending soya protein. Challenge with soya can result in a friable and haemorrhagic sigmoid/rectal mucosa. Reactions to this vegetable protein range from anaphylaxis to respiratory and gastrointestinal symptoms not dissimilar to the features of cows' milk protein intolerance. Halpin *et al.* (1977) described colitis arising from soy protein intolerance; however, unlike ulcerative colitis, here there was no ulceration of the mucosa or disruption of the glandular and epithelial structures of the colon. Clinically, as well as pathologically, the colitis of both cows' milk and soy milk are similar.

Soy protein — atopy and colitis

When a newborn cannot be breast fed from mother or a human milk bank and there is a significant history of atopy, soy milk can be offered in an effort to reduce allergen exposure. If soy protein is as great an antigenic threat as cows' milk proteins then this practice is naive and, even though present-day soy protein isolate is less of an allergenic load than soy flour, reservations about this policy should be made. Although Matthew *et al.* (1977) showed the benefit of removing allergens to avoid eczema, a policy of prophylaxis had been suggested by Glaser and Johnstone (1953) more than two decades earlier. However, others have not demonstrated the benefit of cows' milk avoidance (Halpern *et al.*, 1973; Savilahti *et al.*, 1987) in reducing the incidence of asthma and other respiratory diseases. Early breast feeding clearly is indicated for its immunological virtues, at least until the phenomenon of gastrointestinal 'closure' occurs and the small bowel mucosa abandons the unselective absorption of potential antigens. The combined influence of MALT and GALT hinders the absorption of antigens. Futhermore, topical immunization of the intestine, with the production of secretory IgA and secretory IgM inhibits the uptake of some macromolecules (Walker and Hong 1973). In the post-enteritis situation a soy-based formula should be used with caution because there is an increased risk of soya sensitization. A severe colitis can occur in the recovery phase of an acute enteritis when soy formula is used.

As paediatricians make ever-increasing efforts to recommend cows' milk avoidance, because of a genetic predisposition to atopy, especially in children with the HLA haplotype A1/B8, and the vulnerability of the newborn's bowel to polypeptide absorption, inevitably more cases of soy protein intolerance will be seen.

Diagnostic aids and investigations (including newer biochemical techniques)

1. Small bowel biopsy following soy challenge to exclude villous atrophy. As in coeliac disease serial biopsies are indicated:
   a. $\dfrac{\text{Initial abnormal biopsy}}{\text{soy-free diet}} = \text{no. 1,}$ followed by
   b. $\dfrac{\text{Normal recovered mucosa}}{\text{soy challenge}} = \text{no. 2,}$ followed by
   c. Villous atrophy following challenge = no. 3.
2. Iron-deficiency anaemia.
3. Eosinophilia ($>450 \times 10/\text{dl}$).
4. Presence of blood in stool (micro- or macroscopic).
5. Presence of precipitins to soya in stool.
6. Total IgE raised and positive RAST to soya.
7. Skin (scratch) test to soya.
8. Biopsy material for organ culture studies: revealing altered subcellular structures upon soya exposure.
9. Proctosigmoidoscopy, after soy challenge, to demonstrate proctitis with or without colitis when healed mucosa is systematically challenged with the allergen.
10. Exclude acquired sucrose and fructose intolerance (*see* p. 84) (soy-based formulae may contain sucrose as the major carbohydrate).

Dietary management of soy protein intolerance

Allergic reactions to a soy-based milk substitute are less likely if a preparation based on soy protein isolate is used, rather than one containing soy flour. Where an infant is found not to tolerate either whole milk protein or soy protein isolate type of milk substitute, the alternative formulae are a casein-based hydrolysate, such as:

1. Nutramigen (Appendix IV.5).
2. Pregestimil.

Alternatively, a milk substitute based on a meat protein can be used, such as:

1. Meat Base Formula (Appendix IV.11).
2. Comminuted Chicken.

The diet in older infants and children

Where a soy protein intolerance persists until solid food is introduced into the diet, care must be taken to exclude soy protein. Soy flour is added to many processed foods and any foods which state that they contain soy, hydrolysed protein or textured vegetable protein should be avoided. If exact ingredient information is not available, all processed foods likely to contain soya should be excluded. Meals eaten in restaurants and those from hospital or school meals' kitchens are likely to contain soya in 'made-up' meat dishes.

Food additives, salicylates and hyperactivity

Feingold hypothesis and diet

One of the most controversial and perplexing topics in the realm of child health is that of the Feingold (1975) diet. Paediatricians and nutritionists seem to polarize themselves into either protagonists or vehement opponents of Dr Feingold's theory that postulates hyperkinesis can be managed in 30–50% of children by eliminating additives from the diet. His hypothesis was based on clinical findings and not on a well-controlled research study. The major symptoms of this psychological disorder are overactivity, distractibility, restlessness, impulsive behaviour and a short attention span. Yet these features of movement and impulsiveness are seen at different times and phases of development in all normal children.

At least two important questions must be posed on the subject of behavioural disorders and nutrition. First, is hyperactivity (or hyperkinesis) a disorder unique to the American continent? We are told up to 10% of American children qualify for this label. Or is this abnormal or atypical pattern of behaviour not part of the spectrum of psychological disorders seen in any population of infants? Rutter (1965) identifies this syndrome as a conduct disorder. British practice confines the diagnosis to those with epilepsy, mental subnormality or a recognizable neurological disease (Editorial, 1979).

Secondly, what evidence do we have that food additives, 'natural salicylates' and colouring material can provoke hyperactivity as suggested by Dr Feingold in 1975? Hyperkinesis is probably not a

single entity and the aetiology is multifactorial (Williams and Cram, 1978). A study using double blind challenges with tartrazine and benzoic acid in children with reported behavioural responses to food additives failed to note any changes in behaviour during the tests, and need for objective criteria for diagnosis was pointed out (David, 1987b). Some believe 'minimal brain dysfunction' (MBD) or 'attention deficit disorder with hyperactivity' (ADDH; Weiss, 1983) is the cause and that psychopharmacology is justified. Stimulant medication (amphetamines, methylphenidate, pemoline) is commonly used in Canada and America and, although it can reduce the severity of the overactivity, the drugs bring their own problems: toxicity, long-term dependence and drug abuse. Consequently, safer and more effective help might be achieved using psychotherapy, educational and parent counselling programmes. Those in favour of a pharmacological approach might switch the amphetamines for monoamine oxidase inhibitors (Zametkin *et al.*, 1985); however, there is a clear need for a long-term controlled trial before this approach justifies acceptance (Editorial, 1986).

Minimal brain dysfunction and the evidence

Just as there is much disagreement and scepticism about the existence of 'hyperactivity' as an isolated complex, so others claim data exist upholding the hypothesis (Conners *et al.*, 1976). Two studies published in the same issue of *Science*, one by Weiss *et al.* (1980) and another by Swanson and Kinsbourne (1980) showed objective evidence of behavioural difficulties following a challenge with artificial colouring agents. In a controlled study using a diet containing few antigens (oligoantigenic), Egger *et al.* (1985) demonstrated a relationship between both tartrazine and benzoate with abnormal behaviour.

Much support for Dr Feingold has emanated from parents and the media. However, many experts doubt the justification for an elimination diet [*see* comments by Dwyer (1978)]. Where the diet is manipulated to remove artificial flavourings and colourings a nutritionist must be involved to ensure subsequent difficulties do not arise (Safer *et al.*, 1972). The Nutrition Advisory Committee on Hyperkinesis and Food Additives (USA) has emphasized the numerous problems in testing the Feingold theory. More recently the National Institutes of Health held a Consensus Development

Conference and issued a draft which has not resolved the dilemma (NIH, 1982). Should it be shown ultimately and conclusively that food additives provoke behavioural problems then we need to look at the pathogenesis. Is it a toxic, pharmacological, allergic, non-IgE immune reaction or a combined mechanism that operates? King (1981) clearly demonstrated, but in adults, the development of cognitive emotional symptoms following the sublingual use of allergens in a double-blind study.

In a small group of hyperactive children, Adams *et al.* (1985) detected by high-performance liquid chromatography a significantly higher level of *p*-cresol in faeces than those of controls. Free *p*-cresol, derived from gut microfloral action on dietary tyrosine, is conjugated with sulphate to facilitate urinary excretion and *p*-cresol is the specific substrate for the enzyme phenol sulphotransferase P. Certain foods and drinks inhibit human platelet phenol sulphotransferase P *in vitro* (Gibb *et al.*, 1986). Catechins are present in many foods including tea and anthocyanins are responsible for the colour of some fruits and vegetables. Synthetic food colourants, especially carmoisine (E122), erythrosine (E127), ponceau 4R (E124), amaranth (E123) and sunset yellow (E110) are powerful inhibitors of phenol sulphotransferase P. If catechins, anthocyanins and some specific food additives inhibit conjugation then elevated and circulating *p*-cresol might theoretically result in hyperactivity. It is known that phenols are neurotoxic in the rat. The danger is that dyes or other agents used in the food storage and processing industry become the scapegoat for the child's psychopathology; the diet is examined in depth yet study of the family and child is omitted.

Feingold or Kaiser—Permanente diet for hyperkinesis

The Feingold or Kaiser—Permanente (K-P) diet excludes all salicylates, other artificial colourings, flavourings and food additives. Natural unprocessed foods are allowed (with the exception of those containing natural salicylate), and all processed foods are suspect. Food legislation varies throughout the world: synthetic salicylate is a permitted food additive in the USA, but is not used in the UK. It is necessary, therefore, for parents to carefully scrutinize the label before using any packaged product.

Foods containing salicylate are listed in Appendix IV.35.

Migraine and food intolerance

Migraine is a very contentious subject both in terms of diagnostic criteria and management. The manifestations in children are quite dissimilar to those seen in adults and in the latter classic migraine is readily identified. Furthermore, gastrointestinal features are more prominent in children and neurological complications less evident. This ancient disease was described by Hippocrates (460—377 BC) and the name of this disorder is derived from the Greek *'Hemicrania'* as classically it involves only half (hemi) the skull (kranion).

Features

In children it uncommonly presents with a typical throbbing hemicranial headache accompanied by abnormal visual phenomena. Frequently abdominal pain, rarely headache (in pre-adolescents), nausea, vomiting and marked pallor are the dominant features and occasionally a history of travel sickness. A family history is a useful clue because it is present in 80% of young migraineurs.

Diet and biochemical theories

For two centuries it has been known that certain foodstuffs, particularly those containing vasoactive amines, trigger migraine attacks. Many common provoking dietary agents are known, particularly citrus fruits and drinks, chocolate, coffee, tea, nuts and cheese, but there are many others including pork, onions, alcohol and bananas. Some believe tyramine-containing products are a major cause — yet this was shown to be untrue by Forsythe and Redmond (1974) and Medina and Diamond (1978). The importance of carefully controlled dietary studies is illustrated by an investigation which showed a decreased number of headaches in two groups of children, one of whom was assigned to a high fibre diet and the other received a high fibre diet also low in dietary vaso-active amines (Salfield *et al.*, 1987). A biochemical defect, as opposed to allergy, has been cited as a cause of migraine (Sandler *et al.*, 1974). There are migraine subjects who cannot oxidize tyramine or phenylethylamine. The former is contained in cheese (Appendix IV.36) and the latter in chocolates, as well as in a large number of cheeses and some red wines. An oligoantigenic (few foods) diet resulted in the recovery of 93% of 88 children with severe migraine in a most commendable double-blind study by Egger *et al.* (1983). The diet, which was low in antigenic foods, was comprised of one meat, one carbohydrate, one fruit, one vegetable and vitamin supplements. Furthermore, other symptoms including abdominal pain, behaviour disorders and seizures improved as well.

To give further support to the biochemical theory of the aetiology of migraine Littlewood *et al.* (1982) detected a deficiency of the 'P' variant of the platelet enzyme phenol sulphotransferase in some patients. There are two forms of this enzyme: the phenol inactivating P type and the M enzyme which inactivates monoamines (including tyramine). Littlewood postulated a 'deficit of gut-wall PST-P … the unknown phenols … gain access to the circulation as a consequence'. Moreover, it is known that most red wines inhibit phenol sulphotransferase thus explaining one mechanism of adult migraine induced by the dietary phenols of wine (Littlewood *et al.*, 1985).

Oliver Sacks (1970) put it succinctly when he said, 'Compact and clearly defined at its center, migraine diffuses outwards until it merges with an immense surrounding field of allied phenomena. The only boundaries which exist are those which we are forced to adopt for a nosological clarity and clinical action. We construct such boundaries and limits, for there is none in the subject itself.'

Food allergens and RAST

For some years it has been claimed that allergy to a number of foods can provoke or accentuate migraine. Monro *et al.* (1980) noted that two-thirds of severe adult migraineurs had food allergies. However, the dependence on these results of radio-allergosorbent testing has been questioned because the RAST is said by some authorities to be a semiquantitative test (Speight and Atkinson, 1980) and others have rarely found positive RAST results to food samples from migraine patients (Merrett *et al.*, 1980). Bentley *et al.* (1984) and Katchburian *et al.* (1986) reported a normal IgE level and negative RAST results in a group of children with abdominal migraine. This suggests that the pathogenesis, if immunological, is not reaginic.

Diagnostic aids and research procedures

The following tests should be carried out:

1. Skin testing to foods.
2. Total IgE (*see above*).
3. RAST to specific foods (*see above*).
4. Hydrogen breath test (with or without lactulose test if non-hydrogen producer) to exclude carbohydrate intolerance.
5. Midstream urine (to exclude infection).
6. Erythrocyte sedimentation rate (or plasma viscosity — a more reliable if non-specific marker of disease).
7. Fasting — to see if this provokes migraine as it commonly does.
8. Platelet phenol sulphotransferase ('P' variant) assay.
9. Platelet phenylethylamine oxidase activity (Sandler *et al.*, 1974).
10. Platelet tyramine oxidase activity.

11

Recurrent Abdominal Pain

Peine in the belly is a common disease of childrē.
Thomas Phaire, *The Boke of Chyldren* (1553)

Chronic abdominal pain is not uncommon in childhood. Some investigators claim it is seen in as many as 10–15% of schoolchildren (Pringle *et al.*, 1966; Apley 1975). To qualify for this diagnostic label the pain must recur over a minimum period of 3 months and there should be at least three discrete episodes. How many of these 'tummy-achers' have migraine? Bentley and A. Katchburian (1987, unpublished data) found 30% of children with recurrent abdominal pain to be diagnosed, albeit clinically, as cases of abdominal migraine and all improved with dietary manipulation. This symptom in isolation is stressful for the child, family and, indeed, the paediatrician. Not infrequently the patient will be aware of the uncertainty and procrastination behind the clinician's bland reassurances. The parents may feel stigmatized by a non-organic diagnosis. Moreover recurrent abdominal pain (RAP) might be an unsatisfactory diagnosis for the paediatrician because he is only too aware that an organic disorder such as peptic ulcer (Oderda and Ansaldi, 1988) can be missed and serious pathology go unrecognized. Management of recurrent abdominal pain when due to psychosocial factors is not facilitated by hesitation on the part of doctors. It is prudent for the paediatrician to be reminded of the late John Apley's 'rule': the further the localization of the pain from the umbilicus the more likely is there to be an underlying organic disorder.

Although 70–80 diseases have been cited as causes of RAP (Bain, 1974), there are usually only five predominant reasons for this debilitating problem:

1. Psychogenic abdominal pain.
2. Abdominal migraine.
3. Lactose intolerance.
4. Constipation.
5. A combination of the above.

Psychogenic abdominal pain

A careful history and examination is mandatory. The presence of weight loss and anaemia strongly suggests organic disease. It should be possible to make a positive diagnosis of this cause and not deduce it after extensive investigations of a child have been found to be negative or inconclusive. A group interview usually helps to identify the stresses within the family. Gastric hyperaemia can be produced by emotional factors. A piece of circumstantial evidence is the observation that those with RAP in childhood often come from families with an increased incidence of somatic pains.

Abdominal 'migraine'

There is nothing that is so coueniet for the meygrym as tranquillietie and rest.
The Regiment of Life (1544)

It was in 1765 that Whytt said 'gastralgia' alternated with migraine. Abdominal 'migraine' is seen in as many as one-third of those with RAP. A positive family history and the presence of nausea, vomiting, marked pallor and disturbances of vision, or even transient hemianopia, supports such a diagnosis. Unfortunately, as yet there are no definitive laboratory tests to confirm the diagnosis. Should a diet be unacceptable then the drug ketotifen, a mast cell stabilizer, is frequently helpful. Abdominal migraine is seen by many as synonymous with the periodic syndrome and cyclical vomiting (McCormick, 1980). In a long-term abdominal pain (9–20 years), follow-up study (Apley, 1975) cases of 'typical migraine' were often reported. Abdominal 'migraine' should not be used to describe an extracranial disorder. It seems unlikely that psychosocial factors are the major cause of RAP.

Carbohydrate intolerance

Lactose intolerance should be suspected diagnostically in those who are particularly predisposed because of their ethnic origins. The least invasive diagnostic tool is the hydrogen breath test following a load of lactose 2 g/kg in 250 ml of water (maximum 50 g) (*see* p. 83). Intolerance of this disaccharide has been incriminated as a cause of RAP in children (Barr *et al.*, 1979; Liebman, 1979) but others have not confirmed such findings (Christensen, 1980; Blumenthal *et al.*, 1981; Wald *et al.*, 1982). Many of these contradictory conclusions revolved around the methodology of the investigation, particularly on the criteria for diagnosing lactose malabsorption. A study by Lebenthal *et al.* (1981) showed a similar prevalence of lactose deficiency in the RAP group as in the controls. Sucrase/isomaltase deficiency is a less common cause of RAP, but should be considered where ingestion of sweet foods is associated with abdominal pain.

Constipation

The term 'constipation' describes the hard consistency of a stool and not the frequency of motions. Parents are often more concerned about this common symptom than the infant or child. In the newborn, constipation not infrequently indicates a bowel disorder such as Hirschsprung's disease. This contrasts with the situation found in infants and older children where constipation is not usually associated with any underlying pathology; currently the pendulum is beginning to swing towards the organic lobby and away from the behaviourists (Sondheimer, 1986). Infrequent stools are seen in breast-fed babies. The daily number of stools lessens with maturation.

Constipation is familial in 55% of cases (Abrahamian and Lloyd-Still, 1984) and some infants defaecate only once every 4 or 5 days; however, 94% of pre-school children pass at least one stool a day (Weaver and Steiner, 1984). In many there is a history of soiling which results in or has arisen because of school and/or social pressures. Often a change in diet is the initial cause of the constipation.

Aetiology and investigations

Anal fissures, both internal and external, are commonly the cause of constipation. The anal margins should be carefully inspected and then the internal areas of the anal ring examined. An otoscopic speculum will suffice with the baby or toddler and is less painful when introduced than a paediatric proctoscope.

Neurological diseases which damage the lumbar sacral reflex arc such as spina bifida and myelodysplasia may be responsible by producing sphincter dysfunction, incontinence and constipation. To rule out Hirschsprung's disease rectal suction biopsy for elevated activity of the enzyme acetylcholinesterase and staining for ganglion cells should be carried out. Rectal distension with a fluid-filled balloon normally relaxes the internal sphincter but not in Hirschsprung's disease. However, anorectal manometry is not reliable in the neonate because the reflex is often absent until beyond the perinatal period. In this disorder, large-calibre stools are not produced and the rectum is not full. In many centres it may not be easy to exclude Hirschsprung's disease. Endocrine disorders such as hypothyroidism, congenital adrenal hyperplasia and diabetes insipidus can alter the bowel pattern; metabolic problems, particularly hypercalcaemia and renal tubular acidosis, may also lead to difficulty or delay in passing stools. Even patients with coeliac disease may be troubled by constipation rather than loose stools.

Pathophysiology

There is mounting evidence to show that, in some cases of severe constipation, there is a significant colonic disorder. Manometry alone does not supply all the answers; most investigators have demonstrated a decreased ability of the internal anal sphincter to relax with rectal distension. Findings which perhaps are of greater consequence are those of reduced rectal sensitivity (Meunier *et al.*, 1979) and the increased rectal compliance causing a fall in the intensity of the urge to defaecate (Loening-Baucke, 1984). Meunier *et al.* (1984) noted organic disease in 97% of 63 constipated children — none of whom had Hirschsprung's disease.

Pathological findings of considerable significance were detected in a group of young adult woman with severe idiopathic constipation. By using silver stains abnormalities were shown in the colonic myenteric plexus; these changes were absent in the controls or were not found by conventional haematoxylin and eosin staining (Krishnamurthy *et al.*, 1985).

Management

Anal fissures readily respond to treatment with topical analgesics, stool softeners and laxatives and rarely require anal dilatation. In outpatient departments, dietary advice about constipation coupled with a stool softener (e.g. dioctyl sodium sulphosuccinate or lactulose) and a laxative such as senna are the usual therapeutic measures. In the USA mineral oil is often preferred to laxatives; however, its safety is open to debate (Davidson *et al.*, 1963). If an enema is administered it must be isotonic. Enemas are justified initially when the colon is loaded with faeces. A 'bucket and spade' or 'plumbing' approach to constipation is not advocated, but until impacted faeces are removed diet and laxatives may be ineffectual.

Sometimes infants retain faeces because they are afraid of the lavatory, particularly when switching from a 'potty'. Parents should ensure that their child can sit comfortably on the lavatory with both feet resting on the floor or a platform in order physically to facilitate defaecation. Defaecation depends more on an effective Valsalva manoeuvre than rectal peristalsis. The child may have a fear of falling down the toilet and a simple measure such as providing a special child's seat may resolve the problem. At school, children may avoid the toilet if there is inadequate privacy or sensitivity to dirty conditions.

Some children do not find time to empty their bowels: this may be due to a rushed programme in the morning, or because more interesting pursuits take precedence. In such cases parents and child must devise a regimen, preferably prior to school, so that a few minutes are spent in the lavatory — even if the child takes in a book or toy to alleviate the boredom. Establishment of a routine is of great importance in the re-education of bowel habits. Parents must be helped, however, not to become too obsessive about their child's stools or to make too many enquiries, as this engenders an unhealthy preoccupation which is counterproductive.

Older children

Dietary fibre consists of several different components: the major distinction being the soluble forms (mostly gums and hemicellulose) found in fruits and vegetables, and the insoluble types (bran and cellulose) which are found chiefly in cereal

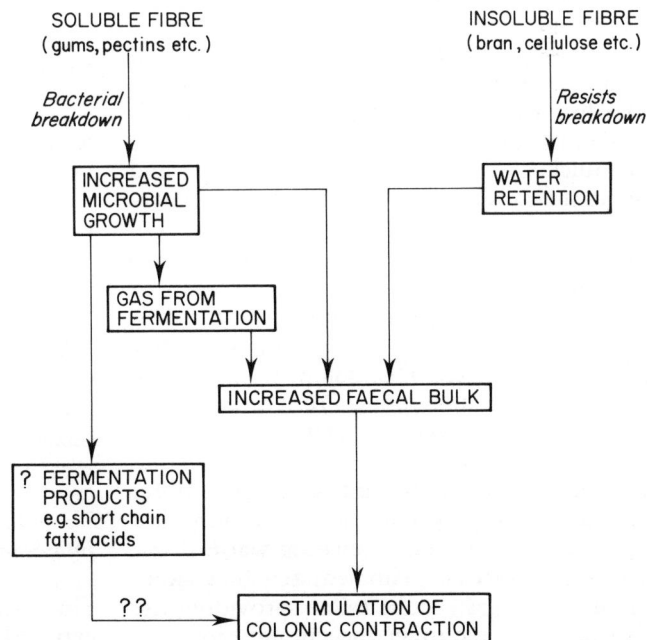

Fig. 11.1 Action of dietary fibre.

foods. The two types of fibre are treated differently in the large bowel. Cereal fibre has a greater effect on increasing stool weight than does fruit and vegetable fibre; however, both types have a part to play in increasing stool bulk and softness and in stimulating colonic movement. The mode of action of fibre is outlined in Fig. 11.1.

High-fibre foods should be encouraged, particularly wholemeal bread and cereals. Children may refuse wholegrain bread because of its colour; but high-fibre white breads are now available. Children are notoriously reluctant to eat vegetables, although peas may be taken; fortunately both these and baked beans are good sources of fibre (Table 11.1). Puréed vegetables can be added to soups or sauces, but are less effective than raw or lightly cooked foods because they are more easily degraded in the gut. The consumption of large quantities of confectionery and sweet foods means that there may be little desire to chew bulky high-fibre items, so refined sugars should be avoided. Instead foods such as crisps, savoury snack items, peanuts, raisins and fruit can be substituted. It should not be necessary to add bran to the diet and there is some evidence that mineral balance is altered when bran is given as a supplement. However, in some stubborn cases of constipation bran may be needed. None of the common forms of bran, wheat, oat or soya, is particularly palatable and usually children who refuse wholegrain bread and vegetables will reject bran. It can be incorporated into home-baked cakes and biscuits, mixed with savoury gravies, sauces and soups. Often it is necessary to give it with a milkshake syrup or evaporated milk in order to disguise the dry texture. A coarse bran is preferable to a finely ground one — large particles are less quickly degraded in the large bowel and thus retain their physical properties, such as water-holding capacity, for longer.

Small children should commence with one teaspoon (approximately 3 g) once daily, increasing to three teaspoons daily, spread throughout the day. If this is ineffective then up to six teaspoons daily (15−18 g) can be given. This quantity should not be exceeded in children under 10 years of age; adolescents can take up to three tablespoons (20−30 g) daily if necessary.

Fluid intake is as important as dietary fibre, because the aim is to produce a soft stool with a high water content. Often a morning warm drink of water or fruit juice taken immediately on waking will stimulate the gastrocolic reflex, providing the child has access to the toilet and enough time.

Table 11.1 Fibre content of foods

Good fibre sources (g fibre/100 g food)		Lesser sources (g fibre/100 g food)	
Cereals			
Bran (wheat)	44.0		
Bread		Bread — white	2.7
wholemeal	8.5		
brown	5.1		
Chapatti — wholemeal		Chapatti — chapatti	
Rice, boiled — wholegrain		flour	3.7
Biscuits/'cookies' —		Rice, boiled — white	0.8
wholemeal, e.g.		Biscuits/'cookies' —	
'Digestive'	5.5	white flour	2.3
Crispbread — rye	11.7	Crackers	3.0
Breakfast cereals		Breakfast cereals —	
bran based	26.7	rice based	4.0
wholewheat	12.7−15.4		
corn based	11.0		
muesli type	7.5		
Fruits			
Berry fruits	4.2−8.2	Strawberries	2.2
Banana	3.4	Apple — raw	2.0
Dates — fresh		Grapes	0.9
Damsons — raw	4.1	Orange	2.0
Prunes — stewed	8.1	Mango	1.5
Raisins, sultanas	7.0	Melon	1.0
Nuts			
Peanuts	8.1		
Peanut butter	7.6		
Coconut — fresh	13.6		
Other nuts	5.2−14.3		
Vegetables			
Potatoes, boiled		Cucumber	0.4
old	1.0	Lettuce	1.5
new	2.0	Tomato	1.5
Potato crisps	11.9		
(1 packet =			
approx 2.0 g)			
Root vegetables	2.8−3.1		
Leafy vegetables	2.5−3.0		
Spinach	6.3		
Beans			
green	3.4		
dried, boiled	5.1−7.4		
Baked Beans	7.3		
Peas — boiled	5.2		
Lentils, boiled — dhal	2.4		

Infants under the age of one year.

Fluid intake should be checked and, if necessary, extra can be given in the form of unsweetened orange juice or other pure fruit juice, diluted 50:50 with water.

Over the age of 4–6 months, fibre can be introduced into the diet in the form of puréed fruit and vegetables. Later cereal fibre such as breakfast dishes based on whole wheat (*see* Table 11.1) can be used.

Encopresis

Encopresis is a serious and disturbing family problem. A difficult but essential task for the paediatrician is to differentiate emotional symptoms secondary to encopresis from those of a primary disorder. It should be ensured there is no soiling as a result of stool impaction with 'spurious' diarrhoea as fluid seep around the rock-like stools.

An intensive, comprehensive programme for encopresis which includes counselling, education, initial catharsis and laxatives can result in almost 80% improvement (Levine and Bakow, 1976). Emphatic early 'potty training' might have induced a negative philosophy manifested later by the withholding of faeces. Often there is no doubt that children are straining to hold on to their stools; parents usually misinterpret the straining as an endeavour to open the bowels. An infant with little control over his parents and his environment may retain his stools, have soiling, and thus cause distress in a very effective if not powerful manner. Not surprisingly, in such situations there is a greater need for referral to a child or family psychiatrist than for the administration of laxatives.

12

Inflammatory Bowel Diseases

Granulomatous colitis (ileo) or Crohn's disease (regional enteritis)

This chronic inflammatory condition of the bowel was first described by Crohn (Crohn *et al.*, 1932) as a terminal ileal disorder (hence 'regional enteritis'). Crohn himself suggested (1967) that his name ought not to be linked to this disease if it was in a non-ileal location; however, as the description 'granulomatous disease' is not satisfactory either because granulomata are not always present, the current eponym continues to be used. In common with ulcerative colitis, there is an increased incidence both in the Jewish population and in whites; however, epidemiologists studying Crohn's disease in Jews claim this observation is suspect because it is based on small numbers (Mayberry and Rhodes, 1984). Any part of the gastrointestinal tract, from mouth to anus, can be involved (Table 12.1), the commonest sites being the proximal colon and the terminal ileum. Although it differs from ulcerative colitis pathologically and in some other respects, both overlap in a number of their features. The incidence of Crohn's diseases appears to be increasing in northern Europe (Miller *et al.*, 1974).

Aetiology

The evidence supporting a genetic and transmissible agent hypothesis is the increased incidence of chronic granulomatous disorder in relatives of patients with Crohn's disease. Granulomata will appear in the footpads of mice after the injection of small bowel or lymph node homogenate from a case of Crohn's disease (Mitchell *et al.*, 1976). This observation supports a transmissible particle theory but not necessarily infectivity. Some investigators have implicated a virus in the pathogenesis. Others have concluded that there is an association between a high dietary intake of refined sugar plus a low raw fruit and vegetable diet with a predisposition to Crohn's disease (Thornton *et al.*, 1979).

Immunological findings could be secondary phenomena and arise as a result of a damaged, ulcerated and permeable gut mucosa.

Clinical features

Often the symptoms at the time of presentation are vague and ill defined. The absence of overt gastrointestinal manifestations may delay early diagnosis by 1–3 years. The major features include:

1. Growth failure in 20–30% (which can precede symptoms, Fig. 12.1).
2. Anorexia.
3. Diarrhoea.
4. Abdominal pain.
5. Fever.
6. Fatigue.

Abdominal pain, diarrhoea and weight loss were the commonest symptom triad in one series (O'Donoghue and Dawson, 1977). Delayed sexual maturation is seen in 20% of children with Crohn's disease.

Perianal signs (abscess, sinus, fistula, tag, fissure) are uncommon in childhood compared with adults. An abdominal mass may be found on palpation.

Table 12.1 Distribution of lesions in children with Crohn's disease (The Hospital for Sick Children, London)

Site of lesion	Percentage of children affected
Small bowel only	65
Ileum only	60
Large bowel only	20
Small and large bowel	15
Ileum involvement in all cases	80
Anal lesions	60

From JAS Dickson (1977) Chronic inflammatory bowel disease. In *Essentials of Paediatric Gastroenterology*, JT Harries (ed.), Churchill Livingstone, Edinburgh.

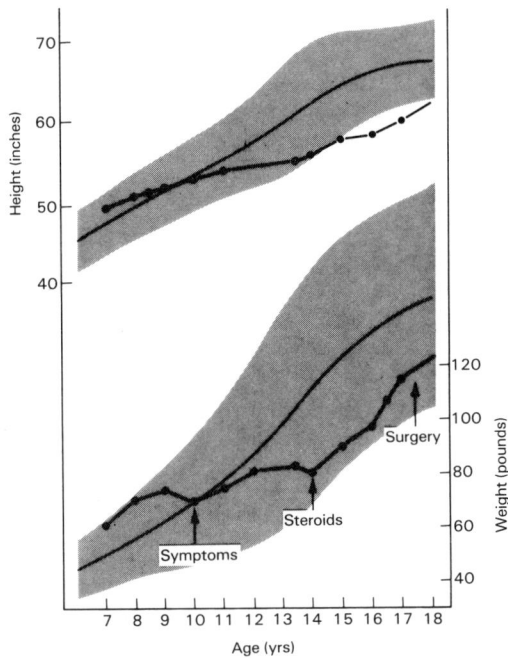

Fig. 12.1 Growth failure in Crohn's disease. (From RJ Grand, 1975, *Pediatric Clinics of North America*, Vol. 22, p. 835.)

Malabsorption and hypoproteinaemia from a protein-losing enteropathy may be the presenting features. Terminal ileal disease or its resection can cause hyperoxaluria. The extraintestinal aspects of Crohn's disease — erythema nodosum, arthritis, digital clubbing, aphthous ulceration, stomatitis and uveitis — should not be forgotten. There appears to be an association between inflammatory bowel disease and abnormalities of the X-chromosome (Arulanantham *et al.*, 1980).

Diagnosis

Barium examination of the small and large bowel with air contrast will determine the sites and severity of the disease. The usual signs include thickened mucosa, ulceration, pseudopolyps, dilatation proximal to any stenosed zones and narrowing of the terminal ileum. If the colon is diseased, there may be difficulty differentiating Crohn's disease from ulcerative colitis. Some histopathologists insist upon the presence of non-caseating granulomata in the bowel mucosa before establishing the diagnosis. When the distal bowel is involved or

there are perianal lesions, a biopsy will confirm the diagnosis. Walker (1978) suggests a biopsy from the buccal mucosa to aid diagnosis. Colonoscopy allows tissue to be sampled by biopsy from any diseased area (Chong *et al.*, 1982).

The differential diagnosis includes other granulomatous disorders such as tuberculosis and sarcoidosis. Lymphomata of the bowel and amoebic colitis also need to be considered.

Investigations

If the disease is active, the ESR (or plasma viscosity) will be elevated. Also there is often iron-deficiency anaemia. Hypoalbuminaemia is frequently seen because of protein loss from the bowel mucosa. Although the terminal ileum may be diseased, the Schilling test is usually normal.

The following may also be found:

1. Circulating immune complexes.
2. Increased plasma cells in lamina propria.
3. Decreased IgA-producing cells in colon (Girardet *et al.*, 1981).
4. Abnormal hypersensitivity reactions (e.g. reduced tuberculin reactivity).
5. Failed dinitrochlorobenzene (DNCB) sensitization.
6. Cytotoxic lymphocytes to colonic epithelial cells.
7. ^{14}C-labelled bile salt breath test (Fig. 12.2).
8. Indium-111−granulocyte scanning. Autologous leucocytes labelled with indium will be shown to congregate at sites of inflammatory bowel disease. There is good correlation with histology and colonoscopy findings (Saverymuttu *et al.*, 1986). A major attraction to the paediatrician is that scanning with this isotope compared with a barium enema involves less radiation exposure.

Pathology

Whereas ulcerative colitis is usually a disease of the gut mucosa, Crohn's disease affects the whole thickness of the bowel wall. The site of distribution of the disease (Table 12.1) differs from that seen in adults. Duodenal and jejunal locations are uncommon but occur more often in children than in adults. When Crohn's disease involves the colon it may be difficult to distinguish from ulcerative colitis.

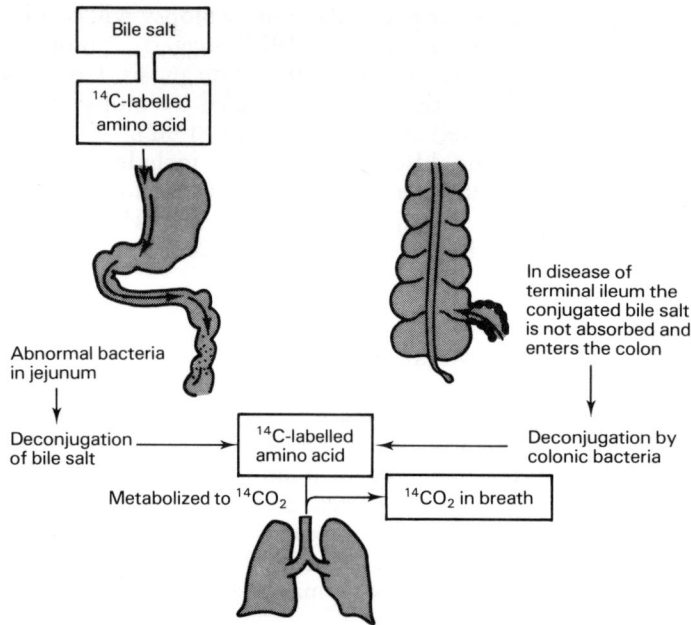

Fig. 12.2 ^{14}C-labelled bile salt breath test. Bile salts can be deconjugated by bacteria. If a conjugated bile salt and an amino acid, labelled with carbon-14, is given orally, the activity of $^{14}CO_2$ in the breath represents the degree of bile salt deconjugation. (From MS Losowsky, 1982, The small intestine, *Medicine*, Vol. 1, pp. 583–588, with permission.)

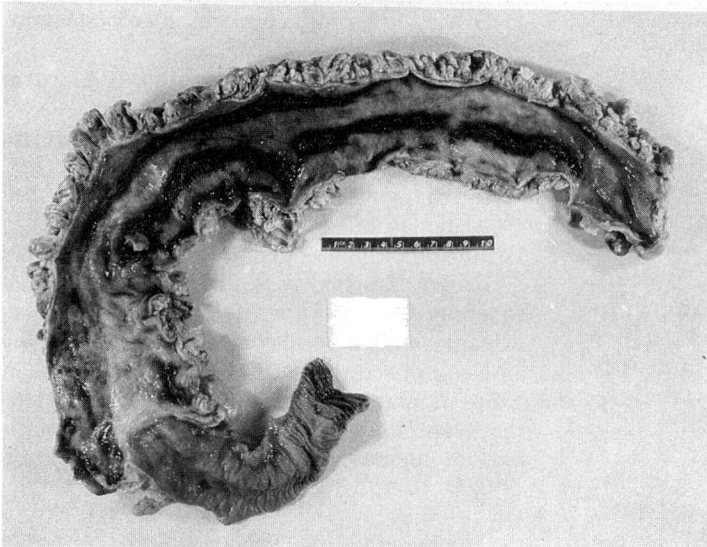

Fig. 12.3 Crohn's disease — part of the colon from a 14-year-old boy who had a total colectomy. The bowel wall is greatly thickened. (Courtesy of Dr BC Morson.)

Features of Crohn's disease

1. Discontinuous areas along the gut (i.e. 'skip' lesions).
2. Thickening of bowel wall (Fig. 12.3).
3. Stricture formation leading to obstruction.
4. Microscopic fissures and ulcers pass from mucosa into the small bowel wall. Granulomata (not always present) are non-caseating and sarcoid like. There is inflammation of the submucosa (Fig. 12.4). The mesentery is thickened and regional lymph nodes are enlarged.
5. Steatorrhoea is present in approximately 40% of patients because of bile loss from the bowel and a reduced bile pool size.
6. Decreased brush border lactase activity.
7. Diminished serum folate.

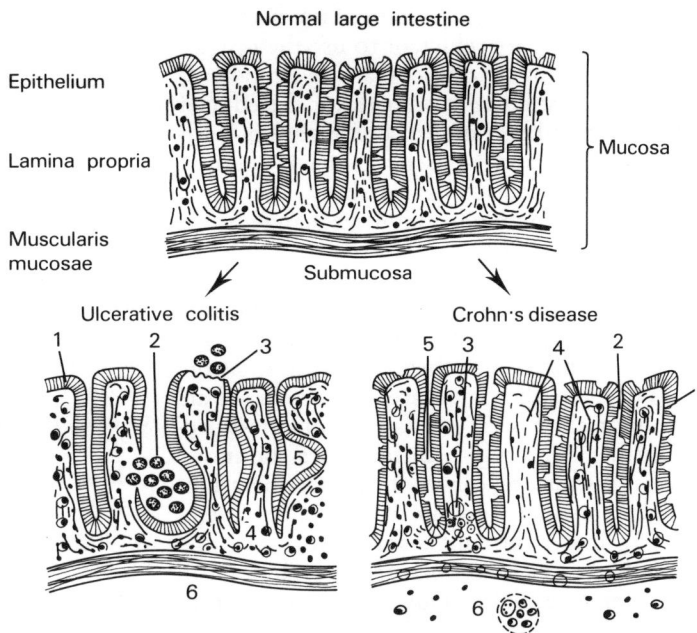

Fig. 12.4 Distinguishing histological features between ulcerative colitis and Crohn's disease. *Ulcerative colitis*: (1) goblet cell depletion; (2) crypt abscesses; (3) ulceration; (4) inflammation of lamina propria; (5) distorted crypts; (6) normal submucosa. *Crohn's disease*: (1) goblet cells preserved; (2) crypt abscesses infrequent; (3) granulomas; (4) patchy inflammation of lamina propria; (5) crypts of normal shape; (6) inflammation involves submucosa. (By permission of Dr PJ Berry and Update Hospital Publications Ltd.)

Complications

Toxic megacolon is less evident than in ulcerative colitis. Intestinal obstruction, fistulae, abscesses, growth retardation, obstructions to the urinary tract, anaemia and reduced plasma proteins can also occur. Symptomatic hypomagnesaemia has been observed in adults (Gerlach *et al.*, 1970). Carcinoma is a risk but the incidence is much lower than in ulcerative colitis.

Management

Satisfactory management can be severely handicapped after any surgery by the tendency for fistulae and wound breakdown to occur at sites of bowel excision. Anaemia (iron, folate or vitamin B_{12}), hypoproteinaemia and malnutrition should be treated if present. An attempt should be made to control diarrhoea.

Medical and surgical treatment

In a small but controlled study in children with proven Crohn's disease, an elemental diet was as effective as high-dose steroids in inducing an improvement (Sanderson *et al.*, 1987).

There is no medication of proven value. Sulphasalazine is recommended but it is not as worthwhile as in ulcerative colitis. To induce a remission the following should be used daily in three divided doses:

1. 2 g/24 hours for children under 25 kg.
2. 3 g/24 hours for those 25−50 kg.
3. 4 g/24 hours for those above 50 kg.

Do not use enteric coated preparations.

Corticosteroids, too, are used to initiate a remission. ACTH 80 units/1.73 m^2 or hydrocortisone 10 mg/kg per day for 7−10 days is a recommended regimen for very severe cases. With improvement, switch to oral prednisolone 1−2 mg/kg per day (maximum 60 mg/day) for 6−8 weeks and then slowly wean off or rarely use maintenance steroids (7.5−15 mg/24 hours) (*see* Silverman and Roy, 1983). Azathioprine may have a role if conventional medical treatment fails (Jewell and Truelove, 1972). However, such an immunosuppressive drug may present major problems both in the short and long term. It is known to be effective in adults in maintaining a state of remission following the withdrawal of steroids. Some advocate disodium cromoglycate but to date there is no convincing evidence of its merit. Metronidazole can help patients with symptomatic perianal or colonic disease (*Drug and Therapeutics Bulletin*, 1986).

Codeine may relieve the severity of the diarrhoea but many clinicians are reluctant to use the opiates diphenoxylate (Lomotil) and loperamide (Imodium) or even the anticholinergic preparations. Reduced small bowel motility favours colonization with pathogens (Grady and Keusch, 1971). If there is terminal ileal disease causing diarrhoea, there is a place for cholestyramine—anion exchange resin which binds bile acids.

A child not attaining optimal growth and chronically ill with a diseased segment(s) might not respond to any treatment including parenteral nutrition. The only course then is surgical excision or bypass of the pathological area which carries an operative mortality of 3%. Also about one-third require further surgery which increases the morbidity risks. Within 15 years of the initial operation there will be a re-operation rate of 89% (Greenstein *et al.*, 1975). It is a difficult disorder for both the child and the family. Support of a psychological nature is almost as important as expert medical advice.

Ulcerative colitis

This is a serious premalignant inflammatory disorder of the large bowel which can be accompanied by a number of non-enteric features. It was known to the ancient Greek physician, Aretaeus the Cappadocian, and was distinguished from epidemic dysentery by Sir Samuel Wilks in 1859.

In the West, the incidence is 3—6 cases per 100 000. Although it is dissimilar from granulomatous colitis (ileo) (Crohn's disease), it is likely that these two disorders are part of a single disease spectrum which overlap in many ways.

Epidemiology

There is a low incidence in the early years of life. Ulcerative colitis is commoner in whites than blacks and perhaps in the Jewish population. In 25—30%, there is a family history of inflammatory bowel disease.

Pathology

Ulcerative colitis may be limited to the rectum or involve the entire length of the large bowel (pancolitis). The lamina propria is infiltrated with inflammatory cells and goblet cell reduction is seen. Mucosal ulceration, crypt abscesses and glandular distortion are characteristic findings of this disease (*see* Fig. 12.4).

Aetiology

Earlier studies suggested the role of bacteria and then of viruses because of the isolation of these enteric pathogens (Cave *et al.*, 1976). An allergic aetiology has been proposed as a result of the presence of eosinophils in the rectal mucosa. This theory is supported by the response of some colitics to oral disodium cromoglycate (Mani *et al.*, 1976).

Truelove (1961) linked milk intake with ulcerative colitis. In a subsequent study, Jewell and Truelove (1972) suggested that if milk had a role in the pathogenesis of ulcerative colitis, it was not mediated by reaginic antibodies. Emotional factors can provoke or exacerbate ulcerative colitis as indeed can purgation but neither is thought to cause the disease. There is increasing evidence to show that several immune mechanisms participate in the pathogenesis of inflammatory bowel diseases:

1. Presence of circulation antigen—antibody complexes and their existence in blood vessel walls (Dixon, 1963).
2. Lymphocytes from patients with inflammatory bowel disease are cytotoxic *in vitro* for colonic cells in tissue culture (Shorter *et al.*, 1968).

Support for an autoimmune mechanism comes from the knowledge that ulcerative colitis may be accompanied by extraintestinal signs, e.g. uveitis, arthritis and chronic active hepatitis.

Clinical features

The commonest symptoms are:

1. Diarrhoea.
2. Blood in stools.
3. Mucus in stools.
4. Abdominal pain (often left-sided).
5. Weight loss.
6. Fever.
7. Tenesmus.
8. Fatigue.
9. Growth failure and delayed puberty.
10. Liver, dysfunction (chronic active hepatitis, primary sclerosing cholangitis, pericholangitis or biliary cirrhosis.

The following are less frequently seen:

1. Erythema nodosum.
2. Pyoderma gangrenosum.
3. Aphthous ulcers.
4. Ocular disease (conjuctivitis, uveitis, episcleritis).
5. Arthritis or arthralgia.

Differential diagnosis

Typically it is not difficult to diagnose ulcerative colitis, but at times the major challenge is to exclude granulomatous colitis (Crohn's disease), particularly as the latter can involve the large bowel (Table 12.2). A number of enteric infections can present with symptoms similar to those of inflammatory bowel disease; for example, *Campylobacter* sp. which has involved the colon as well as its usual site of the small bowel.

In addition the following conditions should be excluded:

1. Amoebiasis.
2. Shigellosis.
3. Salmonellosis.
4. *Campylobacter* sp.
5. *Yersinia enterocolitica*.
6. Tuberculosis.
7. Pseudomembranous colitis.
8. Cows' milk or soy milk colitis.
9. Behçet's disease.

Investigations

Two of the major investigations are barium enema using double-contrast technique to show the nature of the mucosa (Fig. 12.5) and colonoscopy with multiple mucosal biopsies. Tests should include haemoglobin, blood count, erythrocyte sedimentation rate (or plasma viscosity), platelet count (thrombocytopenia is seen in ulcerative colitis), total protein and electrophoresis (hypoalbuminaemia is noted in 50% of cases), agglutinins of amoebae, serum carotene (normal or low), hydrogen breath test or a lactose tolerance test (40−50% of colitics are lactose intolerant). Chromosome studies

Table 12.2 Distinguishing characteristics between Crohn's disease and ulcerative colitis

Characteristic	Crohn's disease	Ulcerative colitis
Incidence	2−4/100 000	3−6/100 000
Onset	30% under 20 years	15% under 20 years
Symptoms		
Diarrhoea	±	+++
Bloody stools	±	+++
Abdominal pain	+	++
Weight	↓↓	↓
Growth failure	++	±
Perianal disease	+	±
Extraintestinal signs	+	+
Pathology		
Site	Small bowel (ileum 80%) Colon (50%)	Colon (100%) Rectum (90%) Ileum (10%) Anus (15%)
Lesion	Transmural and granulomata	Mucosal
Radiology	'Skip' lesions segmental, 'thumb-printing'	Continuous, ulceration, no haustration, shortening
Treatment		
Response to steroids/sulphasalazine	+	++
Response to surgery	Poor — morbidity ↑↑	Very good
Outcome		
Cancer risk	±	+→++→+++ (∝ time)

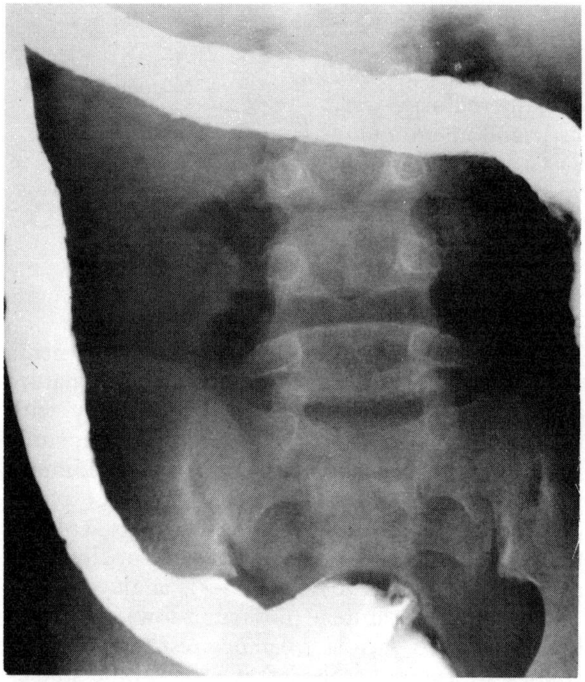

Fig. 12.5 Barium enema in a 14-year-old boy with severe ulcerative colitis showing narrowing of the colon ('lead pipe' appearance), loss of haustrations and fine spicules owing to mucosal ulceration.

should also be considered since there is an association between Turner's syndrome and inflammatory bowel disease (Arulanantham *et al.*, 1980).

Diagnosis

Sigmoidoscopy and rectal biopsy (the suction technique is safer) is the basic method of establishing the diagnosis. Visual examination will demonstrate mucus and friable mucosa with loss of the normal vascular pattern. Swabs should be taken to rule out *Shigella*, *Salmonella*, *Campylobacter* (Bentley *et al.*, 1985) or amoebae. The use of barium enema should be delayed until the bleeding has stopped and for 48 hours after the rectal biopsy. Prepare the colon with saline and not purgatives which can provoke symptoms. Colonoscopy and multiple mucosal biopsy, if executed by an expert, will enable the extent of the disease to be established. In the ill child this procedure is not without risk. Some bowel-scanning techniques, such as technetium-99m, use less radiation than barium studies.

Complications

Acute problems include perforation, fistulae, acute dilatation, strictures, pseudopolyps and, rarely, massive haemorrhage. Long-term complications include carcinoma which is associated with ulcerative colitis after one decade and relates both to chronicity and severity. Devroede *et al.* (1971), using an actuarial analysis, claimed that proctocolectomy improves survival. During the second decade of the disease there is a 20% risk of cancer and by 35 years of the disease the incidence is 43%. Some advocate prophylactic colectomy after 10 years of disease. A less radical alternative is half-yearly rectal biopsies and sigmoidoscopy to detect metaplasia.

Treatment

The aims are management of the symptoms, adequate oral or parenteral nutrition, optimal growth (including 'catch-up') and a state of well-being. The main purpose of the drug sulphasalazine is to keep the child in remission and treat those with mild to moderately active colitis. This drug consists of two components — sulphapyridine and 5-aminosalicylic acid (5-ASA/mesalazine) joined by a diazo bond. Sulphasalazine is not well absorbed in the small bowel and in the colon bacteria split the bond releasing both sulphapyridine and mesalazine. The latter is the active component, sulphapyridine acting as a carrier molecule preventing small bowel absorption. May of the undersirable effects of sulphasalazine are caused by the sulphapyridine moiety and mesalazine (Asacol) may be tolerated. If there are adverse reactions to sulphasalazine, the isolated but active constituent 5-aminosalicylic acid coated with a resin can be given (Habal and Greenberg, 1988). Diseases limited to the rectum can be managed by local steroid enemas but severe disease (more than six stools a day) will justify systemic steroids. The blood loss and protein depletion should be corrected. In the presence of steroid toxicity immunosuppressive drugs, such as azathioprine, have a role but they are not without hazard. A comparative trial in 70 adults with distal colitis demonstrated the efficacy of disodium cromoglycate enemas when compared with prednisolone given rectally, although the patients receiving steroid enemas did achieve a greater reduction of rectal bleeding (Grace *et al.*, 1987). If there is no response to medication after 3 weeks, surgery is indicated.

Some surgeons advocate total colectomy, removal of the rectal stump and ileostomy. New and innovative surgical pull-through techniques may enable continence to be achieved. An operation carried out before puberty or fusion of the epiphyses can reverse growth retardation.

Dietary management of inflammatory bowel disease

Growth failure is a significant feature both of Crohn's disease and ulcerative colitis, even occurring years before the onset of bowel symptoms. Children with inflammatory bowel disease are true 'nutritional dwarfs' according to the criteria set down by Waterlow (1972). This small stature is caused by anorexia, perhaps secondary endocrine abnormalities, increased caloric requirements and excessive gut loss of nutrients. Moreover, reduced somatomedin can also be a feature of malnutrition. Anorexia exists, particularly in the acute phase, resulting in an inadequate nutrient intake. Children may be below their predicted height and weight centiles for age and in order for 'catch-up growth' to occur the total energy intake should be appropriate for chronological age rather than body size.

Treatment of the acute phase

During an acute flare-up of symptoms the main aim is to rest the bowel and improve the chances of early remission.

Total parenteral nutrition, with the withdrawal of all oral feeds, is often advocated. In less severe cases the use of a low-residue diet (Appendix IV.33), avoiding any foods that are noted to cause symptoms, is suggested. A milk-free diet is used in many centres for both Crohn's disease and ulcerative colitis. It is not clear whether benefits ascribed to a milk-free regimen are due to the withdrawal of milk protein or lactose. A proportion of children suffering from Crohn's disease and ulcerative colitis have been shown to malabsorb lactose (20% in Crohn's disease) and bacterial breakdown products of lactose could cause irritation of the bowel mucosa. Milk protein in sensitive subjects causes colitis-like symptoms. It would certainly appear to be wise to avoid the use of large quantities of unaltered milk, used for instance as an energy or

protein supplement, during acute periods. A milk-free diet is described in Appendix IV.19. Fat malabsorption occurs in approximately 40% of children with inflammatory bowel disease and the use of a low-fat regimen, perhaps with the incorporation of medium-chain triglycerides should be considered. Steatorrhoea is more common where there is disease in the upper small bowel. Reducing stool fat will alleviate faecal calcium losses and help reduce the severity of hyperoxaluria which is associated with terminal ileal disease.

Modular feeding regimens tailored to the individual needs of the child should be used during acute periods (Appendix IV.11). Elemental diets have been tried with success and, providing that attention is paid to the osmolality and speed of introduction of these feeds, they can offer a very useful alternative to total parenteral nutrition. In Crohn's disease, their use has been reported to induce remission of symptons and improve linear growth (Sanderson *et al.*, 1987).

Long-term dietary management

The aim in long-term management of inflammatory bowel disease is to ensure a nutrient intake that is tolerated and allows catch-up growth to take place.

Deficiencies of various nutrients have been reported; there is a significant protein loss from the gut due in part to the presence of blood in the stools and as a result a generous protein intake is required. Except in the case of very young children, dietary protein can be calculated according to age as there is little danger of overload.

The energy intake should be at least that which is recommended for the child's age. Excess lactose and long-chain fat may not be well absorbed and a supplement made up using a glucose polymer and MCTs (Appendix III.11) may be useful.

If the child is willing to take a supplement prepared from an elemental formula (Appendix IV.9), in addition to normal diet, this may provide optimum opportunity for absorption. However, most of these formulae are unpalatable.

Metal and vitamin deficiencies have been reported particularly of the vitamin B complex and vitamin D. Severe magnesium depletion can occur in Crohn's disease (Gerlach *et al.*, 1970) and reduced levels of zinc may arise. Hypocalcaemia can be caused by steatorrhoea. A vitamin supplement should be given routinely if it is not included in the energy/protein supplement used. Elements which are likely to be malabsorbed or lost in large quantities from the gut are calcium, magnesium and zinc. It would be advisable to use a mineral/trace element supplement if the child is taking a poor nutrient intake or a supplement which is not fortified. Suitable mineral and vitamin supplements are suggested in Appendix II.13.

There is no evidence that adhering to any particular dietary regimen (e.g. low residue, low fat, milk free) offers any long-term benefit except during the acute phase. Dietary items should only be avoided if there is clear evidence of them causing symptoms or the patient has specific food aversions. There are some advocates of a high-fibre/unrefined carbohydrate diet being of some value in adult Crohn's disease though this benefit has not been demonstrated in children.

A balanced and nutritious diet which is adequate in calories and is unrestricted can be recommended in the absence of active disease.

Necrotizing enterocolitis

This gastrointestinal disorder first described in the last century is still something of an enigma. There have been instances of nursery epidemics while other units have a very low incidence of only 0.3% among their premature babies. Some centres see this large bowel disease in as many as 80% of those less than 1.5 kg at birth.

Presentation

The presenting symptoms commonly include the following:

1. Abdominal distension.
2. Lethargy.
3. Vomiting and regurgitation (commonly blood-stained).
4. Temperature instability.
5. Apnoea.
6. Occult or gross blood in stools.

Early detection is often possible by noting slight distension of the abdomen or a trace of blood in the stool and this may enable prompt measures to be taken to prevent a cascade of downhill events. The average mortality is about 30% (Thomas, 1982), yet is can be as high as 75%.

Vulnerability

Those babies who show the following are particularly vulnerable:

1. Birth weight < 2.0 kg.
2. Those on formula food — especially if hyperosmolar.
3. Significant colonization of baby unit.
4. History of asphyxia/respiratory distress/exchange transfusion/congenital cardiac disease.

Necrotizing enterocolitis is rarely seen in term babies with a weight that is appropriate for the gestational age. Many of the babies have had asphyxia or the other conditions mentioned above.

Pathogenesis

For details of pathogenesis, *see* Fig. 12.6. Animal experimentation has shown that hypoxia, particularly when combined with an artificial feed, can induce the pathological equivalent of necrotizing enterocolitis (Pitt, 1975) by causing a reduction of blood flow in the mesenteric vessels (Touloukian *et al.*, 1972; Alward *et al.*, 1978). It has been postulated that the 'diving reflex' in response to hypoxia deprives the gut of its blood supply so as to protect preferentially the intracranial circulation.

Breast milk is rich in secretory IgA which acts on the gastrointestinal mucosa to prevent bacterial adherence and thus impedes invasion. When breast milk is stored or frozen in a refrigerator, or heat treated (pasteurized or boiled), many of its antibacterial properties are diminished; therefore the milk will be of less help in preventing necrotizing enterocolitis. There is some evidence that the optimal milk is 'raw' human milk (*see* p. 51) fed to a mother's own baby. In a large prospective American study of more than 2000 premature infants, the only perinatal factors associated with the rate of necrotizing enterocolitis, in contradistinction to the findings of other neonatologists, were birth weight and maternal toxaemia (Kanto *et al.*, 1987). Rotbart *et al.* (1988) too has noted a significant correlation between necrotizing enterocolitis and birth weight.

Diagnosis

Good observations combined with note of the

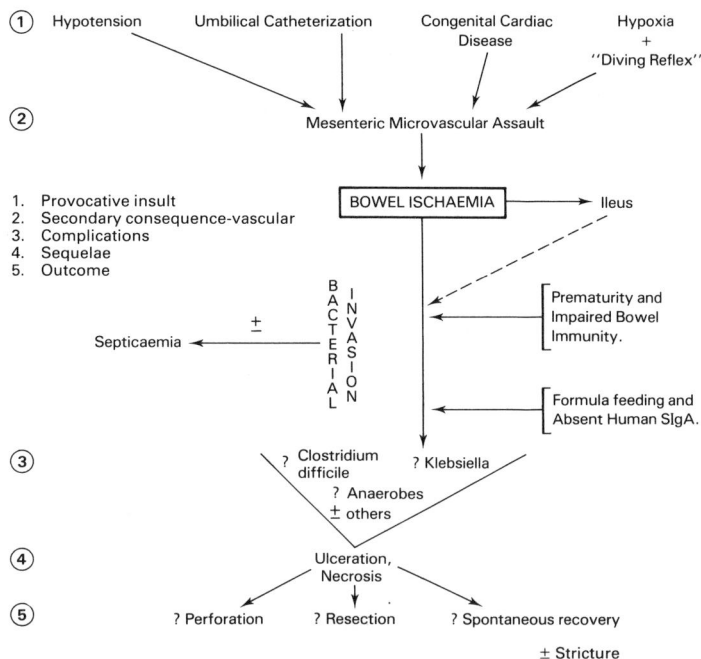

Fig. 12.6 Suspected mechanisms of necrotizing enterocolitis — 'the cascade'. SIgA = secretory IgA.

symptoms and signs will enable an early diagnosis to be made. It can be confirmed by the following:

1. Radiology: X-rays of the abdomen may show pneumatosis intestinalis (intramural gas), ascites, air in the peritoneum or gas in the portal vein. Early films will show dilated loops of bowel.
2. Blood culture and stool may help identify the aerobic or anaerobic organism. Check the platelet count and fibrinogen degradation products to exclude thrombocytopenia and disseminated intravascular coagulation.
3. Viral investigations: serum should be examined for IgM antibodies to rotavirus and rectal swabs can be tested for the same virus by the Rotazyme Assay (Abbott Laboratories, Illinois).

Management

1. Stop all oral feeds and start parenteral nutrition. If dehydrated correct deficit.
2. Keep the stomach empty.
3. Start early antibiotics to cover both aerobic and anaerobic organisms — many advocate aminoglycosides and ampicillin in the absence of any identified gastrointestinal pathogens sensitive to other antibiotics.

If there is evidence of obstruction, suspected bowel gangrene or failure to respond to conservative measures, prompt surgery is indicated.

Complications

Early complications are perforation with or without intestinal resection. Late complications include lactose intolerance and stricture(s) leading to obstruction.

Prevention

Breast feeding should be encouraged (in the absence of contraindications), ideally using the mother's own untreated milk. Attempts should be made to eradicate any colonization within the baby unit and identify those causing cross-infection (usually, but not invariably, doctors).

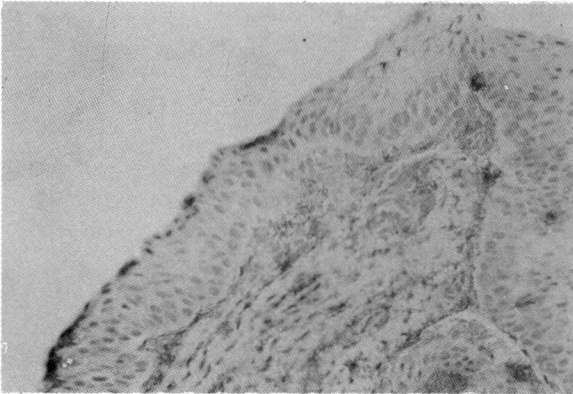

Fig. 12.7 HLA-DR (immunoperoxidase) stain — normal anal cell appearance.

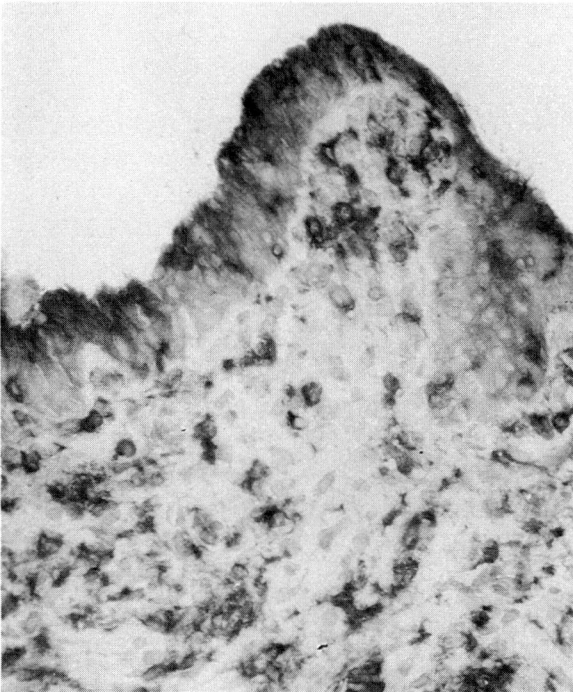

Fig. 12.8 HLA-DR positive stain in food-sensitive colitis in anal cells — note increased darkly stained cells. (By kind permission of Dr I Lampert.)

Milk colitis (soy protein, cows' milk protein and maternal dietary milk protein-induced colitis, food-sensitive colitis)

An enterocolitis caused by soy bean or cows' milk protein is very similar to the clinical situation seen in ulcerative colitis. Milk or soy protein intolerance may cause diarrhoea, fever, failure to thrive, blood and mucus in the stools because of colonic disease. Proctoscopy or colonoscopy will reveal a friable mucosa that bleeds or a zone of hyperaemia around blood vessels. Biopsy may demonstrate changes of an acute colitis with crypt abscesses, depletion of mucus from rectal glands and inflammatory changes within the lamina propria (Halpin *et al.*, 1977). In food-sensitive colitis (FSC), eosinophilia has been reported as well as the presence of IgE-bearing mononuclear cells in the biopsy material. This phenomenon may be due to to the phase of transient deficiency of secretory IgA in the newborn period.

HLA-DR antigens are not normally expressed on oral mucosal lining cells, but have been reported in food-sensitive colitis (*see* Figs. 12.7 and 12.8).

The protein of cows' milk and soy milk can cause comparable clinical and pathological findings. It is postulated that the mechanism is an allergic one (Powell, 1978) and a personal and family history of atopy is often present (Milla, 1986). A reversible small bowel enteropathy may accompany the colitis. Lake *et al.* (1982) described six infants with proctocolitis who were being exclusively fed on breast milk and others have made similar observations. Two of Lake's patients with food-sensitive colitis responded to the withdrawal of cows' milk proteins from the maternal diet. All improved on either soy-based or hydrolysed casein formula. In former years, this was thought to be an uncommon cause of colitis but inevitably will be diagnosed more frequently in future especially where there are facilities for colonoscopy. The diagnosis can be substantiated by the withdrawal of the offending allergen and a repeat rectal biopsy. The prognosis is excellent. Several stools should be examined for viruses and cultured for bacteria to exclude an infectious cause of colitis.

Management

Remove the offending protein and reintroduce breast milk if it is appropriate or, where indicated, withdraw cows' milk from the diet of the nursing mother. If milk, from the mother or a breast-milk pool, is not available use Pregestimil or Comminuted Chicken in place of cows' milk or soy products. Disodium cromoglycate (100 mg) prior to a feed may alleviate the symptoms. For general dietary management, *see* Chapter 10.

13

Pancreatic Exocrine Insufficiency

Cystic fibrosis

Few childhood diseases have seen such momentous and much awaited scientific developments as have been achieved in recent years by geneticists in the field of cystic fibrosis. Cystic fibrosis is the commonest chronic hereditary disease in Caucasians that is potentially lethal. It is a multiorgan recessively inherited disorder due to mutations in a single gene and is seen in about 1:2000 live births in the UK, most western European countries and North America, with a carrier frequency of about 1 in 25. In American Blacks a 10-year survey showed the incidence was only 1:17 000 (Kulczycki and Schauf, 1978). The spectrum ranges from 1:620 in south-west Africa (Super, 1975) to 1:90 000 in Hawaii (Wright and Morton, 1968). The many features of cystic fibrosis include chronic lung disease, pancreatic insufficiency (approximately 85%), liver dysfunction (15−30%) and raised concentrations of sodium and chloride in the sweat (Table 13.1). The typical clinical triad is malabsorption, failure to thrive and chronic suppurative chest disease (Figs 13.1 and 13.2). Although much research has been carried out, the basic biochemical defect remains elusive. However, there is evidence that anion transport across cell membranes is not normal. As yet, the affected fetus cannot be identified with total accuracy in all cases but enzymologists and cytogeneticists are making preliminary claims of modest success (Brock, 1983; Carbarns et al., 1983). However, we now have a much awaited development of colossal significance: — first-trimester prenatal diagnosis by the use of DNA probes in couples with one affected child (Farrall et al., 1986).

Sweat test

The sweat test is still the cornerstone of diagnosis. There is an elevated concentration of sodium and chloride in the sweat of cystic fibrosis patients (both >70 mmol/1) in the homozygotes, but not in the heterozygotes. Although the sweat test is a simple technique, it is essential that it is performed only by experienced staff in a meticulous manner (Littlewood, 1986). The prognosis and genetic implications of this complex disorder are such that any probability of false-negative or false-positive results must be reduced to a minimum. Sweat sodium can be suppressed below 70 mmol/l after 9α-fluorohydrocortisone is given to non-cystic fibrosis children whereas it is not suppressed in cystic fibrosis. This technique does have a discriminatory role in equivocal cases (Hodson et al., 1983; Lobeck and McSherry, 1963).

Prognosis

It is important to remember that the gene for cystic fibrosis has a heterogeneity of expression; thus some patients are seriously handicapped physically while others are not detected until later in adult life. As long ago as 1975, Shwachman reported 70 patients from his Boston clinic who were not diagnosed until over the age of 25 years. This group included six with meconium ileus thus showing that they were not a selected sample of non-severe cases. With better understanding of optimal nutritional management and newer more efficacious antibiotics, the median age of survival has been extended from 12 years in 1966 to 19 years in 1976. (For details of prognosis, see Fig. 13.3.) Bowling et al. (1988) in Brisbane, Australia have shown in a matched study of 28 patients and a cohort of 23 that early diagnosis reduces the morbidity in the first 2 years of life.

In 1985, a mammoth achievement was the identification by several international groups of a DNA marker linked to cystic fibrosis and localized on chromosome-7 (Knowlton et al., 1985; Wainwright et al., 1985; White et al., 1985). Genetic mapping studies represented a crucial milestone and have enabled, in early pregnancy, chorionic

Table 13.1 Features of cystic fibrosis

Feature	Comments
Failure to thrive	
Salty sweat	
Bulky and very malodorous stools	Seen in coeliac disease, Shwachman–Diamond syndrome, lipase deficiency, enterokinase deficiency etc.
Repeated respiratory infections ± reversible airway obstruction	Haemoptysis and spontaneous pneumothorax are common in older patients Common organisms: *Pseudomonas aeruginosa* (mucoid strains), *Staphylococcus aureus* and *Haemophilus influenzae*
Heat stroke	Suggestive of cystic fibrosis — not conclusive in hot climates
Digital clubbing	Present in all toes and fingers; said to start in index finger, can be measured — volume displacement, plethysmography, shadowgram (Bentley and Cline, 1970; Bentley *et al.*, 1976) and other techniques
Bruising and xerophthalmia	Due to deficiencies of fat-soluble vitamins: A, E and K
Oedema	Results from hypoproteinaemia
Ear, nose and throat	Purulent sinusitis, nasal polyps (18%), and mild conductive hearing loss (27%) (Kulczycki *et al.*, 1970)
Male genital tract	Increased incidence of inguinal hernia (15%), hydrocele (4%) and undescended testis (3%) (Holsclaw *et al.*, 1971)

Gastrointestinal/hepatic aspects of cystic fibrosis

Feature	Comments
Meconium ileus	Seen in 15%; presents as bowel obstruction
Meconium peritonitis	± calcified peritoneum; ± calcified testes
Pancreatic insufficiency	Steatorrhoea → failure to thrive
Liver disease	1. Focal biliary cirrhosis → portal hypertension → oesophageal varices 2. Prolonged jaundice in neonate (inspissated bile plugs)
Gall bladder	Small organ, bile acid malabsorption, reduced bile acid pool; cholelithiasis
Rectal prolapse	All children with rectal prolapse need sweat test(s) to exclude CF (but not in less developed countries)
Gastro-oesophageal reflux	Significantly more common (Scott *et al.*, 1985)
Intestinal obstruction	'Meconium ileus' equivalent — seen in bowel atresia, intestinal stenosis and volvulus
Intussusception	1% of patients (Holsclaw *et al.*, 1971)
Vitamin B_{12} malabsorption	Very rare in CF (Deren *et al.*, 1973)
Carbohydrate malabsorption	Lactase deficiency in 25% (Antonowicz *et al.*, 1968)
Glucose intolerance	Present in 40%; diabetes is rare before 10 years of age
Polyarthropathy and hypertrophic pulmonary osteoarthropathy	Uncommon complications
Male infertility	Obstructive azospermia in 97% (Kopito *et al.*, 1973)
Female subfertility	Secondary anovulation, excessive cervical and dehydrated mucus (Oppenheimer and Esterly, 1970; Kopito *et al.*, 1973)

Table 13.1 (Cont'd)

Feature	Comments
Subclinical hypothyroidism	Decreased T_3 and increased TSH common in CF (Azizi *et al.*, 1974)
Delayed puberty	A feature of many serious chronic ailments
Psychological ± sexual problems	Consequences (personal and within family) of a chronic potentially lethal disease

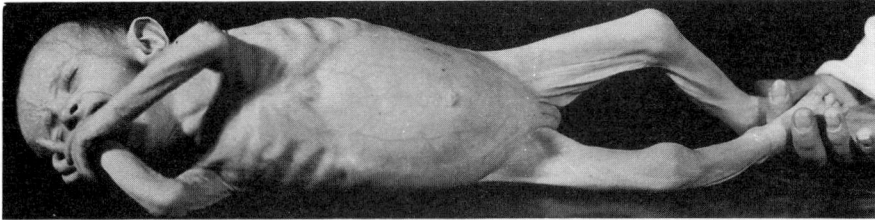

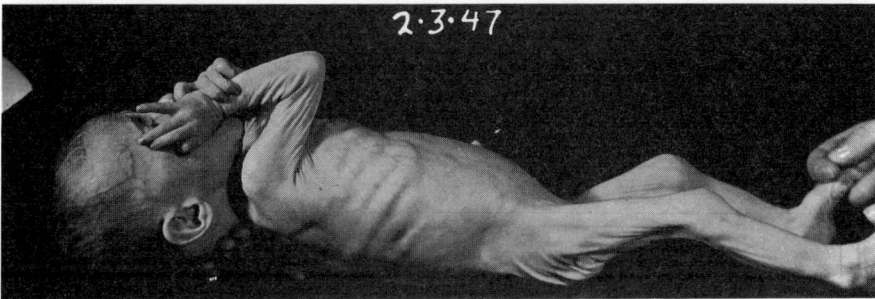

(a)

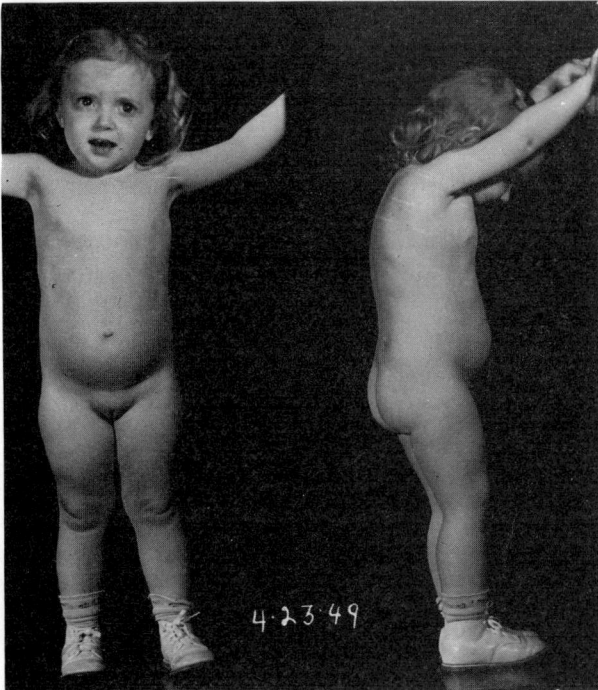

(b)

Fig. 13.1 (a) Child presenting with cystic fibrosis. (b) The same child 26 months later. (Courtesy of the late Dr H Shwachman.)

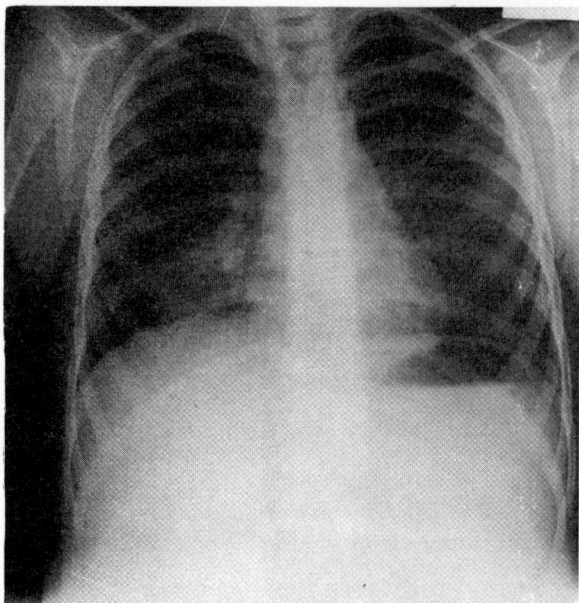

Fig. 13.2   Chest X-ray of 4-year-old girl with cystic fibrosis.

villus biopsy, with DNA probes to detect cystic fibrosis in the fetus (Super *et al.*, 1987). Moreover, Super and his colleagues succesfully predicted and later confirmed the absence of cystic fibrosis in a group of children who had been investigated prenatally.

The mean lifespan in industrialized countries is 20–25 years. However, there are considerable differences both in the international survival rates and indeed those reported from various centres within one country. Of children in England and Wales, 80% survive until the age of 9 years; this contrasts with a level of 78% surviving to 16 years in one Birmingham clinic. Yet in Melbourne, Australia, 80% survive to 20 years. Longevity is seemingly better in specialized centres leading to the World Health Organisation and the International Cystic Fibrosis Association endorsing such establishments in 1983. The advantages, and the few disadvantages, of such a policy were published in the Report of a Working Party on cystic Fibrosis by the British Paediatric Association in 1985.

Presentation

Fifteen per cent of those with cystic fibrosis present in the neonatal period with meconium ileus and they have the worst prognosis (McPartlin *et al.*, 1972); however, following the introduction of the Bishop Koop operation in 1962, there was an improved survival rate. Not all infants with meconium ileus have cystic fibrosis.

The high familial incidence of meconium ileus has suggested there is a genetic predisposition to this complication. Meconium ileus is seen in about 15% of neonates with cystic fibrosis, and yet is present in as many as 30% of affected siblings. Mornet and co-workers (1988) in Paris and London tested cystic fibrosis families both with and without an affected child having meconium ileus and discovered a difference in haplotype between these two groups. Their findings suggest that, as a result of a different mutation of the same locus (multi-allelism), some cystic fibrosis patients are predisposed to meconium ileus.

Diagnosis

Neonates

Diagnosis in neonates is based on:

1. *Serum immunoreactive trypsin* (IRT) is 10 times higher in blood of newborn cystic fibrotics. This is a very sensitive test. The cut-off level is critical; Mastella *et al.* (1984) advises 60 µg/l (99th percentile of normal). The specificity of the IRT test has been improved by a human trypsinogen monoclonal antibody assay.
2. *Stool-screen with BM strip test* (Boehringer–Mannheim Corporation). The test is positive if >20 mg albumin/g meconium present. False-negatives occur in 6–20% (Stephan *et al.*, 1975; Crossley *et al.*, 1977); false-positives occur as well causing the parents unnecessary anxiety. The BM meconium test is very unreliable and now seldom used in the UK.

Infants over 2 months old

Here diagnosis is based on:

1. *Chloride agar plate test* — this is a rapid simple screen but does not replace pilocarpine ionto-phoresis.
2. *Sweat test by the pilocarpine iontophoresis method* — this technique is still the prime diagnostic test (Andersen, 1938; Di Sant'Agnese *et al.*, 1953; Gibson and Cooke, 1959). The mass must exceed 100 mg.

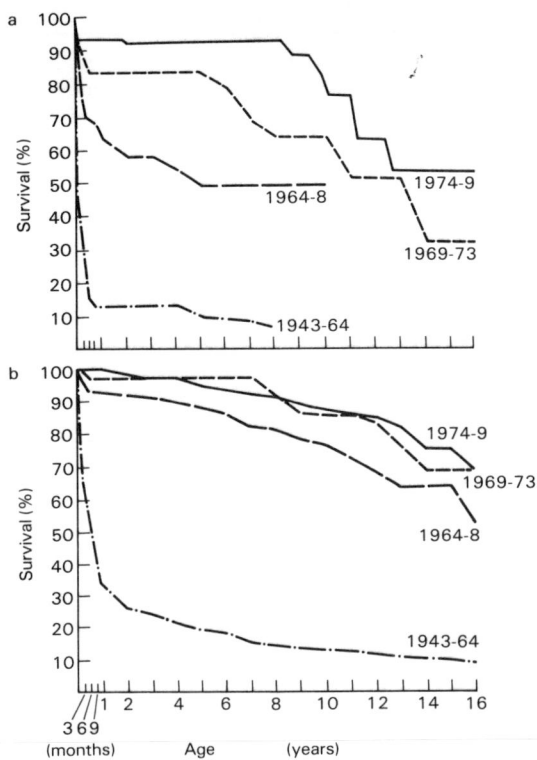

Fig. 13.3 Survival curves of children with cystic fibrosis. (a) Patients with meconium ileus; (b) patients without meconium ileus. Note marked improvement in meconium ileus patients in 1974–79 compared with 1964–68. However, overall survival of cystic fibrosis patients without meconium ileus 1974–79 is disappointing when compared with 1969–73. (Redrawn from RW Wilmott and DJ Matthew, 1983, *Archives of Disease in Childhood*, Vol. 58, p. 836, with permission.)

3. *Sweat osmolality technique* — sweat is collected by Macroduct System (ChemLab Instruments Ltd). Values in cystic fibrosis are 220–416 mmol/kg (Carter *et al.*, 1984). This commendable method has many practical advantages over traditional pilocarpine iontophoresis. Although it is more costly in capital outlay and component expenses, it is rapid and must be less likely to be erroneous due to lack of operator expertise.
4. *Stool trypsin or chymotrypsin test* — this can be carried out on fresh stools or by sending a dried faecal smear to a central laboratory. Stool trypsin < 1/80 supports the diagnosis but cannot be depended upon.

Pancreatic function studies (Table 13.2)

1. *Secretin–pancreozymin (SP) test* — duodenal intubation (ideally with a triple lumen to prevent contamination of pancreatic juices with gastric acid) or a single intraduodenal tube. Give intravenous pancreozymin slowly 1.5 IU/kg then secretin 1.5 IU/kg also by the same slow method. Test for intradermal reactions to both hormones before test. The duodenal aspirations should be analysed for volume, bicarbonate, trypsin, chymotrypsin, lipase and amylase. The duodenal juices must be collected in ice-cooled flasks.
2. *Simpler technique — modified Lundh meal* (McCollum 1977 — fast overnight (4 hours for young infants) and then sedate with chlorpromazine (thorazine in USA) 2 mg/kg. Pass a nasogastric tube for administering test meal (carbohydrate as glucose, protein as milk powder and fat as corn oil) 30 ml/kg to a maximum of 240 ml. Aspirate the fourth part of duodenum (under fluoroscopy); when the collecting tube is in position sample every 10 minutes for two hours using ice-cooled containers.
3. *Chymotrypsin substrate (Bz-Tyr-PABA test)* — N-benzoyl-L-tyrosyl-p-aminobenzoic acid (= Bz-Tyr-PABA) is cleaved by chymotrypsin to benzoyl-tyrosyl releasing p-aminobenzoic acid (PABA). As this is absorbed and then excreted in urine its measurement reflects the activity of the proteolytic enzyme chymotrypsin. The 6-hour urinary excretion is between 60 and 90% in the presence of normal renal function.

Other techniques

1. *Fluorescein dilaurate test* (pancreolauryl test — International Laboratories) (Barry *et al.*, 1982) — fluorescein dilaurate is hydrolysed by pancreatic esterases. The released fluorescein is measured in the urine spectrophotometrically.
2. *Selenomethione (^{75}Se) scanning test* — this test uses an isotope that is taken up preferentially by the pancreas. The pancreas is scanned after an intravenous injection of the radioactive amino acid. Endoscopic retrograde cannulation of the pancreas (ERCP) will allow direct visualization of the pancreas and ultrasound will enable the size and gross morphology to be determined. This is particularly useful for the diagnosis of pseudocysts and abscesses which might rarely follow the complication of pancreatitis.

Table 13.2 Pancreatic function after secretin–pancreozymin tests

	Birth	One month	Normal	Cystic fibrosis	Pancreatic insufficiency
Volume (ml/kg per 50 min)					
Premature	4.4 (4–15)	8.96 (3.4–18.7)	3.9 (1.8–81)	0.3–2.7	1.8–3.9
Term	5.39 (1.6–9.7)				
Bicarbonate (mequiv./l per 50 min)			0.19 (0.08–0.37)	0.001–0.04	0.008–0.19
Trypsin (µg/kg per 50 min)					
Premature	60 (0–482)	196.1 (0.9–660)	765 (215–2100)	0–450	0.9–320
Term	66.1 (1.2–350)				
Lipase (IU/kg per 50 min)					
Premature	77.4 (3–343)	283.6 (11–730)	1464 (350–5000)	0–270	0–68
Term	143.9 (2.2–785)				
Chymotrypsin (µg/kg per 50 min)			860 (252–1900)	0–126	0–105
Amylase (IU/kg per 50 min)					
Premature	0.88 (0–3.6)	1.67 (0–4.6)	665 (160–2150)	0–117	0–31
Term	3.20 (0.1–9.8)				

From J Gryboski and W Allan Walker (1983) *Gastrointestinal Problems in the Infant*, WB Saunders, London.

3. *Three-day fat collection* — determine a sufficient intake during study (35% of dietary energy). Use carmine markers at the beginning and end of 72 hours of collection. Stool fat at >10% is abnormal. Express findings as the coefficient of absorption (CA):

$$CA = \frac{\text{dietary fat} - \text{faecal fat}}{\text{dietary fat}}$$

The CA is related to age:
a. Term infants, 80–85%;
b. 10 months–3 years, 85–90%;
c. Older than 3 years, 95%.

4. *Stool smear* — a quick screen for steatorrhoea is to count fat globules in a stool smear after staining. A count of greater than 100 per high power field is abnormal — diet will obviously influence the number of globules.

5. *Serum carotene* — is low (<20 µg/dl).

6. *Hydrogen breath test* — this is a useful screen for sugar malabsorption (*see* p. 83). If the hydrogen breath test is abnormal confirm with a lactose tolerance test. If the patient is a non-hydrogen producer, repeat but with a lactulose load, to ensure hydrogen producing bacteria are present.

7. *Lactose tolerance test* — see p. 79.

8. *Hair analysis* — useful in neonates for 'postal diagnosis'. Findings are an elevated sodium (93–674 mmol/kg, mean 240 mmol/kg) and elevated potassium (12–75 mmol/kg, mean 38 mmol/kg) (Kopito *et al.*, 1972).

9. *Nail clippings* — this test is also suitable where there are no regional diagnostic facilities and samples can be posted for screening. Elevated sodium (55–350 mmol/kg, mean 140 mmol/kg) and potassium (12–180 mmol/kg, mean 43 mmol/kg) are diagnostic (Kopito *et al.*, 1965).

Nutrition (Table 13.3)

Improvement of the nutritional state of cystic fibrosis is likely to improve the depressed immunological system, increase respiratory muscle strength and enhance appearance and morale. However, as pulmonary function worsens, maintenance of normal nutrition becomes more difficult. In spite of the advantages conferred by good nutritional status, it is unlikely to affect the course of the disease significantly.

The 85% of cystic fibrosis children who have reduced pancreatic function show a similar picture to that of protein–energy malnutrition (PEM) with a decreased body fat content and muscle mass and an increased rate of muscle catabolism (Miller *et al.*,

1982). In addition to the pancreatic insufficiency, abnormalities of bile salt metabolism (Harries *et al.*, 1979) and intestinal lactase deficiency with normal mucosa (Shwachman, 1975) have been described.

Pancreatic enzyme replacement

Steatorrhoea is not totally corrected by pancreatic enzyme preparations. Currently pH-sensitive enteric-coated microspheres of pancreatic enzyme pancrelipase (ECMP) (Pancrease capsules, Ortho-Cilag) and Creon (Duphar) are more effective but more costly than the conventional supplements, e.g. Cotazym (Organon), Nutrizym (Merck), Pancrex (Paines & Byrne). In a few patients ranitidine or cimetidine should be offered 30 min before each meal, where ECMP alone does not correct the fat loss (Gow *et al.*, 1981). These H_2-receptor antagonists will reduce gastric acid activity and thus inhibit acid-peptic inactivation of the supplemented enzymes. However, now there is famotidine, a very potent long-acting H_2-receptor antagonist which can be administered just once a day

Table 13.3 Nutrient requirements in cystic fibrosis

Nutrient	Sources	Requirement
Protein	Diet/ supplement	Generous intake for age or 120–130% RDA per kg body weight
Essential fatty acid	Supplement	1 ml/kg body weight
Energy	Diet/ supplement	Generous intake for age or 130–150% RDA per kg body weight
Sodium	Diet	Adequate intake for age
Calcium	Diet	Adequate intake for age
Iron	Diet	Adequate intake for age
Copper	Diet	Adequate intake for age
Zinc	Supplement	RDA for age
Other trace elements	Supplement	RDA for age
Vitamin A	Supplement	1200–7500 mg daily
Vitamin D	Supplement	100–200 µg daily
Vitamin E	Supplement	100–200 mg daily
Vitamin K	Supplement	300 mg daily
Vitamin B_{12}	Supplement	4 mg daily
Other B vitamins and vitamin C	Diet	RDA for age

and has been used successfully in adults with active duodenal ulcer disease. This new preparation has the advantage over cimetidine and ranitidine of longer anti-secretory activity (Gitlin *et al.*, 1987), but side-effects have been reported and the question has been raised as to whether there are too many H_2-receptor antagonists (Anon, 1988). An alternative option might be to decrease gastric acid secretion by inhibiting the proton pump H^+/K^+ ATPase. This enzyme can be bound by omeprazole which is a substituted benzimidazole (Editorial, 1987). Below a pH of 4.5 lipase is inactivated. It would be prudent to use this pharmacological approach for a short period only because achlorhydria could predispose the patient to enteric infections from ingested pathogens, e.g. salmonellosis. Sodium bicarbonate (15 g/m^2 daily) given with pancreatic enzymes may also improve their efficacy.

For maximum efficiency pancreatic enzyme preparations should be taken with all meals as well as snacks. The preparation should be mixed with a pleasant tasting liquid, such as fruit juice, and sipped throughout the meal. If this is not acceptable then the dose should be divided and taken immediately prior to and slightly after the meal. The preparation should never be mixed with food on the plate as this makes the meal most unappetizing and will result in a diminished food intake.

The quantity of the enzyme preparation given will depend upon the child's size, diet and pancreatic function. The dose should be increased until the consistency and frequency of the stools ceases to improve or the anal area becomes sore owing to the presence of enzyme in the stool. The quantity can be adjusted according to the amount of fat in the diet: parents can increase the dose if the child eats a very fatty meal.

Protein

Faecal losses of nitrogen are as high as 30% in untreated cystic fibrosis patients and the correct usage of a pancreatic enzyme supplement does not result in normal absorption; the greater the amount of fat in the stools the higher the nitrogen loss.

Serum protein levels are generally slightly elevated owing to a raised globulin level while albumin levels are usually low. Body protein stores are decreased with a low muscle mass and increased muscle catabolism (Miller *et al.*, 1982). The requirements for protein in cystic fibrosis are thus greater than normal. Children should receive an

intake of 120–150% of the recommended daily allowance (RDA) on a per kilogram body weight basis. The use of a high protein, moderate fat or MCT drink as a supplement to the diet can improve nutrient intake. If the child will accept a hydrolysed protein preparation, as discussed in Appendix IV.5, then this is likely to be absorbed more completely than whole protein. Recipes for high protein drinks with a low or moderate fat content are given in Appendix III.10.

Fat

Fat malabsorption is the most striking of the gastrointestinal features (Fig. 13.4). Pancreatic enzyme therapy does not restore fat absorption to normal and it may remain as low as 70% of intake. The proportion of absorbed fat remains constant whether the intake is high or low. Some serum essential fatty acids, such as arachidonic and linoleic acid as well as phospholipid and cholesterol levels, are low in cystic fibrosis. The daily administration of essential fatty acids in the form of 1 ml/kg corn or safflower oil has been advocated. This would need to be taken with pancreatic enzyme cover. A significant positive correlation has been found between plasma linoleic acid levels and height in some patients (Yassa, 1983) and supplements of linoleic acid monoglyceride have been used as a supplement (Lloyd-Still *et al.*, 1981).

Advocates of unrestricted quantities of dietary fat maintain that a higher energy intake is achieved. However, the greater the quantity of unabsorbed fat, the more pronounced are symptoms such as abdominal pain, distension and frequent malodorous stools. A balance must be found between acceptability of dietary restriction, achievement of an adequate energy intake and discomfort caused by steatorrhoea.

Parents and children should be encouraged to find a degree of restriction which suits them and advice on the fat content of foods as contained in Appendix IV.25 might be useful. Steatorrhoea is more pronounced during periods of infection and some children prefer to reduce their fat intake at these times.

There are occasions when a low-fat diet, 20–30 g daily, is necessary and only foods with a moderate or low fat content should be taken. These conditions are detailed in Table 13.4. As a low-fat diet is also of low energy content then there should be some kind of supplement. The use of medium-chain triglycerides either to replace milk fat or in recipes

Fig. 13.4 Diagrammatic representation and comparison of the major steps in the digestion and absorption of dietary fat, protein and carbohydrate. These include: the lipolysis of dietary triglycerides (TG) by pancreatic enzymes; micellar solubilization of the resulting long-chain fatty acids (FA) and β-monoglycerides (BMG) by bile acids; absorption of the fatty acids and β-monoglycerides into the mucosal cells with subsequent re-esterification and formation of chylomicrons; and movement of the chylomicrons from the mucosal cells into the intestinal lymphatic system. indicates where it is important in pre-term infants; ■ = block in CF. (Adapted from CC Roy, A Silverman and FJ Cozzetto, 1975, *Pediatric Clinical Gastroenterology*, 2nd edn, CV Mosby Co., St Louis.)

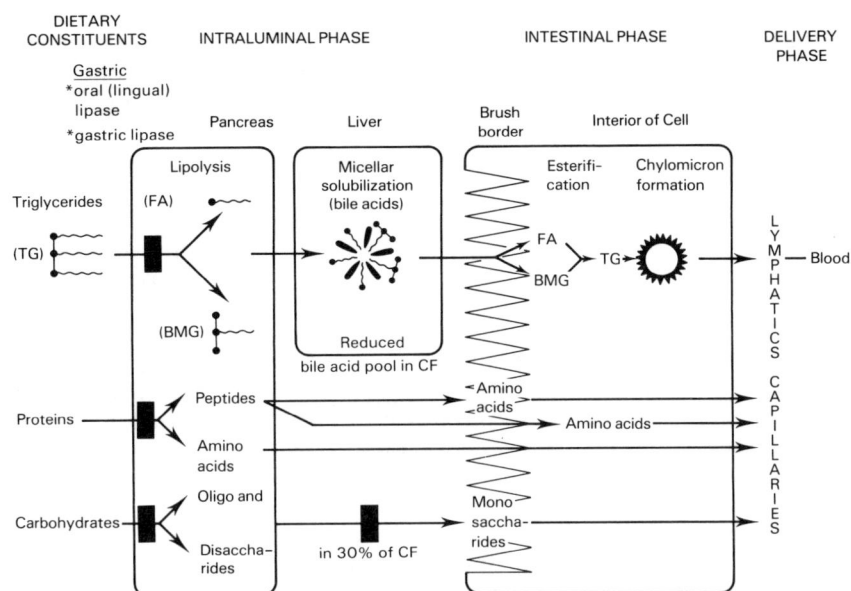

Table 13.4 Conditions which may require a low fat (20–30 g) diet

Postsurgery (particularly infants)
Passing of frequent bulky stools
Failure to thrive
Abdominal pain and distension
Unacceptable passing of flatus
Rectal prolapse
Liver disease

requiring added fat is described in Appendices IV.7 and IV.27.

Carbohydrate

Despite the fact that low disaccharidase activity has been described in a number of children with cystic fibrosis, carbohydrate is probably the most important source of digestible energy in the diet. Lactase deficiency should be suspected in infants if diarrhoea fails to resolve after the introduction of pancreatic enzyme supplements. A low lactose milk, possibly with medium-chain triglycerides in place of long-chain fat, can be used.

Starch in older children can give rise to abdominal pain and distension owing to bacterial fermentation and gas production in the large bowel. It is important that pancreatic enzyme supplements are given with all starchy snacks. A glucose polymer preparation can be used in place of sucrose to improve energy intake. The advantages are that there is less risk of dental caries and the polymer does not have such a sweet taste. It can be used in larger quantities than sucrose to sweeten beverages, desserts and breakfast cereals; in addition, it can be incorporated into high-energy supplements as described in Appendix III.5.

Energy

Because of the inadequacies of digestion, it is generally accepted that children with cystic fibrosis have an energy requirement that is greater than normal. Dietary modifications should be aimed at an overall increase in energy intake. An intake of at least 100% RDA for chronological age or 130–150% RDA for height–age is considered desirable. It would appear that, in spite of apparently large appetites, few children achieve 100% RDA for size.

Fibre

The production of soft, bulky stools, flatus and

reduced bile salt reabsorptions are features of both cystic fibrosis and of a high-fibre diet. There would appear therefore to be no advantage in advising a high fibre intake in cystic fibrosis. However, there is no evidence that cereal or vegetable fibre exacerbates gastrointestinal symptoms and the child should follow the dietetic pattern of the family in this respect.

Minerals

Sodium. In temperate climates there is no evidence that children with cystic fibrosis have an increased requirement for sodium. However, because of their high sweat sodium content, any situation which increases sweating, such as a fever or high environmental temperatures, may necessitate the addition of salt tablets supplying an extra 2—3 mmol/kg daily to older children. Care should be taken in very young infants receiving a whey-based baby milk and supplements of physiological saline may need to be added to the feed to bring the intake up to the normal RDA for weight.

Calcium. Children with cystic fibrosis rarely have the bone abnormalities of rickets but when these do occur they are likely to be due to vitamin D malabsorption. A calcium intake appropriate for chronological age should be ensured.

Iron. Some studies on iron absorption in cystic fibrosis report diminished iron absorption with pancreatic enzyme therapy; others do not support this (Solomons *et al.*, 1981). A similar story exists for body stores of iron. Anaemia is a rare finding in cystic fibrosis although low plasma iron levels are seen. An intake of 100% RDA for chronological age is advised.

Trace metals. Impairment of zinc absorption and retention has been shown (Aggett *et al.*, 1979) and low levels of zinc observed in plasma (Solomons *et al.*, 1981). Although any beneficial effects of zinc supplementation have yet to be proved the normalizing of body zinc levels by the addition of an oral supplement is recommended. High levels of copper in fingernails and plasma have been described, plasma copper levels rising as the disease progresses. The pattern of diminished iron and zinc levels with an increase in circulating copper in ceruloplasmin could be a response to the long-term effects of chronic infection. The requirements of the child with cystic fibrosis are at least normal for height—age. Low blood selenium levels have been described in cystic fibrosis (Dworki *et al.*,

1987). Recent reports indicate that absorption of most trace elements is diminished and that a supplement containing the RDA for all trace metals should be given in addition to the diet.

Vitamins

Because of the fat malabsorption in cystic fibrosis, a supplement of vitamins in a water-miscible form, as described in Appendix II.13, should be given. *Vitamin A.* Decreased vitamin A in 40% and carotene levels in 90% of cystic fibrosis patients have been described (Congden *et al.*, 1981) and symptoms of vitamin A deficiency are seen in untreated cystic fibrosis. Recommendations for vitamin A intake are in the region of 1200—2500 µg daily; the high dose may not be necessary if zinc is supplemented.
Vitamin D. Malabsorption of oral vitamin D and reduced bile salt reabsorption results in low body stores and low plasma levels of 25-hydroxy vitamin D_3 (Hahn *et al.*, 1979). Osteomalacia and demineralization of bone has been demonstrated in cystic fibrosis adolescents and a reduced cortical thickness in younger children. A daily dose of 100—200 µg/day is recommended.
Vitamin E. Plasma levels of vitamin E are low in the majority of children with cystic fibrosis. Although deficiency symptoms attributable to this have not been shown, it is recommended that normal plasma tocopherol levels are maintained by a supplement of 100—200 mg daily. This is particularly important if selenium supplements are not given.
Vitamin K. Hypoprothrombinaemia responsive to vitamin K therapy has been described and the vitamin supplement chosen should provide at least the RDA.
Water-soluble vitamins. These appear to be more readily absorbed than fat-soluble vitamins and, provided an adequate diet containing the RDA is taken, a further supplement should not be necessary. Periods of infection and fever will increase requirements. Vitamin B_{12} absorption has been shown to be impaired (Lindemans *et al.*, 1984). However, absorption can be improved by administration of pancreatic extracts. A supplement equivalent to the RDA in addition to dietary intake is advised.

Feeding children with cystic fibrosis

The maintenance of good nutrition is likely to

improve the quality of life for those with cystic fibrosis. As far as possible children should received a normal diet with the addition of high-energy drinks. It should be remembered that 20% of children with cystic fibrosis have normal or near normal pancreatic function and need no diet modification at all. In general, chest physiotherapy and drainage should be carried out as far as possible from mealtimes as vomiting or loss of appetite may be seen in small children who swallow their mucus. Physiotherapy should be carried out prior to mealtimes, as it will cause vomiting if carried out after a meal.

Infants who present with failure to thrive will have pancreatic insufficiency and need nutritional therapy upon diagnosis. Breast feeding can be continued because human milk fat is well tolerated, but pancreatic enzyme therapy should be commenced. Powdered preparations can be mixed with water, juice or expressed breast milk and given by spoon during the feed. If the infant fails to improve then an energy supplement based on a high-protein low-fat milk described in Appendix III.10 can be given between feeds.

The feeding of infants with meconium ileus may present special difficulty. If the infant has undergone surgery then a regimen as described on p. 72 might be required.

The introduction of solids can be at the same time and of similar type as for non-cystic fibrosis infants unless there is a sugar intolerance where the advice on p. 82 may be followed. Extra pancreatic enzymes should be given whenever weaning foods are offered.

Several regimens have been tried in order to improve the nutritional status of older children and these may have a role in the treatment of cystic fibrosis at particular times. Emergency measures should not be necessary if attention to nutrition is paid from the time of diagnosis. An 'artificial' or elemental diet consisting entirely of amino acids, peptides, MCTs, glucose polymer, vitamins and minerals has been used by several centres in place of ordinary foods. Administration has been either orally or by means of nasogastric tube (Bertrand *et al.*, 1984); total parenteral nutrition has been used (Mansell *et al.*, 1984) and short-term peripheral hyperalimentation (Lester *et al.*, 1986). In general, it would appear that compliance is poor with an oral regimen and that, although increased body weight and muscle mass can be achieved, these improvements are only temporary and an intensive short-term nutrition rehabilitation policy holds a few long-term benefits. As part of a planned protocol with patients automatically receiving aggressive nutritional therapy each time they enter hospital, some long-term advantage may be achieved. The introduction of a self-administered nasogastric tube and a high-energy feed or elemental diet for a given number of nights each week, with the child eating to choice during the day, might also result in nutritional improvement (Bertrand *et al.*, 1984). A feed suitable for such administration is described in Appendix IV.9.

Lung therapy

Nearly all of the mortality and much of the morbidity in cystic fibrosis are the result of chronic lung disease. Just as the cause of this disease is still enigmatic, there is much controversy relating to the optimal philosophy of treatment. Reversible airway obstruction is common and requires bronchodilators. Allergic bronchopulmonary aspergillosis can complicate cystic fibrosis and will need corticosteroids.

Physiotherapy

There is little doubt that this is a major component of the treatment regimen. Parents and patients must be taught to carry out postural drainage, percussion and review their breathing exercise expertise. Vigorous physical exercise, dancing and trampolining can form an important part of the physiotherapy programme. Never presume the adolescent patient nor the parents of a young child have mastered the art of physiotherapy (physical therapy) without constant reassessment of the technique. Older children should be taught to do their own therapy and use the 'forced expiration' technique. Obtain frequent sputum samples for identification of pathogenic organisms and their ever-changing sensitivity patterns. Prior to physiotherapy some patients benefit from a nebulized mucolytic such as acetylcysteine which lowers sputum viscosity.

Antimicrobial therapy

Better survival can be partly attributed to improvements in antibiotic treatment. Some advocate long-term continuous use of antibiotics against staphylococcal (especially in the early years) and

Haemophilus influenzae infections while others are more conservative and are only active when proven pathogens are identified. Increase in intensity and frequency of a cough, especially at night, poor appetite, static weight, malaise and/or deterioration in chest X-ray findings are some of the parameters indicating bacterial infections. Early admission for intensive treatment to deal with *Pseudomonas* is often indicated when signs of deterioration appear. Consider inhaled antimicrobials (Mearns, 1985) and the recent but much awaited oral anti-pseudomonas antibiotics, such as ciprofloxacin (Bayer UK; Hodson *et al.*, 1987) have been used successfully in adults.

Mist tests

Mist tests have not been shown to be beneficial yet some patients claim subjective improvement.

Aerosol therapy

Agents used include antibiotics, bronchodilators, acetylcysteine or disodium cromoglycate. Discourage members of the family from smoking in the vicinity of the patient and consider the role of antiviral agents, viral vaccines and the optimal environment.

General principles of management

Parents, siblings, other close relatives and friends have a heavy burden to bear in their relationship with a cystic fibrosis patient. The physician must not lose sight of the onerous psychosocial and psychosexual problems that a potentially lethal and debilitating disease causes. There will be much parental and perhaps sibling guilt, too, that is not overt. It is easier for the clinician to concentrate on the pathology of the lungs and pancreas as opposed to the psychopathology of a treatable but, as yet, incurable disease. Counselling, be it by a competent social worker, psychiatric social worker or psychiatrist able to deal with an entire family, will reduce some of the bleakness and despair that accompanies this serious disease.

Future trends

Brock (1983) in Edinburgh and other groups have been able to make a prenatal diagnosis of cystic fibrosis by the detection of very low levels of fetal intestinal microvillar isoenzyme of alkaline phosphatase. By the use of monoclonal antibody the specific alkaline phosphatase can be assayed from amniotic fluid. At present only about 90% of cystic fibrosis cases will be detected and there is a false-positive rate of about 5%. This diagnostic technique is the consequence of a secondary effect and will now be supplanted by chorionic villi biopsy which will enable first-trimester fetal diagnosis to be established by DNA probes as opposed to the later identification from the amniotic fluid of abnormal enzyme activity. An earlier diagnostic technique will facilitate termination of pregnancy when it is both indicated and requested.

Using data obtained from DNA probes, Beaudet *et al.* (1988) in Houston and Williamson's group in London have shown that a person with a BB genotype has a one in five chance of carrying the cystic fibrosis gene compared with a one in 500 probability if the genotype is CC. This information relating chromosomes and haplotypes A,B,C, and D by the use of restriction-fragment-length-polymorphisms (RFLPs) will enable cytogeneticists to evaluate the pregnancies of women closely related to patients with cystic fibrosis. Better diagnosis will be achieved when the cystic fibrosis mutation can be tested directly.

Shwachman–Diamond syndrome (pancreatic exocrine insufficiency and bone marrow dysfunction)

This rare multi-organ syndrome constitutes the next commonest cause of pancreatic exocrine insufficiency (PEI) after cystic fibrosis. First described by Shwachman *et al.* (1964), PEI was reported in children with neutropenia or pancytopenia and normal lungs and sweat electrolytes (thus excluding cystic fibrosis). Other observers (Bodian *et al.*, 1964; Burke *et al.*, 1967; Shmerling *et al.*, 1969) expanded the syndrome; currently the major diverse manifestations include:

1. Pancreatic insufficiency.
2. Metaphyseal dystosis (femur, tibia, knees, ribs).
3. Short stature.
4. Susceptibility to infections (chronic or cyclic neutropenia).
5. Haematological anomalies, including anaemia,

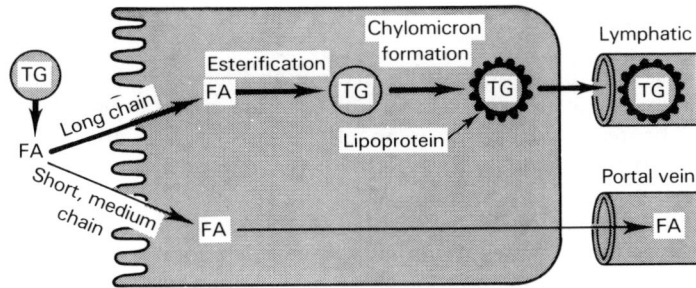

Fig. 13.5 Lipid transport in the mucosa.

FA = Fatty acids   TG = Triglycerides

thrombocytopenia, elevated HbF and bone marrow hypocellularity.

Symptoms

Infants of both sexes present with steatorrhoea and failure to thrive in the first year of life. The fat loss in the stools decreases with age because of an increase in lipase secretion (Hill *et al.*, 1982). The gastrointestinal symptoms may appear by 3 months of age and not infrequently are noted at birth. In as many as half of the patients eczema is seen. The common haematological features are neutropenia, seen in almost all patients, anaemia and thrombocytopenia. In addition, Brueton *et al.* (1977) described hepatic dysfunction. Mental retardation was reported in 85% of cases reviewed in a series of 21 patients (Aggett *et al.*, 1980). Galactosuria is seen in some children. Hip dysostosis can cause coxa vara with an abnormal gait. As many as 25% die (one series reported nine deaths from a group of 36 cases — chiefly from infections). The protean findings in this syndrome have included myeloproliferative and lymphoproliferative neoplasia.

Investigations

The following investigations are used:

1. Faecal fat studies over 3 days.
2. Enzyme studies (Shwachman and Holsclaw, 1972):
   a. Measure tryptic activity in duodenal fluid — reduced;
   b. Measure amylase activity in duodenal fluid — reduced;
   c. Measure lipase activity in duodenal fluid — reduced.
3. Pancreozymin-secretin function testing (p. 119).

4. Reduced amount of pancreatic enzymes and bicarbonate (Lundh test meal, p. 119).
5. Small bowel biopsy — normal histology and mucosal disaccharidases and enterokinase activity.
6. Triolein breath test — non-invasive technique, stool collection not required.
7. Fluorescein dilaurate test (Barry *et al.*, 1982).
8. [^{75}Se]Selenomethionine scanning (Braganza *et al.*, 1973).

Treatment

At present results are unsatisfactory. Steatorrhoea can be improved with a high dose of pancreatic extracts (preferably microencapsulated enteric-pH-coated preparations).

Other measures include: offering at least 30 000 units of lipase with sodium bicarbonate and H$_2$-receptor antagonists (e.g. ranitidine, cimetidine) to abolish steatorrhoea; aim at maintaining intragastric pH above 4. However, hypochlorhydria combined with neutropenia could make an infant very vulnerable to an ingested pathogen.

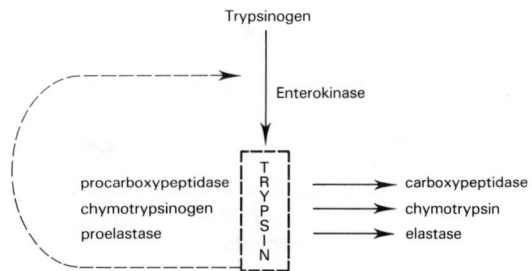

Fig. 13.6 The activation of pancreatic zymogens.

Dietary treatment

Because the absorption of fat, protein and lactose is likely to be impaired an infant formula based on a protein hydrolysate is an effective form of dietary management. A formula such as Pregestimil (Appendix IV.5) meets the requirements as the components are readily absorbed with little need for digestive enzymes. Alternatively an elemental or modular regimen can be designed (Appendix IV.9).

Older children will need to obtain a proportion of their nutrient requirements from drinks based on a protein hydrolysate or elemental formula; many of these have an unpleasant taste. The remainder of the diet needs to be fairly low in fat (about 20 g daily) with foods selected from those that are moderate or low in fat (Appendix IV.25). MCTs can be used in cooking for this diet (Appendix IV. 27).

It is important to prescribe a water-miscible form of the fat and water-soluble vitamins together with iron and vitamin B_{12}.

Isolated enzyme deficiencies

Trypsinogen deficiency

The presence of trypsinogen in the pancreas is essential for proteolytic activity. Inactive trypsinogen is converted to an active form (trypsin) by the intestinal enzyme enterokinase (*see* Fig. 13.6). Then activated trypsin is able to activate other proenzymes — procarboxypeptidase (to carboxypeptidase) and chymotrypsinogen (to chymotrypsin) and, furthermore, converts more of the proenzyme trypsinogen to trypsin.

Trypsinogen deficiency is an inborn error of metabolism associated with hypoproteinaemia, oedema, failure to thrive and/or anaemia.

Treatment

Treatment is with pancreatic extracts combined with a hydrolysed protein formula in infants (e.g. Pregestimil). Older children tolerate a fairly normal diet, but growth is improved if a supplement of an elemental or predigested drink is given.

Congenital enterokinase deficiency

Enterokinase is a duodenal mucosal enzyme which activates trypsinogen. The clinical features of the deficiency (Tarlow *et al.*, 1970) are similar to cystic fibrosis: loose, frequent stools from birth and failure to thrive. To confirm the diagnosis duodenal trypsin/chymotrypsin are assayed before and after the addition of enterokinase. Small bowel biopsy reveals normal mucosal histology but the enzyme enterokinase is lacking in the homogenate. Replacement treatment is not used as yet but an adequate response is seen with pancreatic preparations.

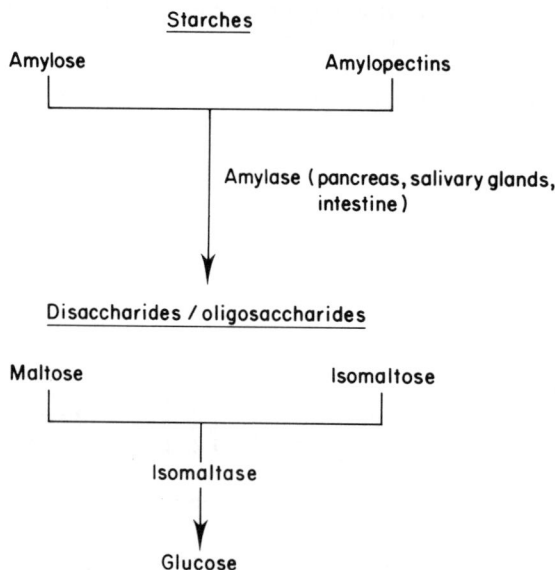

Fig. 13.7 The metabolism of starches.

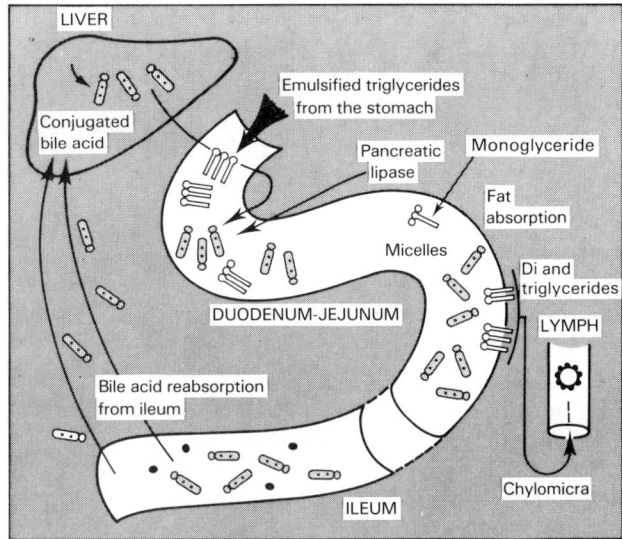

Fig. 13.8 Intraluminal micelle formation, fat and bile salt absorption.

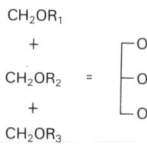

(*a*)

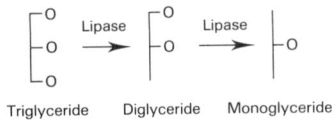

(*b*)

Fig. 13.9 (*a*) Fatty acids; (*b*) the action of lipase.

Pancreatic amylase deficiency

This very rare enzyme disorder is a physiological phenomenon seen in immature newborns and a potential problem in infants given a disproportionately large intake of starch for their amylase capacity (Fig. 13.7) (Lowe and May, 1951; Lilibridge and Townes, 1973).

Congenital pancreatic lipase deficiency

In this condition (Sheldon, 1964) steatorrhoea is present from birth and a characteristic feature is the passage of oil from the bowel. Although pancreatic lipase but not co-lipase is deficient, a functioning gastric source of this lipolytic enzyme is present (Figarella *et al.*, 1972; Muller *et al.*, 1975; Borgström *et al.*, 1979) (Fig. 13.8). There is also evidence of lingual/pharyngeal lipase activity. The differential diagnosis includes cystic fibrosis and the Shwachman—Diamond syndrome.

Neutral fats (triglycerides) are composed of the carbohydrate glycerol and three fatty acids (R_1, R_2, R_3) (Fig. 13.9a). Lipase releases fatty acids from glycerol by hydrolysis (Fig. 13.9b).

Treatment

Large amounts of pancreatic extracts should be used for the lipase deficit. A low-fat diet will reduce the steatorrhoea.

14

Hepatobiliary Disease

Acute neonatal hepatic necrosis

Neonatal hepatic necrosis is a very uncommon disorder which presents in newborn infants during the first month of life. Jaundice is not always evident but all develop severe haemorrhagic problems. There is marked necrosis in the liver. Aetiological agents include herpes virus, echovirus, adenovirus and the Epstein–Barr virus. Some of the cases arising beyond the first month of life are due to hepatitis B virus.

Chronic liver disease (Fig. 14.1)

Chronic persistent hepatitis

This disorder arises when hepatitis develops, often due to type B infection, and lasts beyond the usual 10-week period of viral hepatitis (Novick and Thomas, 1984). However, hepatitis types A, non-A and non-B can also cause chronic persistent hepatitis. It is characterized by fatigue, anorexia

and liver tenderness. Biopsy shows hepatic inflammation primarily within the portal tracts. The lobular architecture is preserved. Also, the diagnosis is suspected when serum transaminases fail to fall or return to normal. Both the serum bilirubin and γ-globulin may be elevated. Hepatitis B surface antigen (HBsAg) may be found in the serum. Since the clinical and laboratory findings do not help classification of the various forms of chronic liver disease, the histopathological features determine the diagnosis. Treatment is not needed because the outcome is usually benign.

Autoimmune chronic active hepatitis

The differences between chronic persistent hepatitis and chronic active hepatitis are shown in Table 14.1. This is a severe form of disease and a history of recurrent hepatitis should suggest the diagnosis (Mowat, 1980). The major characteristics of autoimmune chronic active hepatitis (ACAH) include chronic aggressive hepatitis with or without

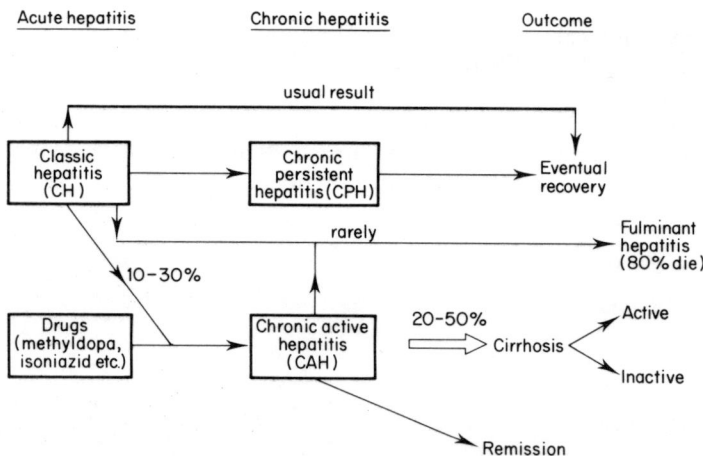

Fig. 14.1 Spectrum of chronic liver disease.

Table 14.1 Features of chronic hepatitis

Feature	Chronic persistent hepatitis	Chronic active hepatitis	
		HBsAg$^+$	HBsAg$^-$
Incidence in children	Uncommon	Rare	Common
Extrahepatic manifestations	Rare	Uncommon	Common
Symptomatology	Mild	Moderate	Severe
Jaundice	Rare	Uncommon	Common
Cirrhosis	Rare	Common	Less common
Prognosis	Good	?	Poor
Associated risk factors, e.g. transfusion, drug abuse etc.	Common	Unusual	Rare

Adapted from Silverberg (1979).

cirrhosis, increased serum transaminases, hyper-gammaglobulinaemia and the presence of autoantibodies (Mowat, 1987a). The clinical features are usually those of acute hepatitis but often the presentation is insidious and non-specific with anorexia and lethargy combined with enlargement of the liver and spleen. Alternatively the signs may be those complicating cirrhosis (e.g. ascites) or hepatic coma. In this disorder there is a dominance of young females and in the majority of them there is the presence of the HLA antigen B8 DR3. A biopsy (Fig. 14.2) is necessary to distinguish between CPH and ACAH and this is indicated because the latter can lead to cirrhosis or liver failure (Redeker, 1981).

Liver biopsy shows necrosis, blurring of the

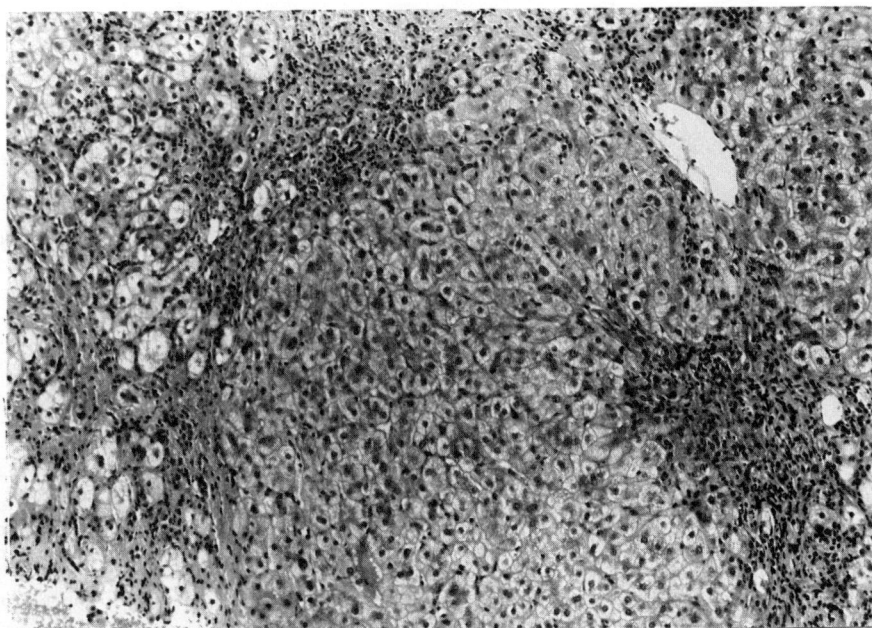

Fig. 14.2 Chronic active hepatitis — needle biopsy of liver. Note portal inflammatory infiltrate, with mild fibrosis, eroded margins of hepatocyte lobules, and preserved architecture. Haematoxylin & eosin, x 150. (Courtesy of Dr P Lewis.)

limiting plate (limiting plate separates the portal tract from hepatic parenchyma) and 'bridging' between portal tracts and the hepatic veins and lobules. The necrosis bridges adjacent portal areas and the central vein or portal areas of other lobules.

Other disorders which can produce the same changes include Wilson's disease, α_1-antitrypsin deficiency and hepatotoxic drugs.

The cause of this chronic hepatitis is unknown but the markedly elevated IgG and the presence of autoantibodies as well as reduced complement would suggest an impaired immunoregulatory mechanism. Early diagnosis is important because of the need to introduce prompt immunosuppressive therapy as this disease has a significant mortality. (Silverberg, 1979). The main therapeutic agents are prednisolone and/or azathioprine. A combined drug regimen might give the best results (Mowat, 1981).

Once clinical and biochemical remission has been achieved an alternate day steroid programme will avoid some complications (uncontrolled study by Arasu, 1979).

Classic hepatitis

Classic hepatitis (Table 14.2) is the common form of acute liver disease and usually resolves. At times it leads to fulminating hepatitis which is life threatening and has a mortality as high as 80%. The liver architecture reverts to a normal pattern in most instances.

Hepatitis A is caused by an RNA agent that is a member of the picornavirus family. It is transmitted by person-to-person contact generally via faecal contamination and like hepatitis B virus through

Table 14.2 Viral hepatitis screening profile: interpretation of results

IgM-specific anti-HAV	Assays HBsAg	Anti-HBc	Interpretation
Positive	Negative	Negative	Recent acute hepatitis A infection
Negative	Positive	Negative	Early acute hepatitis B infection; confirmation required to exclude non-specific reactivity
Negative	Positive	Positive	HBV infection, either acute or chronic[a]
Negative	Negative	Positive	Active HBV infection cannot be excluded. Test for anti-HBs and anti-HBe. A positive anti-HBs test indicates a previous HBV infection and usually signifies immunity to hepatitis B.[b] Consider testing the sample for IgM anti-HBc if HBV of recent onset is suspected. A negative anti-HBs and a positive anti-HBe indicate recent HBV infection. Confirm by demonstrating anti-HBs seroconversion in 2–6 weeks or by examining the sample for IgM-specific anti-HBc
Negative	Negative	Negative	Possible non-A, non-B hepatitis, other viral infections, or toxic (drug-induced) liver disease
Positive	Positive	Positive	Recent acute HAV infection in an HBV carrier

[a] Differentiate acute from chronic hepatitis by examining the sample for IgM-specific anti-HBc. The presence of HBeAg indicates those specimens that exhibit the potential for enhanced infectivity. HBeAg is found only in the presence of HBsAg. Other serological markers that may be present at the same time include HBV (Dane) particles. By disrupting the virion, HBcAg and viral DNA polymerase can be measured.
[b] Exclude recent transfusions, immune globulin administration, or a maternal antibody source within the previous 6 months.
Adapted from *Hospital Practice*, Vol. 22, No. 2, p. 104, 1987, by permission of F. Blaine Hollinger, Houston and HP Publishing Co., New York.
HAV, hepatitis A (an enterovirus); HBV, hepatitis B (human hepadnavirus); IgM-specific anti-HAV, IgM — specific antibody to HAV; HBsAg, hepatitis B surface antigen present on the surface of the virus and the unattached tubular and spherical particles; HBcAg, hepatitis B core antigen; anti-HBc, antibody to the core antigen; HBeAg, an antigenic component of the capsid (core) of the hepatitis B virus; anti-HBe, antibody to the 'e' antigen; DNA polymerase, a component of the core; Dane particle, the complete hepatitis B virion.

Consider Reye's
Reye's Syndrome is a disease of infants and children of all ages

Suspect Reye's in a Patient with:

- Signs of Disturbed Brain Function
  Characterised by lethargy; staring; stupor; agitated delirium and screaming; rapid respiration; extensor spasms; decerebrate rigidity; involuntary movements; coma
- Unexpected Vomiting following a prodromal flu-like upper respiratory infection or chickenpox or gastroenteritis
  Infants and children under 3 years may have minimal vomiting and no clear prodrome
- Hypoglycemia and hepatomegaly which are sometimes present
- Elevated serum transaminases and blood NH_3 in the absence of jaundice

For Early Diagnosis
- Consider Reye's
- Emergency liver function tests
- Prothrombin time
- Blood NH_3

Initial Treatment
- 10% Glucose to provide 70% of maintenance fluid requirements
- Check blood sugar values
- Maintain air-way and normalise abnormal blood gases
- Institute measures to control Intracranial pressure while arranging transfer to a Paediatric Intensive Care Unit with facilities for measuring intracranial pressure

British Reye's Syndrome Register
- Please report cases to British Reye's Syndrome Register:
  PHLS Communicable Disease Surveillance Centre,
  61 Colindale Avenue, London NW9 5EQ. Tel: 01-200 6868

EARLY DIAGNOSIS AND TREATMENT MAY PREVENT DISABILITY AND DEATH

Reg. Charity No: 288064

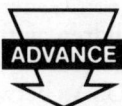

National
Reye's Syndrome*
Foundation
of the United Kingdom
*A disease that affects
the liver and brain

22 Wellands,
Wickham Bishops, Witham, Essex.

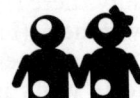

Fig. 14.3 Awareness campaign issued by the National Reye's Syndrome Foundation (UK).

blood or blood products. Immunoglobulin given before exposure or during the incubation period of hepatitis A (15–50 days) is protective against clinical illness. Water-borne, milk-borne and food-borne epidemics (especially raw shellfish) have been reported. Improved sanitation and socioeconomic conditions will result in a decreased exposure to hepatitis A. Although an attack of hepatitis A produces immunity there is no protection against subsequent hepatitis B infection.

Hepatitis B (HBV), a DNA virus, is a major cause of acute and chronic hepatitis, cirrhosis and primary hepatocellular carcinoma. Hepatitis B infection may appear as rapid fulminant liver disease or it may produce no clinical symptoms. The combined use of hepatitis B vaccine and immunoglobulin will result in greater than 90% protection in children born to mothers of high infectivity (i.e. 'e' antigen positive, HBsAg carriers). In newborns the risk of becoming a carrier is as high as 80–90% and an infant may remain infected indefinitely with only about 1–2% reverting to HBsAg negativity. Previously the classic treatment for preventing the carriage of hepatitis B from mother to child was the use of hepatitis B immune globulin which conferred a reduction in infant carrier status by 70–80%.

The incidence of hepatitis B virus infection is increasing. There were almost 2000 cases reported in England and Wales in 1984 which resulted in 40 deaths. A major obstacle to immunization is the high cost of the vaccine for a course of three injections and availability as well as the expense of hepatitis B immune globulin (Finch, 1987). However, now there is an opportunity to significantly reduce the likelihood of vertical transmission of hepatitis B by using an immunization regimen (Table 14.3).

Reye's syndrome

In 1963 Reye, an Australian pathologist, described a new syndrome characterized by acute non-infectious encephalopathy and hepatomegaly (Reye *et al.*, 1963). Pathologically there is fatty infiltration of the liver and other organs. Because of the previous high mortality there is heightened professional and parental awareness (Fig. 14.3). Early diagnosis is associated with a better prognosis. The age range is 3 months to 16 years and invariably there has been an antecedent or accompanying illness such as a

Table 14.3 Hepatitis B vaccine immunization regimen in infants born to HBsAg positive mothers

	Initial	1 month	6 months
0.5 ml[a] (10 µg) (at birth + immunoglobulin[b])		0.5 ml (10 µg)	0.5 ml (10 µg)

[a] Merck Sharp and Dohme H-B-Vax (paediatric) is a 0.5 ml dose containing 10 µg of vaccine.
[b] Administer the vaccine and immunoglobulin at different sites.
In the UK specific dosage details of the immunoglobulin are available from the Public Health Laboratory Service.

mild respiratory infection (influenza like) or chickenpox. Any child with severe vomiting, drowsiness and an enlarged liver must be regarded as a possible case. In the American National Reye Syndrome Surveillance Study for 1982 the overall incidence was only 0.33 cases per 100 000 population (Rogers *et al.*, 1985). During the year 1983–84 there was an incidence of 0.7 per 100 000 in the UK.

Aetiology

Many outbreaks have been associated with influenza A or B epidemics and also with varicella. Other viruses including parainfluenza, Coxsackie and adenovirus have been linked to this syndrome. In Thailand, aflatoxin B_1 was recovered from 22 out of 23 autopsied cases (Shank *et al.*, 1971) and in Mississippi in six out of seven livers at necropsy with proven Reye's syndrome (Ryan *et al.*, 1979).

Acetylsalicylic acid may play a role in the development of Reye's syndrome and is significantly higher in those with a fatal or a bad outcome than in those who recover with a good prognosis (Partin *et al.*, 1982). Salicylates may disturb mitochondrial function.

In the UK, the Department of Health and Social Security in June 1986, following the advice of the Committee on Safety of Medicines, advised that aspirin should not be given to children under 12 years of age unless specifically indicated. Yet, as early as 1982 the US Surgeon General warned that aspirin be avoided in children with influenza or chickenpox. Moreover, a decreasing trend in Reye's syndrome in Michigan, USA, between 1979 and 1984 had been related to a fall in the use of aspirin

(Remington *et al.*, 1986). In a mouse model, influenza B virus in combination with a chemical emulsifier (Toximul MP8) has produced hyperammonaemia, changes in hepatic urea cycle enzymes and liver morphology consistent with human Reye's syndrome (Crocker *et al.*, 1986). However, numerous environmental toxins, either alone, or in synergism with a virus, have been thought, by some hepatologists, to play a role in the aetiology.

Pathology and pathophysiology

Liver biopsy will show diffuse, severe, microvesicular fatty infiltration. Although necrosis and inflammation are absent or minimally present, there are significant ultrastructural changes within the mitochondria.

Symptoms

Typically the disease presents acutely in a previously well child who is recovering from an upper respiratory tract infection or varicella. Vomiting is the dominant feature. Usually the infant is anicteric but there is hepatomegaly. Tachypnoea or apnoea may occur. Hyperventilation of central origin can result in respiratory alkalosis. Neurological sequelae range from lethargy to coma. Seizures, particularly in young children, may develop.

Clinical staging:

1. Grade 1 — lethargic.
2. Grade 2 — agitated.
3. Grade 3 — decorticate.
4. Grade 4 — decerebrate.
5. Grade 5 — flaccid.

Diagnosis and laboratory findings

In addition to the findings of an encephalopathy and enlarged liver the following are required for the diagnosis:

1. Sterile cerebrospinal fluid (<10 white cells/ml).
2. Elevated serum hepatocellular enzymes (aspartate aminotransferase; alanine aminotransferase).
3. Blood ammonia over 1.5 times normal (well above 100 µg/dl).
4. Prolonged prothrombin time (greater than two standard deviations from the mean).
5. Hypoglycaemia is commmon and the serum bilirubin is usually <68 µmol/l (4.0 mg/dl).

If the diagnosis is in question a liver biopsy will confirm the syndrome (*see above*).

Treatment

Supportive measures include correction of hypoglycaemia and of the hyperammonaemia. Exchange transfusion and peritoneal dialysis have also been used successfully.

Diet in Reye's syndrome

Cerebral perfusion pressure (which is the difference between mean arterial blood pressure and intracranial pressure) must be monitored in stages III—IV of coma by an intracranial device and maintained above a critical level of 40 mmHg in an endeavour to reduce the morbidity rate (Jenkins *et al.*, 1987).

Measures should be taken to provide a diet which will decrease the blood ammonia and raise the blood glucose level. A high-energy, high-carbohydrate, low-protein diet is discussed in the section on dietary management of cirrhosis.

Prognosis

When first described there was a mortality of over 50%; now it is 30—37%, but in one centre of expertise the figure was only 7%. Cases of Reye's syndrome must be managed in highly specialized, preferably paediatric, units. Of survivors, 34—61% have a permanent neuropsychiatric disorder (Brunner *et al.*, 1979). If a recurrence arises it is important to exclude ornithine transcarbamylase or carbamyl phosphate deficiency because these biochemical disorders have caused Reye-like syndromes. There is a relationship between outcome with the depth of coma as well as blood ammonia levels. Few who reach stage IV coma will survive (i.e. deep coma unresponsive to painful stimuli).

Wilson's disease (hepatolenticular degeneration)

This rare inborn error of copper metabolism is an autosomal recessive disorder which results in a potentially fatal liver and nervous system disorder. The carrier rate is 1:200—1:500 with a disease frequency of 1:66 000 — 1:100 000. Although a very uncommon illness, paediatricians need to be aware of it because a delay in referral is associated with the development of cirrhosis (Mowat, 1981). It is seen mainly in Caucasians.

Dietary copper is essential for a variety of enzymes such as cytochrome oxidase, dismutase and ceruloplasmin; however, if excessive, this metal inhibits ATPase and may be found in many tissues especially liver, brain and kidneys. The liver is the main organ for storage. Ceruloplasmin is the major binding protein of copper. In Wilson's disease copper is deposited in the caudate—lenticular nuclei and in the cornea forming Kayser—Fleischer rings which are green-brown in colour. There are also renotubular defects.

Symptoms

The onset of symptoms is rare under 6 years of age, but can present as early as 2 years. Modes of presentation are variable and include acute hepatitis, chronic liver disease, cirrhosis, hepatic failure, haemolytic anaemia or neurological signs. A fulminating form can present as ascites and advance to hepatic coma. Central nervous system features can be clumsiness, poor handwriting, tremor, slurring of speech and athetosis. Any child presenting with a deteriorating scholastic performance at school must be considered as a possible case of Wilson's disease. Some children find their way to the psychiatrist because the organic diagnosis has eluded the clinician.

Diagnosis

1. Abnormal liver function tests are to be expected.
2. Ophthalmoscopic examination by slitlamp to show Kayser—Fleischer rings within the limbus of both eyes.
3. Chelation challenge: measure 24-hour urine copper excretion with 1 g of penicillamine. Collect urine in copper-free containers. Controls excrete <30—50 μg copper/24 hours. Values above 50 μg/24 hours are abnormal and frequently reach 1000 μg (12.5 μmol)/day in Wilson's disease.
4. Serum ceruloplasmin normally 25 mg/dl, low in Wilson's disease (< 20 mg/dl; 1.25 μmol/l). Ceruloplasmin can be normal in this disorder.
5. Serum copper normally 60—160 μg/dl, low in Wilson's disease (< 20 μg/dl) but as normal or

high values are observed serum copper is of limited use in establishing the diagnosis.
6. Liver biopsy: histopathology will show cirrhosis and copper content normally < 250 μg/g dry weight. If there has been no chronic cholestasis, hepatic copper concentration > 400 μg/g dry weight is diagnostic (Perman et al., 1979).
7. Radiolabelled copper studies with ^{64}Cu or ^{67}Cu to determine copper incorporation into ceruloplasmin demonstrate prolonged whole-body turnover of this metal.

Treatment

Drinking water should be analysed because of copper pipes. If the content is greater than 0.1 mg/l distilled or bottled water should be used. Alternatively, potassium sulphide 30—40 mg three times a day will bind intestinal copper. Chelation therapy is very effective and must be continued indefinitely.

D-*Penicillamine* 10 mg/kg per day increased after 2 weeks to 20 mg/kg per day in divided doses before meals will cause copper and zinc to be excreted in the urine. Patients intolerant of penicillamine can be chelated with triethylene tetramine hydrochloride 25 mg/kg per day in three divided doses (Walshe, 1969). Other options are zinc sulphate which is seemingly non-toxic (Cossack, 1988; Scheinberg and Sternlieb, 1988) or Unithiol (Konovalov et al., 1957). Penicillamine can cause leucopenia, immune complex nephritis, nephrotic syndrome, a lupus-like syndrome and haemolytic anaemia. Pyridoxine (5—10 mg/24 hours) should be given to prevent vitamin B_6 deficiency. Supplemental iron is indicated because chelation will remove iron as well as copper, zinc and other metals.

Diet in Wilson's disease

The dietary management is similar to other chronic hepatic conditions. There is a need for a moderate amount of protein based on the size of the child given there are no signs of impaired ammonia handling. A generous energy intake is important. The dietary copper should be restricted to the safe and adequate quantity recommended by the National Academy of Sciences (Appendix I.7). This ranges from 0.5—1.0 mg for infants to 1.0—3.0 mg daily for older children. In practice this means that during chelation therapy a fairly normal diet can

Table 14.4 Foods with a high copper content

Wheatbran	Peas	Dried	Cocoa	Malted	Egg yolk	Meat and meat
Wholemeal bread	Beans	fruits	Chocolate	milk-type	Shellfish	extracts
Wholegrain	Lentils	Olives	Liquorice	beverages	Game meats	Stock cubes
cereals	Mushrooms	Nuts	Fruit gums		(pheasant, hare,	Sauces and
			and		venison etc.)	ketchup
			pastilles			

Note: block salt, iodized and sea salt may contain copper; table salt should be used instead.
Water from copper pipes (or other sources likely to be contaminated) containing more than 0.1 mg/l should be avoided and distilled or mineral water used.

Table 14.5 Copper content of milk and formulae

Milk	Copper content (mg Cu/100 ml milk)
Human breast milk (mature)	0.04
Cows' milk	0.02
Infant formula (whey-based)	0.05
Premature formula	0.07

be recommended but avoiding foods with a particularly high copper content. Examples of such foods are given in Table 14.4. The copper content of milks and formulae is given in Table 14.5. It should be noted that infant formulae, particularly those designed for premature infants, have a high copper content and also may need to be avoided in neonates who are suspected of having the disease.

Prevention

Siblings of patients should be investigated.

Prognosis

If untreated all patients will eventually die unless given a liver transplant (Anon, 1987a).

Cirrhosis

Cirrhosis describes a histopathological change and is the end-stage of chronic hepatic disease in which there is widespread irreversible liver damage, fibrosis and the presence of regenerating nodules to replace normally arranged hepatocytes.

Often the cause is unknown but cirrhosis may be secondary to hepatitis, Wilson's disease, galactosaemia and α_1-antitrypsin deficiency.

Clinical features

Signs of chronic liver failure and portal hypertension are the chief features. Physical signs will depend upon the underlying cause, e.g. Kayser–Fleischer rings in Wilson's disease, bronchiectasis in cystic fibrosis, acne and striae in chronic active hepatitis. Hepatic coma (portal systemic encephalopathy) can be precipitated by:

1. Gastrointestinal bleeding.
2. Renal failure.
3. Excessive dietary protein.
4. Infection.
5. Constipation.
6. Diuretics.
7. Sedation.

Diagnosis

Biopsy is the principal means of diagnosis. Although liver function tests may be normal, elevation of the transaminases and γ-globulin with hypoalbuminaemia are commonly seen in cirrhosis. The most sensitive yet currently uncommon measure of liver function is the bromosulphthalein test (BSP). BSP clearance is a sensitive means of detecting slight hepatocellular damage but fatalities have occurred with this technique; therefore, this test should only be used in special circumstances. Extravasation of BSP into tissues must be avoided. The test involves injecting 5 mg/kg body weight in a fasting state of BSP intravenously as a 5% solution over 2 minutes. Results are expressed as a retention percentage at 45 minutes:

1. Newborn infants up to 15% (normal).
2. Older babies and children less than 5% (normal).

Management

An attempt should be made to define the cause of cirrhosis because specific therapy will be indicated in particular situations, e.g. lactose-free diet in galactosaemia, chelation in Wilson's disease. In the presence of active liver disease, prednisolone is indicated.

Large doses of vitamin D may be required to correct osteomalacia (rickets) such as 1.25–5 mg a day. Iron or blood is indicated if hypochromic anaemia is present secondary to blood loss.

Bleeding from oesophageal varices demands urgent attention. In the presence of hypersplenism, thrombocytopenia may arise. Because of this and impaired coagulation resulting from reduced activity of vitamin-K-dependent factors, vitamin K (5–10 mg/dose) as well as platelet concentrates should be considered. If ascites is present an aldosterone antagonist, such as spironolactone 3 mg/kg per day will mobilize the ascitic fluid. In the presence of tense ascites paracentesis will reduce both the respiratory and abdominal distress.

Biliary atresia and intrahepatic biliary hypoplasia

Extrahepatic biliary atresia accounts for at least 50% of all cases of prolonged obstructive jaundice in the neonate. Also absence or hypoplasia of the intrahepatic bile ducts is responsible for persistent obstructive jaundice of less than 10% of such affected neonates.

It has been suggested (Landing, 1974) that biliary atresia and hepatitis are different stages of one disease process and that they be grouped under one heading (Table 14.6).

Nutritional management of chronic liver disease

Energy

The energy intake in all forms of liver disease needs to be generous in order to protect the damaged liver from the effects of tissue catabolism. The UK or USA energy recommendations for age should be used, even if the child is small for chronological age. Lipids may be malabsorbed and the use of

Table 14.6 Histological features of the hepatitis syndrome of infancy and biliary atresia

Hepatitis	Biliary atresia
Disorganization of liver cords (lobular disarray)	Bile duct proliferation
Cholestasis	Bile stasis/bile lakes
Hepatocellular necrosis	Normal hepatic architecture
Inflammatory cell infiltrate in parenchyma and portal tracts	Inflammatory cells (portal)
Giant cell transformation	Giant cell transformation
Portal duct proliferation	

An epidemiological survey in south-east England by Cottrall showed that the neonatal hepatitis syndrome occurred in 1:2000 live births.

medium chain triglycerides (MCTs), whose absorption is independent of bile salts, can be used to replace up to 75% of ordinary dietary fat. The introduction of MCT as a milk formula for infants is described in Appendix IV.7. For older children a water-miscible MCT emulsion can be used in drinks or MCT oil in cooking, though care must still be taken to introduce these products slowly in order to avoid gastrointestinal symptoms. A recipe for a suitable high energy drink incorporating MCTs is given in Appendix III.11. If there is portal hypertension and shunting of the products of digestion into the systemic circulation then MCTs should be used with caution as it might induce ketosis.

Carbohydrate is generally well tolerated and should be used as the major energy source; generous carbohydrate should also help alleviate hypoglycaemia. Glucose polymers can be incorporated into drinks and food or can be given as a drink on its own (Appendix IV.14).

Protein

The protein intake should depend upon the clinical findings. Where there is a low serum albumin, a moderately high protein intake may be indicated using UK/USA recommendations for age. A higher protein load should be used with caution and reduced if the blood ammonia rises or hepatic coma develops. When tissue catabolism is increased then a low protein diet may be necessary and intakes similar to the WHO recommendations for weight (Appendix V.1) can be followed. As a last resort a minimum protein diet as described in Appendix V.10 can be used for short periods.

For adults with hepatic failure, a measure of success has been reported by the supplementation of low protein diets with branched-chain amino acids. Some of the symptoms of encephalopathy are thought to be due to the passage of aromatic amino acids crossing the blood–brain barrier; branched-chain amino acids inhibit the transport of aromatic amino acids. While few improvements in psychometric parameters have been described it has been suggested that nutritional status is benefited by this type of supplementation, due to the increase in the total nitrogen intake. As most children with long-standing liver disease are malnourished, there may be advantages in their use but this is unproven in children.

Sodium

If ascites is present then reduction of the dietary sodium intake to 10–20 mmol daily may be indicated. Details of the sodium content of foods is given in Appendix V.2. However, children with advanced liver disease are usually anorexic and there may be difficulty in persuading the child to consume any food if salt restriction is severe. Children with ascites require frequent small feeds or meals throughout much of the day and night where practical, due to the discomfort caused by gastric distension.

Vitamins and minerals

The problems of children requiring a modified diet for hepatic disease are very similar to those of children with chronic renal failure and the increased requirements and supplements are discussed in the section on p. 175. Fat-soluble vitamins are poorly absorbed if there is lipid malabsorption and double the normal supplement of vitamins A and D may be needed. Vitamin K supplements may also have a place. The requirement for vitamin D is increased, not only as a consequence of impaired absorption, but also because much of the vitamin is converted into the inactive hydroxylated cholecalciferol; in addition, if barbiturates are used, requirements are further elevated.

Oesophageal varices

Where these are present care must be taken to ensure that the diet is of a soft consistency and does not include sharp items such as potato crisps or apple which may cause physical damage if inadequately chewed. For young children, the diet may need to be given in a liquidized or semisolid form.

Infantile obstructive cholangiopathy

1. Neonatal hepatitis.
2. Biliary hypoplasia.
3. Biliary atresia.
4. Non-correctable biliary atresia.

Following the developments of newer surgical techniques and a policy of early intervention it is important to distinguish biliary atresia from hepatitis. In former years the outlook for children with biliary atresia was bleak. Since the introduction of methods involving the anastomosis, within the first 60 days of life, of the porta hepatis to the bowel (the Kasai portoenterostomy), the survival has risen to 60%.

However, it is imperative that expert surgery is offered no later than 8 weeks of age. By 60 days from birth 90% of those operated on are anicteric and 10-year survival for those free of jaundice is 90%. Earlier detection and diagnosis of jaundice would be facilitated if the 'well baby' review was at 4 weeks, as in Japan, and not 6 weeks as is common elsewhere. If paediatricians saw all infants who were jaundiced at 14 days from birth biliary atresia (1 in 12 000–14 000) would be picked up and treated promptly in specialized centres and thereby reduce the probability of subsequent liver transplantation (Mowat, 1987b).

There is no single test as yet that will separate cases of biliary atresia from hepatitis (intrahepatic cholestasis). Standard liver function tests and liver biopsy, unless examined by an expert histopathologist, are frequently unhelpful.

The following diagnostic tests are suggested to those in appropriate centres:

1. γ-Glutamyl transpeptidase is usually elevated (Wright and Christie, 1981).
2. Lipoprotein-X (abnormal, low-density lipoprotein found in sera of patients with obstructive jaundice) (Campbell *et al.*, 1974).

3. Modified[131]I-rose bengal excretion test, using cholesytramine — a non-absorbable resin which binds bile in the bowel (Poley *et al.*, 1972). Faecal excretion less than 10% suggests cholestasis.
4. Biliary scintigraphy with DISIDA (Dick and Mowat, 1986). ^{99m}Tc-diisopropyliminodiacetic acid given intravenously after oral phenobarbitone is as accurate as the rose bengal faecal excretion test.
5. Red-cell peroxide haemolysis test (Lubin *et al.*, 1971).
6. Vitamin E absorption test (Melhorn *et al.*, 1972).
7. Serum α-fetoprotein (Zeltzer *et al.*, 1974).
8. Serum 5′-nucleotidase is increased in extrahepatic biliary atresia (Yeung, 1972).
9. Ultrasound to exclude choledochal cysts.

Dietary management

The nutritional consequences of diminished bile flow reaching the intestinal tract include fat malabsorption, caloric deprivation and fat-soluble vitamin deficiencies. Preparations containing medium chain triglycerides have been used to replace ordinary fats in the management of disorders in which fat is malabsorbed. Failure of bile to neutralize the low pH of gut contents may result in inactivation of proteolytic enzymes causing protein malabsorption. A formula containing a protein hydrolysate (Appendix IV.5) may be beneficial.

Table 14.7 Neonatal hepatitis syndrome — King's College Hospital Study 1970–1974 (classification by aetiology and structural abnormality)

Syndrome	No. of patients
Extrahepatic biliary atresia	32
Choledochal cyst	2
Neonatal hepatitis of known cause	32
α₁-Antitrypsin deficiency	24
Galactosaemia	1
Tyrosinosis	1
Hepatitis B virus infection	2
Rubella	2
Toxoplasmosis	1
Rhesus isoimmunization	1
Idiopathic hepatitis	71

From AP Mowat, 1976, *Topics in Paediatric Gastroenterology*, p. 99, London, Pitman Books Ltd, with permission.

The hepatitis syndrome of infancy

This syndrome (Table 14.7) of conjugated hyperbilirubinaemia is characterized by the features of an obstructed biliary tract, i.e. jaundice, pale stools, dark bile-containing urine and often an enlarged liver. Inflammatory disease is present within the hepatic parenchyma and portal tracts but the cause need not be due to infection and can be the result of a metabolic disorder. Indeed there are many causes of this syndrome, e.g. idiopathic hepatitis, biliary atresia, hepatitis caused by infection, inherited inborn errors of metabolism, gallstones, hypothyroidism, cystic fibrosis, choledochal cyst, sepsis and haemolysis. The most appropriate disease title is controversial which, in part, relates to our ignorance of its pathogenesis.

Infections that may be accompanied by jaundice are listed in Table 14.8. *Listeria* sp., *Toxoplasma* sp. and syphilis are important to diagnose as they can be treated. Urinary tract infections and septicaemia due to Gram-negative organisms not uncommonly cause jaundice. Multinucleated giant cells may occur in biliary tract obstruction or in hepatitis.

Dietary management of hepatitis and acute liver disease

In the absence of hyperammonaemia or ascites, the aim of dietary treatment is to maintain the nutritional status. Because of anorexia, infants may

Table 14.8 Infectious causes of hepatitis syndrome in infancy

'TORCH'[a]	Causative organism
T	*Toxoplasma gondii*
O	Hepatitis B virus
	Coxsackie B virus
	Varicella virus
	Herpes simplex
	Zoster virus
	Treponema pallidum
	Listeria sp.
R	Rubella virus
C	Cytomegalovirus
H	Herpes simplex

[a] In the 'TORCH' syndrome, the 'O' stands for other diseases.

require nasogastric tube feeding and older children dietary supplements in the form of drinks.

The provision of an adequate energy intake is of prime importance with carbohydrate providing at least 60% of the energy. In some cases galactose is not well tolerated, leading to high blood levels and the presence of reducing sugars in the urine. An infant formula with a low lactose content (Appendix IV.1) may be used. In the presence of steatorrhoea, a low fat diet is indicated. Jaundice in itself does not mean that a low fat diet is needed.

Fat intake should only be reduced if feeding gives rise to abdominal pain or if steatorrhoea is so severe that the patient is unable to gain weight. If a low fat diet is prescribed, the energy deficit should be compensated for by an increased use of glucose polymer or by the introduction of medium chain triglycerides (MCTs).

Some infant formulae, such as Portagen (Appendix IV.7), have both a low galactose content and include MCTs. The protein intake in hepatitis should be moderate for the size of the child based on the UK/USA recommendations for weight. Hypoalbuminaemia is not an indication for a high protein diet because of the risks of hyperammonaemia or hyperaminoacidaemia. A moderate protein intake with a high energy content should result in the correction of low albumin levels.

Whenever possible, infants should continue to be given unheated breast milk from their mothers because of the immunological benefits. Examples of drinks for older children are given in Appendix III.11 and those providing an energy supplement in the form of glucose are listed in Appendix III.5

Defects of tyrosine metabolism

Tyrosine in plasma is derived from the amino acid phenylalanine and dietary proteins (Fig. 14.4). Disorders of tyrosine metabolism may arise from inherited enzyme deficiencies or as the result of liver damage. Secondary disturbances of tyrosine metabolism can result from untreated galactosaemia or fructosaemia.

Neonatal tyrosinaemia

Neonatal tyrosinaemia is a disorder due to reduced hepatic p-hydroxyphenylpyruvate oxidase activity and is seen in pre-term infants. A high protein

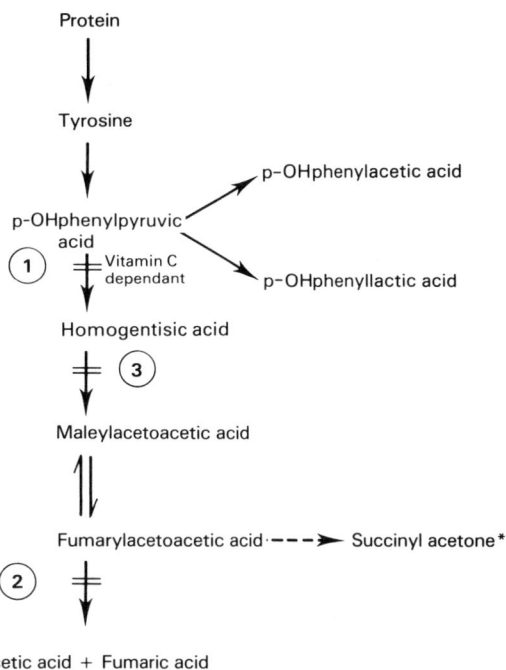

Fig. 14.4 Inborn errors of tyrosine metabolism. (1) p-Hydroxyphenylpyruvate oxidase deficiency in transient neonatal tyrosinaemia. Overcome in premature infants with vitamin C and a reduction in protein intake. (2) Fumarylacetoacetase deficiency present in hereditary tyrosinaemia together with block (1). The accumulating metabolites are marked*. (3) The block in alkaptonuria — the first inborn error to be studied and described by Garrod (1909).

intake (more than 5 g/kg per day) represents too large a tyrosine load. This phenomenon is usually transient and will respond to a lower protein intake (2–2.6 g/kg per day) or to ascorbic acid, the cofactor of p-hydroxyphenylpyruvate oxidase (50–100 mg/day). Although the outlook is very good, impaired mental development has been described.

Hereditary tyrosinaemia

Hereditary tyrosinaemia (a better term than 'tyrosinosis') may present in an acute or chronic manner. In the acute type, which is seen in the first year of life, there is often hepatomegaly, anorexia, vomiting and diarrhoea. Later jaundice may develop and progressive liver failure occur. Hepatomata may arise in those who do not die from liver failure.

The chronic type is seen later in infancy or childhood with cirrhosis and renal tubular lesions causing hypophosphataemic rickets. Plasma concentrations of tyrosine and phenylalanine are elevated with or without increased levels of methionine. Excessive amounts of tyrosine metabolites will be found in the urine (mainly *p*-hydroxyphenyl-lactic acid and succinyl acetone). Renal tubular damage causes generalized aminoaciduria, glycosuria, proteinuria and phosphaturia. Hypoglycaemia is common. The site of the enzyme block is not completely understood. The accumulating metabolites imply two distinct enzyme deficiencies. It is thought that the fulminating neonatal presentation may occur with a relatively larger deficit of the distal enzyme (from tyrosine) while the chronic disorder may be accompanied by a greater deficiency of *p*-hydroxyphenylpyruvate oxidase (much closer to tyrosine), which limits the amount of substrate reaching the second block (fumarylacetoacetase). The diagnosis can be established by assaying one of the compounds such as succinyl acetone, which has accumulated because of the metabolic block. Prenatal diagnosis is now possible by determination of fumarylacetoacetase in cultured amniotic fluid cells (Kvittingen *et al.*, 1985).

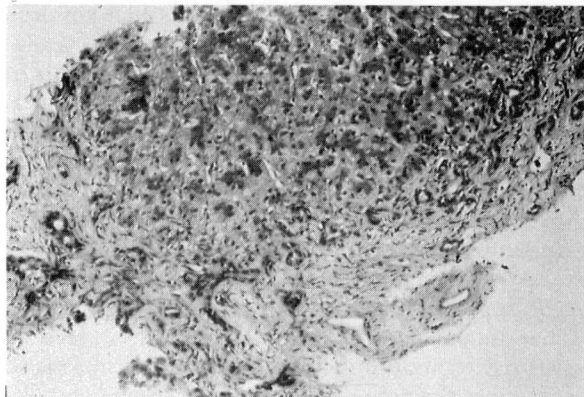

Fig. 14.5 α_1-Antitrypsin deficiency: percutaneous liver biopsy from an infant 4 months of age who had been jaundiced from the third week of life (Pi phenotype PiZZ). Occupying part of the lower figure is a broad band of relatively acellular fibrous tissue which contains prominent bile ducts. No distinct portal tracts or hepatic veins are seen. The hepatoctyes, in double cell plates which is normal in this age group, are deranged and cholestatic. The picture is compatible with cirrhosis. The infant died of liver failure at 9 months of age. With liver transplantation the infant might have survived. Haematoxylin and eosin. (By kind permission of Alex Mowat, London.)

Nutritional management

The principles of dietary treatment are similar to that of phenylketonuria (p. 148). The diet consists of a measured amount of protein which is adjusted in response to plasma tyrosine levels. A nitrogen supplement low in phenylalanine, tyrosine and methionine is used to maintain an adequate nutrient intake (*see* Appendix V.9).

Inherited and metabolic hepatocellular disorders

α_1-Antitrypsin deficiency

This inherited disorder accounts for a significant number of infants with obstructive jaundice in the newborn period (Sharp *et al.*, 1969). α_1-Antitrypsin (αlAT) is a glycoprotein which is synthesized in the liver and inhibits several proteolytic enzymes that can destroy certain tissues (Fig. 14.5). Its specificity is directed against elastase.

αlAT is a major α_1-globulin that has been studied by various electrophoretic techniques. Fagerhol (Fagerhol, 1964; Fagerhol and Laurell, 1967) showed that αlAT migrates before albumin, using acid starch gel electrophoresis, forming eight distinct bands. These bands have different speeds of migration depending on the protease inhibitor system. The pattern seen in 95% of the normal population is that of an intermediate speed. Abnormal protease inhibitor (Pi) systems can move faster or slower. The phenotype nomenclature uses letters relating to the velocity of migration, e.g. PiMM for a homozygous normal, M being letter from the center of the alphabet. F, S and Z are used for fast- or slow-moving zones so we have patterns of abnormal αlAT deficiency such as PiFF, PiSS and PiZZ or any heterozygous combinations of these with the normal or with each other, e.g. PiSZ.

The most serious liver disease appears to be linked with the Z band. Yet in a large Swedish screening survey Sveger (1976) found only 47% of those with the PiZ (or Pi nul) expression had abnormal liver function studies. Hence deficiency of αlAT may lead to transient liver injury and, rarely, cirrhosis. More recently Sveger (1984) showed in the 8-year follow-up that the prognosis for PiZ infants with neonatal liver disease is more optimistic than was previously thought. His investigation in Sweden was prospective and involved screening 200 000 newborns. A major new development was the technique of prenatal diagnosis by analysis of the mutation site (Kidd *et al.*, 1984).

Prenatal diagnosis has been achieved by analysis of material obtained at amniocentesis or chorionic villus biopsy. Until 1984, prenatal diagnosis of α_1-antitrypsin deficiency could be accomplished only by Pi typing of the fetal blood obtained during the second trimester by fetoscopy, a potentially hazardous technique with a significant risk of pregnancy loss. The recombinant DNA technology made it possible to develop synthetic probes specific to the M and Z alleles. Liver disease in PiZZ children shows a strongly positive intrafamilial correlation so that, if one sibling is severely affected, the risk to subsequent siblings is such that prenatal diagnosis would be justifiable (Anon, 1987b).

The dietary management is similar to that for cirrhosis (p. 138). In infancy the use of a protein hydrolysate milk formula has been found to be beneficial (Appendix IV.5).

Galactosaemia

Galactose-1-phosphate uridyltransferase deficiency

Galactosaemia is a rare inherited disease in which galactose is not converted to glucose but accumulates together with its metabolites. Galactose is derived from the hydrolysis of lactose which, after it is phosphorylated, becomes converted into glucose by the enzyme galactose-1-phosphate uridyltransferase. Galactosaemia should be considered in any newborn presenting with jaundice and hepatomegaly; however, the incidence is only 1:40 000 births. Infants lacking the red cell enzyme galactose-1-phosphate uridyltransferase are unable to utilize galactose. This sugar then accumulates in various body tissues (liver, kidney, red cells). Galactosaemia can readily be screened for in ill and jaundiced neonates by detecting reducing substances in the urine, given that they are drinking milk which is not free of lactose. However, to avoid a delayed diagnosis, many American states carry out an assay on all newborns for galactose (and galactose 1-phosphate) using the Paigen *E. coli*-phage assay.

Children are normal until given lactose- or galactose-containing formulae or breast milk. The symptoms and signs presenting in the first week of life are: vomiting, failure to thrive, hepatomegaly, jaundice, sepsis — particularly *Escherichia coli* infections and cataracts. Female galactosaemics may have delayed puberty as a result of hypergonadotropic hypogonadism (Clothier and Davidson, 1983). In any case of unexplained jaundice, screening should be carried out for this disease by examining the urine for reducing substances (test with Clinitest and not Clinistix or Labstix — galactose is a reducing monosaccharide sugar). The precise diagnosis requires the assay of the red cell enzyme galactose-1-phosphate uridyltransferase.

If untreated, many galactosaemics will die. The mean IQ is low even when patients are on a well-controlled diet.

Galactokinase deficiency

Galactokinase deficiency is a very rare inborn error due to galactokinase deficiency with a normal galactose-1-phosphate uridyltransferase. The condition causes cataracts but no mental retardation or hepatic enlargement. Galactitol formed from galactose is responsible for the cataracts. Also this disorder is characterized by galactosaemia and galactosuria.

Dietary treatment of galactosaemia

Lactose and galactose are excluded by removing milk (of all species) and milk products. Normal baby milks are avoided and the infant can be placed on a very low lactose formula as described in Appendix IV.1. The diet is essentially the same as a low lactose diet (except that offal meats should be avoided) and only foods known to be free of lactose (Appendix IV.19) may be eaten (Clothier and Davidson, 1983). Great care is necessary when manufactured foods are eaten or tablet (pill) type of drugs are prescribed, because lactose is frequently used as a filler, e.g. antipyretics, analgesics. Flavour enhancer, texture modifier or sweeteners are often derived from hydrolysed whey and should likewise be avoided.

Galactose occurs naturally in some plant polysaccharides but because the α-galactosidase necessary for the release of free galactose is absent in the human gut, this source is generally disregarded. An insignificant amount of galactose may be derived from bacterial fermentation of galactosides in the small intestine. As a precaution infant formulae based on whole soy beans are best avoided, though those from soy protein isolate are considered safe.

Foods containing galactosides, mainly peas, beans, lentils, peanuts, coconut, cocoa and chocolate should not be consumed during the first year of life. (Anon, 1982).

Dietary treatment needs to be lifelong because intellectual ability can deteriorate when the diet is de-restricted (Brandt, 1980). Furthermore, adolescents and adults should avoid alcohol because galactose elimination is inhibited by ethanol. Monitoring of erythrocyte galactose 1-phosphate levels must be carried out regularly on all galactosaemic individuals to ensure that dietary compliance is adequate. Levels of substrate must be maintained below 3 mg/100 ml.

A homozygous mother should be receiving a low galactose diet prior to her pregnancy and dietary advice must be reinforced. In addition, erythrocyte galactose 1-phosphate levels have to be checked early in pregnancy because free galactose and galactitol can damage the fetal eye. It is also thought that galactose in the heterozygous mother's blood can cause damage to a homozygous fetus; therefore many centres place the heterozygous mother on a low galactose diet. However, the value of this procedure has been questioned (Donnel et al., 1980).

The long-term outcome of early diagnosed and treated galactosaemic children is disappointing because of impaired intellect and visual–perceptual difficulties. The reason for this may include damage occurring *in utero*, delayed diagnosis, poor dietary compliance which remains undiscovered due to infrequent biochemical monitoring and the possibility that galactose is a semiessential nutrient in the neonate (Anon, 1982). Perhaps our dietary management is too rigid — or it is not strict enough! Further research is needed to find the optimum regimen for galactosaemia.

Enterohepatic circulation of bile salts

Bile salts, synthesized within the hepatocytes from cholesterol, play a major role in the solubilization and absorption of dietary lipids. The two primary bile acids (cholic acid and chenodeoxycholic acid), when present in duodenal juice above a certain concentration ('critical micellar concentration'), form micelles, i.e. aggregates with the products of lipolysis (*see* Fig. 13.8), and function as carriers. Bile salts promote water excretion and help to

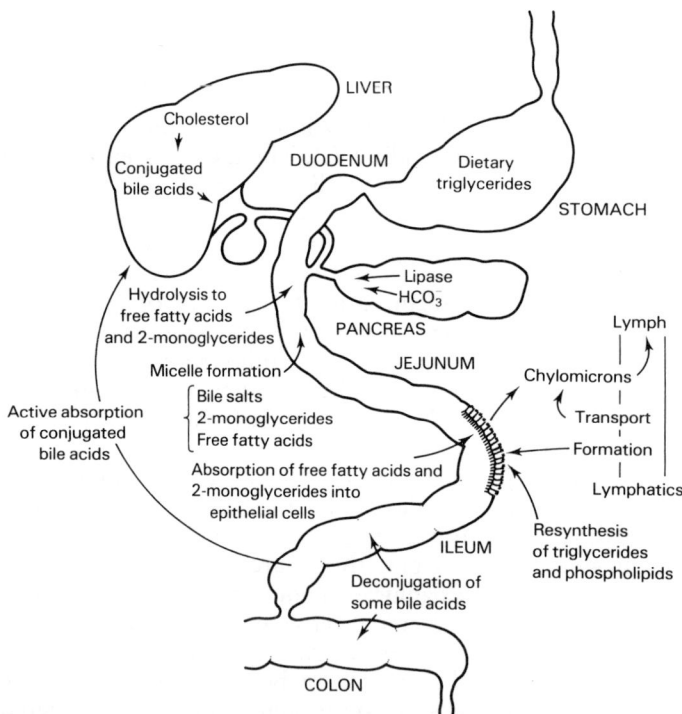

Fig. 14.6 Enterohepatic circulation of bile salts. (Redrawn from Hofmann, 1973, *Mayo Clinic Proceedings*, Vol. 48, p. 617).

emulsify fat, assist pancreatic lipolysis and solubilize the products of lipase. Also bile salts release gatro-intestinal hormones. A third bile acid component of bile is deoxycholic acid which is a product of bacterial hydroxylation of cholic acid in the bowel. Bile acids are secreted into the bile and stored in the gallbladder. The primary bile acids, cholic (trihydroxy) and chenodeoxycholic (dihydroxy) in a ratio of about 2:1 are conjugated with glycine and taurine and thus acquire detergent properties.

Bile salts cycle within an efficient enterohepatic circulation (Fig. 14.6). The level is maintained by synthesis from hepatic microsomes. Absorption of the salts takes place in the ileum and only a small faecal loss of less than 10% occurs. There are six to eight complete cycles in 24 hours. A fall in total concentration of conjugates below the critical micellar concentration results in malabsorption of dietary triglycerides. Deconjugation of bile salts by bacteria in the distal small bowel and large bowel converts the primary bile acids (cholic and chenodeoxycholic) to secondary bile acids (deoxycholic and lithocholic) which is less efficiently reabsorbed.

15

Selected Inborn Errors of Metabolism

Disorders of amino acid metabolism

Phenylketonuria

Phenylketonuria (PKU) is a recessively inherited inborn error of metabolism in which the amino acid phenylalanine cannot be metabolized normally. This disorder, which is seen once in about every 11 000 births, is caused by a deficiency or absence of the hepatic enzyme phenylalanine hydroxylase (Fig. 15.1). There is a marked variation in the frequency of the condition; in Belfast it is as high as 1:4500 and in both Finland and Japan it is only 1:100 000. Deficiency of this enzyme is almost unseen among Negroes and Ashkenazi Jews.

As a result of the disorder, alternative catabolites are produced which include phenylpyruvate, phenyl-lactate and phenylacetate (Fig. 15.1). Since all pyruvate metabolites contain a 'keto group' (−C=O) which is easily detected chemically by ferric chloride, the disease bears the name 'phenyl-ketonuria' after the urinary metabolite.

Unless phenylalanine is restricted in the diet, children with PKU will become mentally handicapped. However, as the amino acid is an 'essential' one, i.e. it is also required for normal growth, it must therefore be included, in strictly limited quantities, in the low phenylalanine diet. Blood levels of the amino acid should be monitored throughout childhood.

There are several variants of this disorder: benign or transient hyperphenylalaninaemia; persistent mild hyperphenylalaninaemia; and the rarest but most severe variant is due to abnormalities in the dihydropteridine reductase system. For a review of the biochemical background, see Smith (1985). In the last group they lack the cofactor tetrahydro-biopterin (BH$_4$), there is complete absence of any response to a low phenylalanine diet and although these patients do not have phenylalanine hydroxylase deficiency, the disease runs a more malignant course. The same cofactor is required by tyrosine

and tryptophan hydroxylase for the production of the important neurotransmitters dopamine and serotonin (5-hydroxytryptamine). The liver has a major role in modulating plasma phenylalanine concentration and elevation of this amino acid can be the result of impaired hepatic function or, in the neonate, from too high a protein intake.

Clinical features

Infants with PKU if untreated present with severe mental retardation and may have an IQ of less than 30. Ultimately only 3% of untreated PKU patients achieve an IQ above 50. Many are both fair-haired and fair-skinned with blue eyes and some have eczema; however, a dark complexion does not exclude the diagnosis. There is a characteristic mousy or musty odour due to the metabolite phenylacetic acid. About one in four have seizures and approximately one-third are hypertonic. In some infants there are typical features of spastic cerebral palsy. This clinical heterogeneity might be the result of genetic variation — namely different haplotype cofiguration (DiLella *et al.*, 1987).

Diagnosis

In the early 1930s, Asbjörn Fölling added ferric chloride to the urine of two mentally retarded siblings and noted a green colour reaction. Eventually he isolated phenylalanine and measured its high concentrations in the blood and urine of his cases.

Following this the diagnosis was suspected from a screening test made on the nappy by using 'Phen-istix'. This technique gave an unacceptably high rate of false-negatives because the unstable pyruvate metabolite is only present in freshly voided urine. Guthrie (Guthrie and Susi, 1963) devised a screening method for an elevated blood phenylalanine by a bacterial inhibition assay. In 1968 the Phenistix screening test was abandoned and by 1974 the

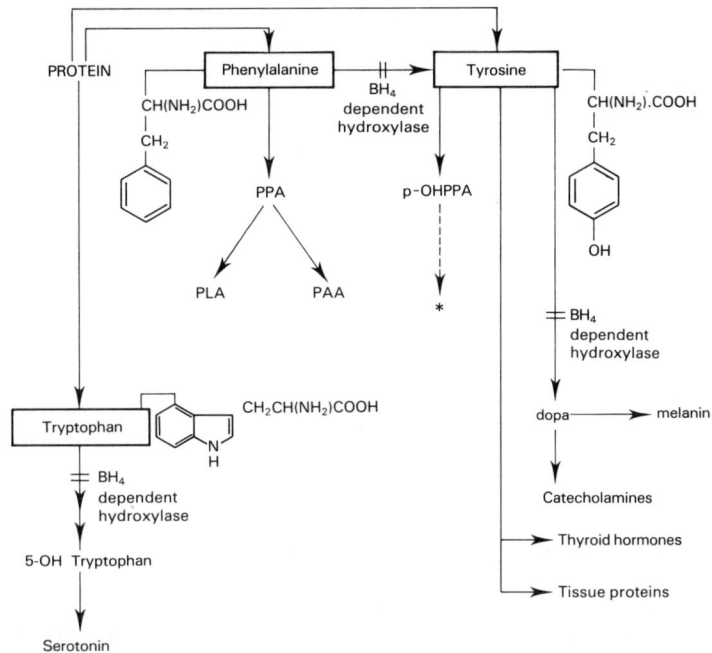

Fig. 15.1 Metabolism of phenylalanine, tyrosine and tryptophan. ╫ is the enzyme dependent on biopterin cofactors (BH₄). PPA, PLA and PAA = phenylpyruvate, phenyl-lactate and phenylacetate from phenylalanine. *p*-OHPPA = corresponding *p*-hydroxymetabolite from tyrosine. * = tyrosine pathway.

whole of the UK had a national programme using the Guthrie test on a small blood specimen obtained from a heel prick.

PKU is diagnosed as persistent hyperphenylalaninaemia of at least 480 μmol/l on a normal diet and should be confirmed by a careful laboratory study of phenylalanine metabolites in freshly passed urine using gas chromatography or another suitable technique.

Prenatal diagnosis of classic PKU has been made by DNA analysis of amniotic fluid cells. Furthermore it is suggested that carriers can be identified by a technique of enzymatic amplification of a subgenomic DNA fragment (DiLella *et al.*, 1988).

Management

The evidence that a phenylalanine-restricted diet is essential at the time of diagnosis in the newborn period to avoid mental retardation is not disputed. However, there is controversy about the age at which the protein intake and level of phenylalanine should become less rigidly controlled. Waisbren *et al.* (1980) recommend that the following psychological and physical characteristics be noted:

1. Emotional well-being on and off diet.
2. Visual motor coordination.
3. The relationship between the electroencephalogram pattern and differing levels of phenylalanine.

4. Changes in intelligence quotient (IQ) following diet treatment.

The Collaborative Study Group at the University of Southern California (Koch *et al.*, 1982) recommends caution and advised a low phenylalanine diet be maintained until adolescence or later.

The other important dietary management issue relates to maternal PKU during pregnancy or perhaps before conception and damage to the non-phenylketonuric offspring (Smith *et al.*, 1979). Smith attempted to avoid an embryopathy by monitoring the diet of the pregnant mother with PKU — but this failed despite a well-controlled diet from the fifth week after conception.

A malformed baby was born with microcephaly and severe cardiac malfunction. Since then further cases have been described. By 1980, 110 PKU mothers in the USA had given birth to more than 200 damaged children according to figures presented at a meeting of the US Collaborative Study (Bickel, 1980).

More recently, mothers who had begun a low phenylalanine diet between the first and fourth months after conception and who had maintained good control throughout pregnancy had better outcomes in terms of the infant's physical development (Watchel, 1986; Rohr *et al.*, 1987). A survey of 64 infants born to women with phenylketonuria showed good results in women with blood concentrations below 600 μmol/l prior to conception, and concluded that only a strict diet started before conception is likely to prevent fetal damage (Drogan et al., 1987).

If the infant's or child's phenylalanine level is kept consistently below 600 μmol/l (10 mg/dl) children will have a satisfactory development. Although there is controversy regarding the management of those with levels between 600 and 1200 μmol/l (10−20 mg/dl) there is a consensus of opinion that values exceeding 900 μmol/l require a low phenylalanine diet.

Aims of management. From 0 to 10 years plasma phenylalanine concentrations should be maintained between 180 and 480 μmol/l (3−8 mg/dl). From 10 years onwards a level of 900 μmol/l (15 mg/dl) is acceptable. Preconceptual management in women with known PKU should be to return to a strict low phenylalanine diet and reduce the amino acid level to less than 600 μmol/l (10 mg/dl) (Collins and Leonard, 1985).

Some claim that to terminate the special diet before mid-childhood will lower the IQ by as much as 8−10 points; in addition behavioural difficulties such as reduced attention span are commonly seen in some (though not all) children who de-restrict the diet early.

Nutritional management of phenylketonuria

The aim of treatment in phenylketonuria (PKU) is two-fold: to provide adequate nutrients and energy for normal growth and development and to ensure that phenylalanine is not given in quantities greater than the capacity of the body to metabolize it.

Principles of treatment. Dietary phenylalanine must be adjusted in accordance with blood levels. Since all natural proteins contain phenylalanine, it is difficult to construct a diet that will provide adequate protein and safe amounts of phenylalanine, so a protein substitute with adequate nitrogen must be used. Details of these products are given in Appendix V.5.

Nutrient requirements. The nutrient requirements for a child with PKU are not significantly different from the normal recommendations. Phenylalanine tolerance will depend upon the nature and severity of the enzyme defect, the child's age and growth velocity. Requirements given in Table 15.1. are theoretical, i.e. correct amount of phenylalanine for an individual is one that results in normal growth and development. Because of the nature of the enzyme deficiency, tyrosine becomes an essential amino acid and must be supplemented. The exact requirement for tyrosine in PKU is not known, but it has been shown to be a limiting amino acid in some regimens during periods of rapid growth (Shortland et al., 1985). Where synthetic amino acids are used in place of dietary protein, intestinal hydrolysis of the peptide bond results in 1.0 g intact dietary protein becoming equivalent to 1.2 g amino acids. Consequently, 100 g pure amino acids is taken to be 83.0 g intact protein. Only L isomers are used in amino acid preparations, because the D forms are not metabolized. Where a hydrolysate is used the product will contain some short-chain peptides, so the amount of water incorporated

Table 15.1 Nutrient requirements in phenylketonuria

Age	Phenylalanine (mg/kg body wt)	Total protein[a] (g/kg body wt)	Energy (kcal/kg body wt)
Premature infants	90[b]	3.2	125−130
0−3 months	60−90	3.0	120−125
3−6 months	50−80	2.5	115−120
6 months−1 year	40−50	2.4	105−110
1−3 years	30−40	1.9	90−105
4−6 years	25−30	1.7	80−90
7−9 years	15−25	1.6	70−90
10+ years	10−20	1.5	70−80
Pregnancy	15−30	1.3	40−50

[a] Total protein consists of the natural protein plus the protein equivalent provided by the substitute as stated by the manufacturer.
[b] From Shortland et al. (1985).

during digestion is not known. In addition, there is racemization of between 2 and 10% of L into D isomers (Clayton *et al.*, 1970; Kindt *et al.*, 1983), thus rendering them unavailable. Despite these uncertainties the same correction factor has been used for the protein equivalent figure in Table 15.1, i.e. 100 g hydrolysate protein is equivalent to 83.0 g intact dietary protein.

PKU children fed on the FAO/WHO recommended daily allowance (RDA) for protein have been shown to exhibit a lower growth velocity than those fed a higher quantity (Kindt *et al.*, 1983). The higher protein intake recommendation (i.e. the USA figures — Appendix I.2) should be used. Because the RDAs are based on intact protein, it is important that the phenylalanine allowance is given at the same time as the protein substitute so that a full range of amino acids is taken.

It is most important to avoid weight loss and other catabolic states, because the breakdown of body protein will release phenylalanine. The provision of an adequate energy intake is vital so the recommendations for infants and children with PKU are a little above the RDA for the average population (Acosta *et al.*, 1977). The rate of weight gain should be monitored to ensure that the intake is not excessive. In the older child, receiving an amino acid preparation, it is important to include special proprietary products, based on wheatstarch or cornstarch, to achieve the energy requirements. Such products include low-protein breads, biscuits (cookies) and pasta, and are available in the UK, USA and most European countries. The artificial nature of the diet is such that vitamins, minerals and trace elements will be inadequately supplied as a result of the limited amounts of natural foods allowed. Supplements are either integrated with the protein substitute or manufacturers recommend their use. The optimum balance of micronutrients in such supplements has not been determined. Decreased retention of trace elements has been described (Taylor *et al.*, 1984) and vitamin deficiencies were common in the early days of dietary treatment.

Practical management of a restricted phenylalanine diet

Infants. The theoretical quantity of phenylalanine, protein and energy should be calculated for the individual. The type and amount of natural protein which will provide the phenylalanine is decided. The remaining protein and energy is derived from the selected substitute. The calculated volumes of protein replacement and milk are each divided into five or six equal portions according to the feeding pattern. Ideally the bottle containing milk should be offered prior to the protein substitute to ensure that none is rejected. A certain amount of flexibility is allowed over the consumption of the protein substitute, because it is impossible to predict individual protein and energy requirements.

Infants who are breast fed. It is generally possible for mothers of PKU infants to continue breast feeding but this presents problems to the mother, the paediatrician and the dietitian and they should be aware of these difficulties before a decision on feeding a PKU infant is made. The phenylalanine content of mature breast milk varies but it is generally lower than other milks (Table 15.2). If the protein requirements of the infant can be met by breast milk, i.e. if at least 100 ml milk/kg is consumed and the serum phenylalanine levels can be maintained between 0.2 and 0.5 mmol/l, then all that may be needed is the addition of a protein-free energy supplement such as a 10 or 15% solution of glucose polymer. The intake of breast milk must be varied in response to blood levels and this can be achieved by altering the quantity of protein substitute offered and by attempting to adjust the period of breast feeding. In infants with a low phenylalanine tolerance, it is necessary to use a protein substitute to 'top up' protein requirements. A measured quantity is offered prior to breast feeding as a supplementary feed.

Solid foods. Weaning foods or Beikost should be introduced at the normal time, from about 4 months of age. Initially very small quantities of low-protein, low-phenylalanine foods can be offered, such as fruits and vegetables. The phenylalanine contribution to the dietary intake at this stage is

Table 15.2 Phenylalanine contents of milks

Product	Content per 100 g			
	Protein (g)	Phenylalanine (mg)	Energy (kJ)	(kcal)
Human milk, mature	1.3	46	293	70
Cows' milk	3.4	180	280	67
Regular baby milk (reconstituted liquid)	1.9	100	275	65
Dialysed whey baby milk (reconstituted liquid)	1.5	56	275	65

negligible but, when larger amounts of solid food are consumed, then phenylalanine must be counted as part of the daily allowance.

Because all protein-containing food also contains phenylalanine, an exchange system similar to that used for diabetic diets has developed. In the UK, the exchange system is based on 1 fluid ounce (30 ml) milk, which contains 50 mg phenylalanine; fruit and vegetables with a protein content of less than 1.5 g protein per 100 g are either measured as a 20 mg phenylalanine exchange or are allowed freely without being measured. In the USA, exchanges of food are based on 30 mg and 15 mg portions. If the phenylalanine content has not been determined, it can be calculated for a food, provided the protein content is known, from Table 15.3. A list of foods and their phenylalanine content is given in Appendix V.7

Foods which are very high in protein, such as meat, fish, cheese and egg, are not normally included in a low-phenylalanine diet as the quantity allowed for an exchange would be very small and difficult to measure. Some naturally occurring foods are low enough in protein to be included in the diet without their phenylalanine content being counted. A list of forbidden foods and those which can be allowed freely is shown in Appendix V.7. It is important in older children that the phenylalanine allowance and the protein substitute are given at the same time; the quantity of natural protein and protein substitute should be divided into three equal doses throughout the day.

Problems with diet. The three major problems with the dietary management of PKU are persistently low or high blood levels and intercurrent infection.

It is important that very low levels, below 0.06 mmol/l, are treated immediately because the effects of insufficient phenylalanine are as hazardous as high serum values. Dietary phenylalanine should be increased by approximately 100 mg increments daily and a blood test should be repeated within the next 5–7 days. If levels remain below 0.2 mmol/l for a period of some weeks then the possible explanations should be sought. Misdiagnosis of PKU is one possibility; often a transient benign hyperphenylalaninaemia has been managed with an overly restricted diet. Where this is suspected, a phenylalanine load of 50 mg/kg body weight should be administered. If levels rise to 1.2 mmol/l then the diagnosis of classic phenylketonuria is confirmed. If levels rise to between 0.9 and 1.2 mmol/l then the child has a mild or variant type pf phenylketonuria which still requires a low phenylalanine diet, but the amino acid tolerance is likely to be higher than in the classic form.

If levels do not reach 0.9 mmol/l on loading, then the child should be placed on a moderately restricted diet giving 2.0 g protein/kg daily; if serum phenylalanine levels still fail to rise above 0.9 mmol/l after one week, then a normal diet can be commenced.

A further cause of persistently low levels is an inadequate phenylalanine allowance — a response should be made to each low level by increasing the daily phenylalanine allowance by 30 or 50 mg. This is particularly important in periods of rapid growth when the need for phenylalanine is high. The child may not be consuming the full phenylalanine allowance, either because of food rejection or parental misunderstanding. A careful diet history and discussions with the parent should elucidate the source of the difficulty. The timing of the blood test needs to be examined — ideally, specimens should be taken fasting or at least 4 hours after a meal. Changes in the timing of tests may account for swings in blood levels. If a microbiological assay of phenylalanine is carried out, falsely low levels will appear when the child is on antibiotics.

The commonest cause of persistently high levels of phenylalanine is non-dietary compliance. This is seen frequently in children who attend kindergarten or school where uninformed staff or other children offer inappropriate foods or milk drinks. The parents themselves may be overestimating the size of phenylalanine exchanges. Another common cause of high serum levels is failure to provide an adequate energy intake. This, in turn, results in a reduced growth velocity and a low phenylalanine requirement. If the energy deficit is such that weight loss

Table 15.3 Phenylalanine content of proteins

Food	Phenylalanine content (mg/g protein)	
Milk, dairy products, meat, poultry, fish		
Cereals, pulses, peas, beans lentils, nuts	50	(5%)
Potato		
Dark-green leafy vegetables	40	(4%)
Other vegetables, fruits	30	(3%)

occurs, then phenylalanine will be released by catabolic activity. Energy in the low phenylalanine diet is largely provided by the inclusion of the special low-protein starch products. Other ways of increasing the energy intake is by the use of low protein 'milk' shakes or fruit-flavoured drinks supplemented with 15–20% carbohydrate, such as glucose polymer or proprietary products as described in Appendix III.5.

Parents should be instructed to provide the protein substitute evenly throughout the day and to do the same with the phenylalanine allowance ensuring that both are given at approximately the same time. Blood tests for phenylalanine levels should not be within 2 hours of a meal or transient elevation will be misinterpreted.

Infection or intercurrent illness usually results in high serum phenylalanine levels. To minimize this, high-energy, low-protein drinks should be encouraged, as described above. If the protein substitute is not accepted, it is safe to omit this for a few days; but when re-starting the preparations it is best to begin with a half-strength concentration to avoid the danger of vomiting and further rejection. The vitamin, mineral and trace element supplement may be safely omitted for a few days.

De-restriction of diet

Because of the risk of damage to the nervous system it is probably safer to continue the strict low phenylalanine diet, maintaining blood levels between 0.2 and 0.5 mmol/l until the early teens. After this a low-protein diet (1.0–1.5 g protein/kg body weight) has been used and blood levels are kept between 0.9 and 1.2 mmol/l. This is the same regimen as described for renal disease on p. 173. The special wheatstarch breads and flours are not required and the child can eat a limited amount of cereals and animal products. Although nutritionally the protein substitute is not required, there may be advantages in its retention in small quantities (0.5–1.0 g/kg daily) for girls in order to prepare them

for the controlled regimen strongly indicated during pregnancy.

Diet during pregnancy

Maternal levels of phenylalanine should be below 0.6 mmol/l prior to conception. Women should resume a precise low phenylalanine diet prior to conception. The principles of dietary treatment are the same as for children; estimated requirements are given in Table 15.1.

Diet in tetrahydrobiopterin deficiency

A low phenylalanine diet does not prevent abnormal features developing. Nevertheless, the diet is necessary because high phenylalanine concentrations limit neurotransmitter synthesis. Often the serum phenylalanine levels are not as elevated and the infant has a high tolerance to the amino acid. The diet is the same as for classic PKU and the overall aim is to keep the blood levels between 0.2 and 0.6 mmol/l. Phenylalanine tolerance improves with age and the child can often accept a moderately low protein diet (i.e. WHO recommendations for age) without the need for supplements by the age of 2 years (Dhondt, 1984).

Histidinaemia

This is an autosomal recessive and questionable disorder of histidine metabolism, first described by Ghadimi *et al.* in 1961, with an incidence range of 1:10 000 (Japan), 1:14 000 (Massachusetts) and 1:37 000 (Sweden). It is characterized by an elevated level of histidine in both the blood and urine. Histidinaemia is due to an inherited deficiency of histidase activity. This defective enzyme normally converts histidine to urocanic acid (Fig. 15.2).

Some patients have a speech defect and/or intellectual handicap while others have normal speech and intelligence. No favourable effects of dietary

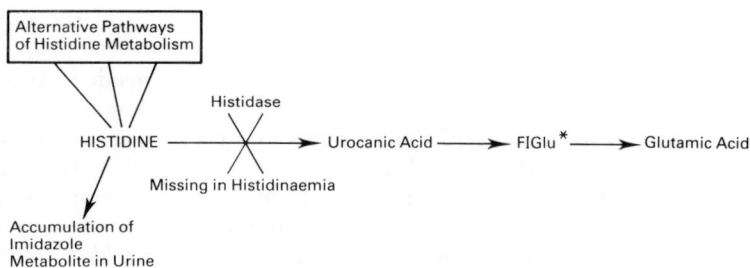

Fig. 15.2 Metabolism of histidine.
* = formiminoglutamic acid.

treatment have been observed, although biochemical control has been seen. Histidinaemia may be a benign biochemical finding and not a disorder needing dietary treatment (Levy *et al.*, 1974; Scriver and Levy, 1983). There are no specific clinical features that are pathognomonic of this particular disease.

Laboratory findings

1. Elevated blood histidine — 0.27–1.47 mmol/l.
2. Elevated urinary histidine (seen in other conditions, e.g. pregnancy).
3. Skin histidase absent or very low (not in all cases).
4. Abnormal urinary metabolite present — imidazolepyruvate.
5. Sweat composition — no urocanate present.

Treatment

If treatment is contemplated then the principles of management are as for phenylketonuria (p. 148); a low histidine nitrogen supplement can be used (Appendix V.9).

Homocystinuria

In the classic form of the disorder there is a deficiency of the enzyme cystathionine β-synthase which partly or totally blocks the conversion of homocysteine to cystathionine (Fig. 15.3). Consequently there is a build-up of homocystine and methionine in the plasma and tissues with an elevated urinary excretion. The enzyme defect has been noted in the liver, brain, skin fibroblasts and amniotic fluid cells. One form of homocystinuria is pyridoxine responsive.

Homocystinuria is a recessively inherited disease leading to an accumulation of some sulphur-containing metabolites as well as a rise in plasma methionine but with reduced cystine and cystathionine levels. The incidence is about 1:100 000 in the UK.

Symptoms

Patients tend to be tall with long fingers and toes and it may be mistaken for Marfan's syndrome. Mental retardation is seen in two-thirds of cases. Other features include osteoporosis with genu valgum, anomalies of the spine and thorax, a malar

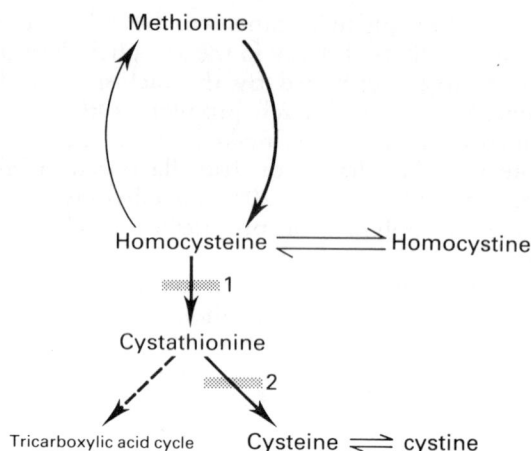

Fig. 15.3 Degradation of methionine: (1) cystathionine synthase; (2) cystathionase.

flush, lens dislocation and vascular thromboses. Thromboembolic attacks are common particularly of the coronary, renal and cerebral arteries. Early atherosclerosis is the usual cause of premature death. There are metabolic variants of homocystinuria including deficiencies of tetrahydrofolate methyltransferase and reductase.

Diagnosis

To avoid confusion with Marfan's syndrome, a quantitative serum amino acid analysis is essential whenever homocystinuria is suspected. A delay in establishing the diagnosis and instituting dietary manipulation may be associated with the development of thromboembolic episodes and other complications in homocystinuria. The urinary cyanide–nitroprusside test (Brand test) can give both false-negative as well as positive results.

Management

The aim of treatment is to remove homocystine from the urine and reduce plasma methionine to below 80 μmol/l. A daily supplement of cysteine is needed. As a result of the metabolic block, cysteine becomes an essential amino acid. Also a trial of pyridoxine 100–500 mg/day (Collins and Leonard, 1985) is indicated for all to help identify the 40% who are vitamin B_6 responders. Homocystinurics do have an increased folate requirement (10–20 mg/day) as a result of the elevated homocysteine which consumes methyltetrahydrofolate. Methionine is supplied by measured amounts of natural protein foods as described for phenylketonuria, folate and a nitrogen supplement low in methionine are also given (*see* Appendix V.9). Plasma methionine, cystine, homocystine and urinary homocystine levels should be monitored to ensure that the dietary methionine intake is suitable. Betaine is a methyl donor which remethylates homocysteine back to methionine and thus lowers the plasma homocystine concentration (Fig. 15.4). However, this treatment is not recommended by some investigators (Sardharwalla, 1980) because it can produce high levels of methionine. The other pathways for remethylations are via folate or vitamin B_{12}. Wilcken *et al.* (1983) recommend betaine in homocystinurics who are not responsive to pyridoxine.

The nutritional management of inborn errors of protein metabolism

There are two major methods of dietary manipulation for the treatment of inborn errors of metabolism. In one the total nitrogen intake is decreased as in some organic acidurias and urea cycle defects where accumulations of toxic products of protein metabolism occur, but plasma levels of amino acids remain normal. In contrast, the amino acid pattern of the diet can be altered if the metabolic error has resulted in elevated plasma levels of one or more essential amino acids or their direct metabolites. Furthermore, some amino acids may become essential as a result of a metabolic block and these must be added to the diet in adequate quantities. The diet must also contain sufficient nitrogen, minerals and vitamins for normal growth and development. Energy is particularly important in all these regimens to prevent tissue breakdown and release of toxic metabolites.

Low-protein diets

Where a life-threatening condition is suspected, infants should be placed on a protein-free feed as a temporary measure after blood and urine samples to establish the diagnosis have been collected. The feed should consist of a high concentration of carbohydrate, preferably glucose polymer, with added vitamins and minerals. A suggested regimen is given in Appendix V.11) and an energy intake of at least 100 kcal/kg body weight (420 KJ/kg) should

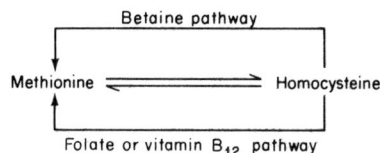

Fig. 15.4 Conversion of homocysteine to methionine.

be aimed for. In the initial stages fat should be avoided as it can exacerbate ketosis.

Because intercurrent infection causes breakdown of body protein leading to an accumulation of harmful metabolites, a protein-free diet should be commenced directly the child begins to become anorexic or to deteriorate.

If diagnosis or recovery from infection and commencement of a suitable feeding regimen is delayed beyond 4 or 5 days, then a minimal protein intake of 0.5 g/kg body weight should be given to prevent muscle wasting. This type of regimen will not support life for more than a short period. Additional minerals and vitamins must be given as well as an energy intake of at least 100 kcal/kg body weight (420 kJ/kg).

For the long-term treatment of infants and children who are not receiving additional amino acid therapy, the protein intake must at least equal that recommended (Appendix I.2), and the energy derived from protein in the diet should not fall below 6% of the total energy intake (Collins and Leonard, 1985). Treatment of older children is based upon protein exchanges (*see* Appendix V.1), low-protein food products, e.g. breads, such as those used in phenylketonuria (Appendix IV.30), and high-energy supplements.

Urea cycle disorders

Known metabolic disorders are associated with each of the hepatic enzymes involved in urea synthesis (Fig. 15.5). Because the sole function of the urea cycle is to convert ammonia to the non-toxic compound urea all disorders of urea synthesis cause ammonia intoxication, but this varies in proportion to the proximity of the block to the entry of ammonia into the cycle. Disturbed amino acids may be detected in the urine in citrullinaemia, argininosuccinic aciduria and hyperargininaemia. Clinical symptoms common to all urea cycle disorders usually include vomiting, intermittent ataxia,

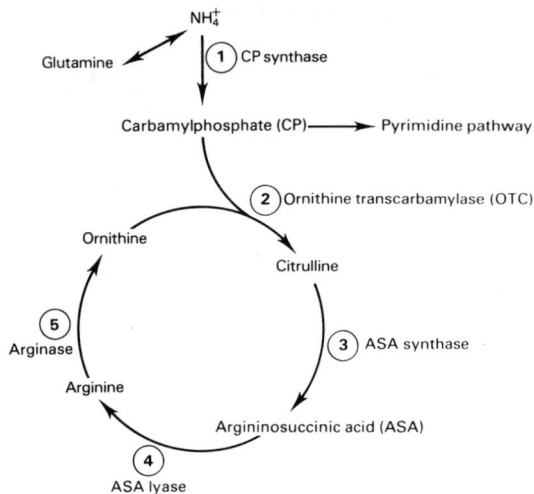

Fig. 15.5 Enzymes in the urea cycle; (1) carbamylphosphate synthase; (2) ornithine transcarbamylase; (3) argininosuccinic acid synthase; (4) argininosuccinic acid lyase; (5) arginase.

irritability, lethargy, mental retardation and aversion to a high protein diet. The accumulated ammonia is particularly toxic to the central nervous system.

Carbamylphosphate synthase deficiency

No orotic aciduria or aminoaciduria is detectable. Carbamylphosphate synthase (CPS) needs to be differentiated from ornithine transcarbamylase deficiency and organic acidaemias which cause secondary hyperammonaemia.

Ornithine transcarbamylase deficiency

This was the first of the urea cycle disorders to be described and was formerly known as primary hyperammonaemia. Many cases of this disorder were described before CPS deficiency was known but it differs from the latter because metabolites of carbamyl phosphate accumulate, resulting in the increased excretion of pyrimidines and its precursor orotic acid. Diagnosis can be established by hepatic enzyme assay.

Citrullinaemia

This is an extremely rare, recessive disease due to a deficiency of argininosuccinate synthase. There is raised blood, cerebrospinal fluid and urine citrulline but the ammonia levels will not be so high as in CPS and ornithine transcarbamylase (OTC) deficiencies. The plasma amino acid profile is diagnostic.

Argininosuccinic aciduria

This disorder is associated with mental retardation and friable tufted hair (trichorrhexis nodosa). In argininosuccinic aciduria there is an absence of argininosuccinase. The amino acid argininosuccinic acid is detectable in the urine but does not accumulate in the blood. In the plasma there is a characteristic amino acid chromatogram that establishes the diagnosis.

Hyperargininaemia

Hyperargininaemia is characterized by mental retardation, spastic diplegia and elevated blood and cerebrospinal fluid arginine levels. There is reduced arginase activity in the erythrocytes. This neurodegenerative condition distinguishes arginase deficiency from the other urea cycle disorders. The metabolic block results in the accumulation of an amino acid profile that is typical.

Nutritional management of hyperammonaemia

Most defects resulting in primary hyperammonaemia respond to sodium benzoate therapy. This is conjugated with glycine in the liver and, by providing an alternative pathway for the excretion of nitrogen, removes glycine from the metabolic pool. The basis of dietary treatment is a low protein diet. However, in defects of the urea cycle, with the exception of hyperargininaemia, arginine becomes an essential amino acid, since it cannot be synthesized from precursors in the pathway. It must therefore be included as a supplement to the diet.

Organic acidaemias

The enzyme blocks involved in these diseases occur widely throughout metabolism. The particular organic acid is not an amino acid but a substance that accumulates anywhere along catabolic pathways in fat, carbohydrate or protein metabolism; in fact, at any site in intermediary metabolism. This heterogeneous group of disorders includes lactic acidosis, ketosis or, very rarely, an inability to make ketones when they are appropriate.

The pinpointing of these enzyme disorders started with isovaleric acidaemia (IVA) by Tanaka *et al.* (1966) followed by non-ketotic hyperglycinaemia (Childs *et al.*, 1961). This was shown to be two distinct entities — methylmalonic aciduria and propionic aciduria. Fig. 15.6 shows the increasing rate of discovery of organic acidurias per year over the last two decades. Maple syrup urine disease is one of the commonest organic acidaemias and has an amino acid profile that is diagnostic. Vomiting, dehydration, metabolic acidosis and ketosis are some of the commonest clinical features. Often these infants are profoundly floppy. Failure to thrive, hypoglycaemia and fulminating infection can be the presenting signs. Intravenous feeding or clear feeds can reverse the picture as the protein intake ceases but, before such an improvement is achieved, it is essential to send blood and urine to the laboratory while there are sufficient metabolites to identify. The clinical suspicion of metabolic disease is of paramount importance. Some hospital laboratories can provide thin layer chromatography of amino acids but specialist biochemical help will be needed as many organic acids can only be identified by gas chromatography or mass spectrometry.

Many organic acid disorders have a vitamin-responsive and a non-responsive form. For example, methylmalonic aciduria can be due to a deficiency or mutation of methylmalonyl-CoA mutase or cobalamin coenzyme synthesis (Mahoney and Bick, 1987). Propionic acidaemia can be biotin responsive because this is the cofactor for propionyl-CoA carboxylase, the defective enzyme in this disorder. It is important to start vitamin therapy before laboratory confirmation is obtained, as several different organic acidurias are dependent on the same few vitamins.

Nutritional management

Where the condition is not completely responsive to cofactor therapy (e.g. vitamin B_{12}), then some form of dietary manipulation is required. Infants and children with organic acidaemias often show poor appetite and so frequently require intermittent nasogastric feeding for several years before they can

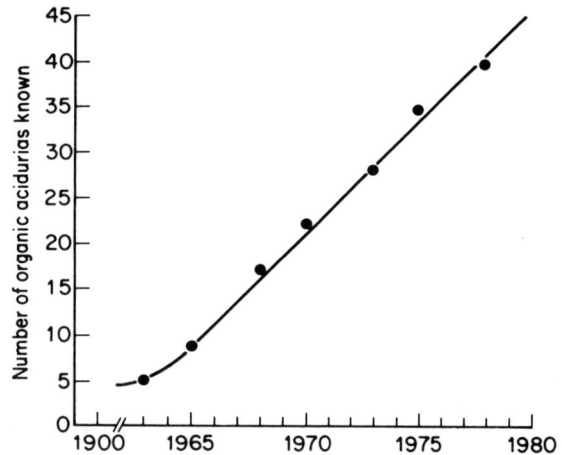

Fig. 15.6 Rate of increase in identification of organic acidurias. (Redrawn from RA Chalmers and AM Lawson, 1982, *Organic Acids in Man: Analytical Chemistry, Biochemistry and Diagnosis of the Organic Acidurias*, p. 3. Chapman and Hall, London.)

accept an adequate oral intake. There is evidence that patients with methylmalonic acidaemia have a secondary carnitine deficiency, and this should be supplemented (Mahoney and Bick, 1987).

The dietary treatment of maple syrup urine disease (MSUD) differs from the treatment of other organic acidaemias because the condition results in elevated plasma levels of the three essential branched-chain amino acids, leucine, isoleucine and valine. The principles of treatment are essentially as described for phenylketonuria (p. 148) with measured amounts of natural protein administered as 'exchanges' which are varied in response to the blood amino acid pattern. Since infants and children with classic MSUD have a small tolerance for natural protein (0.2–0.6 g/kg daily) a nitrogen supplement, low in branched-chain amino acids, is required. Examples are shown in Appendix V.9.

Elevated plasma amino acids are not a feature of the other organic acidaemias and a low protein diet is the method used to control the metabolic disturbance. The amount of protein tolerated depends upon age, size, growth velocity and degree of responsiveness to cofactor therapy. Plasma and urinary organic acids should be monitored to ensure that the protein intake is not excessive; plasma amino acid pattern and levels, and also weight and height velocity, should be studied to confirm the adequacy of protein for growth. Protein supplements tailored for individual inborn errors can be used to increase the minimal protein intake

Table 15.4 The familial hyperlipidaemias

	Type	Biochemical properties	Clinical features*
I	Familial hyperchylomicronaemia (familial lipoprotein lipase deficiency)	Cholesterol N/ ↑ ↑ Triglyceride ↑ ↑ ↑ Lipoprotein electrophoretic pattern: heavy band at origin — chylomicrons ↑ ↑ LDLs and HDLs ↓ ↓	Very rare autosomal recessive disease due to a lipoprotein lipase deficit which affects less than 1 : 10⁶ people. Abdominal pain, recurrent acute pancreatitis, hepatosplenomegaly, xanthoma, lipaemia retinalis, creamy serum. No premature atherosclerosis or ischaemic heart disease
IIa	Familial hypercholesterolaemia (familial type II hyperlipoproteinaemia, familial hyperbetalipoproteinaemia)	In heterozygous: Cholesterol ↑ ↑ Triglyceride N/ ↑ Electrophoretic pattern: increased β band LDLs ↑	Autosomal dominant: 0.1–0.5% in USA Heterozygous form: tendon xanthomata, xanthelasma, arcus senilis, premature atherosclerosis ± splenomegally Homozygous form: very rare, poor prognosis. Death before 20 years of age. Defect in LDL receptor sites on cell membranes
IIb	Familial combined hyperlipidaemia	Cholesterol only ↑ in 1/3 Triglyceride only ↑ in 1/3 Both ↑ in 1/3 Electrophoretic pattern: increased β and pre-β bands VLDLs ↑	Autosomal dominant. No xanthomata. No acute pancreatitis. Premature atherosclerosis. ? due to abnormal triglyceride transport (Goldstein *et al.*, 1973)
III	Familial broad beta (broadened β band) disease (familial type III hyperlipoproteinaemia)	Cholesterol ↑ or ↑ ↑ Triglyceride ↑ or ↑ ↑ Electrophoretic pattern: broad β band LDLs N/ ↓	Autosomal dominant and rare disorder. Skin xanthomata are deep orange and prominent on palms and fingers, arcus senilis, abnormal glucose tolerance test and hyperuricaemia. Obesity common. Atherosclerosis present. ? due to disorder of VLDLs conversion to LDLs (West and Lloyd, 1979)
IV	Familial hypertriglyceridaemia (familial type IV hyperlipoproteinaemia)	Cholesterol N/ ↑ Triglyceride ↑ in 1/3 Electrophoretic pattern: increased pre-β band LDLs N VLDLs ↑	Autosomal dominant. No xanthoma. Obesity, hyperuricaemia, abnormal glucose tolerance test and acute pancreatitis. Premature atherosclerosis
V	Familial type V hyperlipoproteinaemia	Cholesterol ↑ or ↑ ↑ Triglyceride ↑ or ↑ ↑ Chylomicrons ↑ Electrophoretic pattern: heavy band at origin and increased β and pre-β bands VLDLs ↑	Very rare — gene present in 0.2% of population. Acute pancreatitis is major complication. Increased incidence of coronary heart disease in type I adults

N = Normal
↑ = slight increase, ↑ ↑ = moderate increase; ↑ ↑ ↑ = marked increase.
↓ = slight decrease; ↓ ↓ = moderate decrease.
* = VLDL, LDL, IDL, HDL = lipoproteins (*see* text).

(Appendix V.9), but the usefulness of such products has been questioned (Leonard *et al.*, 1984).

Lipoprotein disorders

The topic of hyperlipidaemia (Table 15.4), especially hypercholesterolaemia, has attracted the attention of many investigators because of its known association with atherosclerosis. Cholesterol esters, triglycerides and phospholipids are the predominant lipids found in human plasma. All are esters of long-chain fatty acids. Some of the lipids are present in a bound state with apolipoprotein or apoprotein to form lipoproteins (Fig. 15.7). Cholesterol can be either in a free (non-esterified) or esterified form and is found in all classes of lipoproteins. The lipoprotein categories can be determined by electrophoresis of the serum (Table 15.5).

Electrophoresis on agar gel, polyacrylamide gel or other media will produce separate bands because of their distinctive mobility and differing compositions in respect of lipid and protein (apoprotein) content and their ratios (Fig. 15.8). It is essential to emphasize that a specific type of hyperlipoproteinaemia only describes a particular electrophoretic lipoprotein pattern and does not in itself establish a diagnosis. In a fasting subject, the chylomicrons will not be seen as bands on electrophoresis. The mobility rates of the various lipoproteins also relate to the type of media used in electrophoresis. Classification can also be determined by the density of the lipoproteins upon ultracentrifugation (Table 15.5 and Fig. 15.9).

Chylomicrons

Chylomicrons are large lipoprotein particles in the intestinal absorptive cells (enterocytes) which transport exogenous dietary lipids and cholesterol in the lymph and blood. The lipoprotein lipase

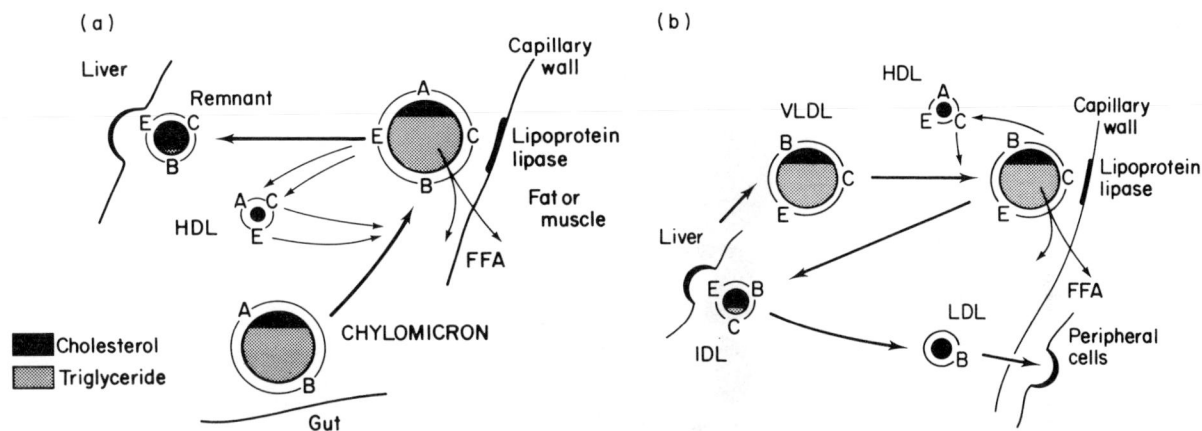

Fig. 15.7 (a) Metabolism of exogenous lipids. (b) Metabolism of endogenous lipids; lipoprotein core containing cholesterol and triglycerides, surrounded by phospholipids and apoproteins (clear areas). A, B, C, E = apoproteins. FFA = free fatty acids. (Redrawn from JF Zilva and PR Pannall, 1984, *Clinical Chemistry in Diagnosis and Treatment*, 4th edn, with permission of Lloyd-Luke, London.)

Table 15.5 Classification of lipoproteins according to electrophoretic mobility and ultracentrifuge sedimentation

Lipoprotein	Electrophoretic mobility (agar gel)	Ultracentrifuge (S_f)
Chylomicron	Nil	$10^3 - 10^5$
Very-low-density lipoprotein (VLDL)	Slow (pre-β)	20−400
Low-density lipoprotein (LDL)	Intermediate (β)	0−20
High-density lipoprotein (HDL)	Fast (α)	

S_f = Svedberg flotation units.

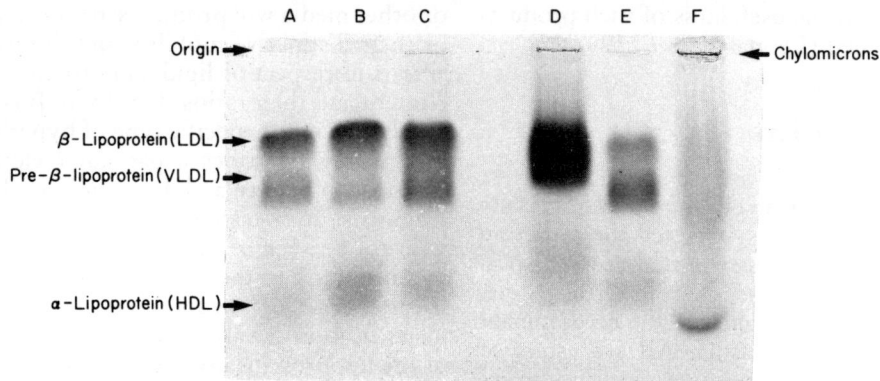

Fig. 15.8 Lipoprotein electrophoresis on agarose gel allows phenotyping of various forms of hyperlipoprotein-aemia (Frederickson/WHO system of classification). (A) Normal fasting serum; (B) type IIA showing increased β-lipoprotein; (C) type IIB with increased β- and pre-β-lipoprotein; (D) type III showing deeply stained chylomicrons at the origin and a 'broad β' band, composed of an abnormal pre-β-lipoprotein which is cholesterol rich and has the mobility of β-lipoprotein; (E) type IV showing increased pre-β-lipoprotein but normal β-lipoprotein; (F) type V grossly elevated chylomicron band at the origin. Very wide, diffuse pre-β-band with trailing lines back to the origin. Note that type I, hyperchylomicronaemia, is a very rare lipoprotein pattern, showing a heavily stained chylomicron band at the origin only. This phenotype is not shown in the photograph. (Courtesy of Dr IM Trayner.)

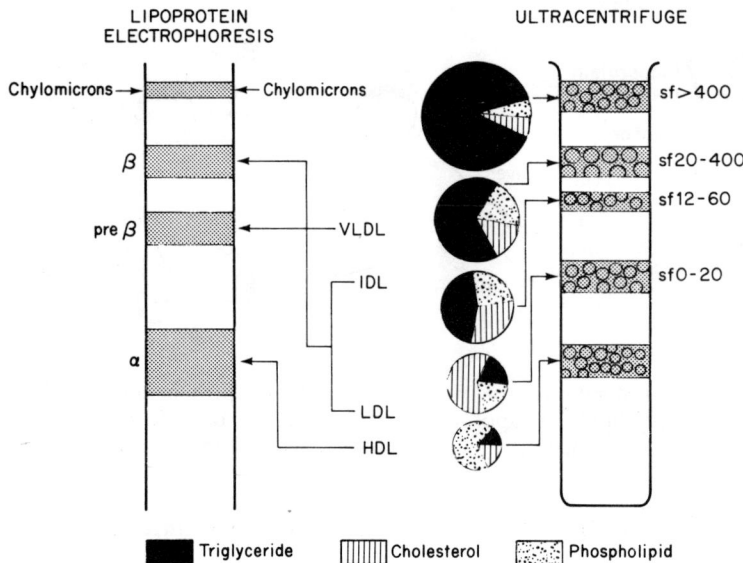

Fig. 15.9 Diagrammatic representation of the separation of lipoproteins by electrophoresis and ultracentrifugation. (Courtesy of Dr IM Trayner.)

located in the capillary walls of adipose tissue hydrolyses the triglycerides to glycerol and free fatty acids. Finally, the remnant of the chylomicrons is catabolized in the liver.

Very-low-density lipoproteins (pre-β-lipoprotein)

Very-low-density lipoproteins (VLDLs) transport endogenous triglycerides and cholesterol in a chiefly esterified form from the liver to the cells. The triglyceride is hydrolysed by lipoprotein lipase to a transient intermediate lipoprotein (IDL; *see* Fig. 15.7). Further modification of the IDL with loss of triglycerides results in the formation of LDL (low-density lipoprotein; β-lipoprotein) which is present in the plasma.

Low-density lipoproteins (β-lipoproteins)

Low-density lipoproteins (LDLs) derived catabolically from VLDLs are the major transport proteins for cholesterol and are important in the development of atheromatosis. Excess cholesterol has to be incorporated into high-density lipoprotein (HDL) if it is to be excreted in the bile. Endogenous cholesterol synthesis can be reduced by a feedback mechanism of enzyme inhibition. There is a finely balanced arrangement for controlling cholesterol uptake and synthesis.

High-density lipoproteins (α-lipoproteins)

High-density lipoproteins (HDLs) in essence are transporters of cholesterol to cells. This lipoprotein is a small phospholipid complex encircled by apoproteins A, C and E (*see* Fig. 15.7). HDLs are synthesized in hepatic and intestinal cells. Free cholesterol derived from cell membranes and other lipoproteins is taken up by HDLs and esterified – the enzyme for this catabolism is lecithin:cholesterol acyltransferase (LCAT). Much of the esterified cholesterol is transferred to IDLs, LDLs and remnant particles of chylomicrons.

Normal values

Fasting serum cholesterol and triglyceride levels above the 95th percentile are regarded as abnormal (Table 15.6). A large number of genetic and environmental factors influence the serum lipoprotein level and therefore the 95th percentile value will differ in various societies and, indeed, within a given population at different times. Serum cholesterol before puberty is 4.6 ± 0.65 mmol/l $= 180 \pm 25$ mg/dl (1 s.d.). The mean for girls is higher than for boys (0.13–0.26 mmol/l $= 5$–10 mg/dl) at all ages (Hames and Greenberg, 1961; Godfrey *et al.*, 1972) (Tables 15.6 and 15.7).

The hyperlipoproteinaemias were categorized by Fredrickson *et al.* in 1967. However, this classification has since been amended (Table 15.8). In addition, the classes reflect electrophoretic lipoprotein patterns according to the electrical charge of the apoproteins and not specific diseases. Elevated lipoprotein may be due to genetically heterogeneous determined disease or arise as a secondary phenomenon to a number of disorders (e.g. nephrotic syndrome, diabetes mellitus).

High density lipoprotein and atheroma

Lipids within the atheromatous plaque of vessels are derived from lipoproteins. As ischaemic heart disease is a major, if not epidemic, cause of death in the industrialized world, correction of lipid abnormalities is an essential prophylactic need. However, a number of prospective studies have not shown an inverse correlation between HDL cholesterol and ischaemic heart disease (Pocock *et al.*, 1986). In families where a member has died under 45 years of age, because of ischaemic heart disease or premature atherosclerosis, familial hypercholesterolaemia (FH) should be excluded in the children.

The renowned and oft-quoted Framingham study in America demonstrated an association between an elevation in LDL cholesterol and coronary heart disease. Moreover, other clinical data, namely premature atheroma in familial hypercholesterolaemia, also support the study findings. Epidemiological investigations have shown that risk factors for coronary heart disease include low HDLs. The

Table 15.6 Plasma total cholesterol (mmol/l) in white children (data modified from Tamir *et al.*, 1981)

Age (years)	Mean	95th centile	Mean	95th centile
	Males		Females	
6–7	4.0	4.9	4.2	4.9
8–9	4.0	4.8	4.3	5.2
10–11	4.2	5.4	4.2	5.2
12–13	4.1	5.2	4.2	5.4
14–15	4.0	5.1	4.0	5.1

Plasma triglycerides (mmol/l) in white children (data modified from Tamir *et al.*, 1981)

Age (years)	Mean	95th centile	Mean	95th centile
	Males		Females	
6–7	0.56	0.78	0.72	1.60
8–9	0.62	1.12	0.73	1.31
10–11	0.68	1.08	0.82	1.28
12–13	0.70	1.21	0.82	1.38
14–15	0.79	1.45	0.81	1.38

Data from the American Lipid Research Clinics Program Prevalence Study. (Modified by G. R. Thompson, London.)

Table 15.7 Suggested upper limits of normal for fasting serum cholesterol and triglyceride

Fasting serum lipid (mmol/l)	Age 0– 1 year	
	Mean + 1 s.d.	Mean + 2 s.d.
Cholesterol	2.1 (83)	2.6 (102)
Triglyceride	1.4 (53)	1.8 (68)

Values in parentheses are mg/dl.
From Drash (1972) and Andersen and Friis-Hansen (1976).

higher the plasma HDLs the lower the risk — this is not surprising in view of the role of HDL as a carrier of cholesterol from peripheral tissues for excretion. Factors associated with a high risk of cardiovascular disease and linked to low HDL levels include smoking and carbohydrate-rich diets — in contrast to exercise which increases HDLs. The alleged link between hypertriglyceridaemia and vascular disease is probably explained by the established inverse relationship of LDL triglycerides and HDL cholesterol. It is the low HDL level which represents the risk factor and not the hypertriglyceridaemia.

Prevention

There is evidence that reducing LDL cholesterol and increasing HDL cholesterol by dietary manipulation is effective in preventing atheroma (Hjermann et al., 1981). The Lipid Research Clinics Coronary Primary Prevention Trial showed the advantage of lowering cholesterol by cholestyramine and the fall in both LDL cholesterol and coronary heart disease (Lipid Research Clinics Program, 1984a,b). Theoretically, all children should be screened and, indeed, some selected fetuses.

Antenatal diagnosis of homozygous familial hypercholesterolaemia has been made by culturing amniotic cells and incubating them with labelled LDLs. In the newborn, HDL cholesterol can be measured in cord blood. Total newborn screening is as yet unrealistic because of the high incidence of false-positive in those with normal LDL levels and of false-negatives in babies with familial hypercholesterolaemia — quite apart from the colossal cost of providing such a screening service. Thompson (1985) suggests screening all children before school-leaving age. Children at particular risk of developing arterial disease should be identified and fasting blood taken on at least two occasions. Risk factors include a family history of coronary heart disease, hypertension or obesity.

Hypolipoproteinaemic disorders

These are disorders in which there is a deficit of the low density lipoprotein: abetalipoproteinaemia Bassen–Kornzweig disease; *see* p. 73; and familial high density lipoprotein deficiency (Tangier disease).

The latter is a rare disorder named after the Chesapeake Bay Island home in America of the first two patients recognized. It is characterized by large tonsils and adenoids, which are greyish-orange in colour, as a result of the presence of cholesterol esters. Many of the patients have a peripheral neuropathy. There is a severe deficiency of normal HDLs in the plasma and an accumulation of cholesterol esters in many tissues. The plasma cholesterol is low and the triglycerides normal or elevated.

Familial lecithin: cholesterol acyltransferase deficiency

This metabolic disorder is characterized by corneal

Table 15.8 WHO classification of hyperlipoproteinaemia

Type	Plasma cholesterol	LDL cholesterol	Plasma triglyceride	Lipoprotein abnormality
I	Raised	Low or normal	Raised	Excess chylomicrons
IIa	Raised or normal	Raised	Normal	Excess LDLs
IIb	Raised	Raised	Raised	Excess LDLs and VLDLs
III	Raised	Low or normal	Raised or normal	Excess chylomicron — remnants and LDLs
IV	Raised	Normal	Raised	Excess VLDLs
V	Raised	Normal	Raised	Excess chylomicrons and VLDLs

opacities from early childhood, anaemia and pro-teinuria with eventual renal failure. Also the cholesterol esters and lysolecithin are very reduced (*see* Fig. 15.10) and the LCAT absent or deficient. Foam cells are sometimes seen in bone marrow and/or the kidneys. Premature atherosclerosis takes place.

Treatment of familial hyperlipidaemias
(Table 15.9)

Familial lipoprotein lipase deficiency — type I

All fat should be restricted. If the child suffers from acute abdominal pain and vomiting then fat ought to be reduced temporarily to less than 10 g daily. Once the acute episode has passed fat can be re-introduced slowly. Usually only about 25–30 g daily can be taken without abdominal symptoms recurring. Foods that have a low or moderate fat content only should be selected (Appendix IV.25). Because medium chain triglycerides (MCTs) are not absorbed through the chylomicron route, they may provide a useful alternative source of energy. They should be introduced with caution as described in the section on MCTs in Appendix IV.7. Care must be taken to ensure that the child receives an adequate energy intake from carbohydrate and protein foods and that supplements of the fat-soluble vitamins are given. If dietary carbohydrate includes unrefined sources such as fruit, vegetables and wholemeal cereals, then abdominal discomfort associated with fat ingestion seems to be improved,

possibly due to delayed or reduced fat absorption; this type of regimen may not be possible in the younger child because they need a diet with a high energy density. As this condition is not associated with premature atherosclerosis the diet is only to relieve symptoms and, although plasma triglycerides often remain raised, there appears to be no advantage in correcting the hypertriglyceridaemia.

Familial hypercholesterolaemia — type IIa

Total energy from dietary fat should not exceed 30–35% of the complete energy intake of the child. Cholesterol needs to be restricted to 100–200 mg daily. High cholesterol foods should be avoided. All animal fats contain cholesterol; some items such as egg, offal and shellfish are particularly high. A list of the cholesterol values of some foods is given in Table 15.10. The amount of polyunsaturated fatty acids (PUFAs) relative to saturated fats (SF) should be increased so that the polyunsaturated: saturated (P:S) ratio is 1.5. If fat is used in cooking a polyunsaturated oil is preferable and a PUFA margarine should be used in place of butter or other spreading fat. The P:S ratio of some vegetable oils is given in Table 15.11. As much of the carbohydrate as possible should be of the unrefined type rich in natural fibre. In the long term this diet can prove monotonous and poor compliance is a problem particularly in adolescents. Regular monitoring of plasma cholesterol and frequent counselling about the diet is essential to maintain the interest of both the child and the family. The long-term effects of both diet, alone and combined with bile

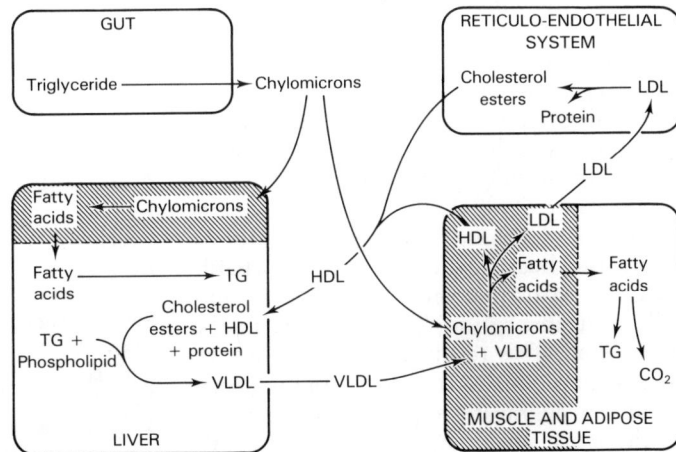

Fig. 15.10 The origin and fate of lipoproteins. TG = triglyceride. Cross-hatching represents the extracellular portion of the liver, muscle and adipose tissue. (Redrawn from EA Newsholme and C Start, 1973, *Regulation of Metabolism*, p. 211, with permission of John Wiley and Sons Ltd, Chichester.)

Table 15.9 Diets for hyperlipidaemias types I—V

Type	Diet	Fat	Cholesterol	Carbohydrate
I	Low fat	25—30 g daily Type not important MCT can be used	Not restricted	Sufficient to provide adequate energy; preferably high fibre
IIa	Low saturated fat	30—35% energy from fat. Decrease sat. fat. Increase PUFAs P:S 1.5	Low 100—200 mg daily	55% energy from carbohydrate High fibre
IIb & III	Restricted energy Low sat. fat	Normal quantity for energy requirement Decrease sat. fat, increase PUF. P:S 1.5	Moderate < 300 mg daily	Normal quantity for energy requirement High fibre
IV	Restricted carbohydrate Restricted energy	Normal quantity for energy requirement P:S 1.5	Moderate <300 mg daily	45% energy from carbohydrate. No added sucrose High fibre
V	Low fat	30% energy from fat P:1.5	Moderate—normal approx. 300 mg daily	50% energy from carbohydrate High fibre

acid binding resins has shown that this therapy is safe, effective and achieves normal growth (Glueck *et al.*, 1986).

Familial combined hyperlipidaemia — type IIb

The need for strict dietary intervention in children with this disorder has yet to be established because plasma lipid patterns are dissimilar from the adult. If there is obesity, then a weight-reducing programme is necessary, otherwise a prudent diet as commended for the general paediatric population (p. 165).

Both type IIa and IIb, diet may not correct the hypercholesterolaemia and, therefore, drug treatment will be indicated. Drug compliance in children with familial hypercholesterolaemia is poor (West *et al.*, 1980). In addition, the fibric acid agent, clofibrate, does not significantly reduce the hypercholesterolaemia. Currently, cholestyramine or colestipol are used because they are non-absorbable anion-exchange resins that bind bile acids. By impeding bile acid absorption, the synthesis in the liver is stimulated. This results in increased catabolism and a fall in plasma LDLs. Both drugs increase VLDLs and can aggravate hypertriglyceridaemia. They are therefore unsuitable for type III or IV

hyperlipoproteinaemia. Nicotinic acid and nicofuranose (a fructose ester of nicotinic acid), especially when combined with an anion exchange resin and also aspirin, have been recommended for familial hypercholesterolaemia. Probucol, if given with a resin, will decrease both LDL and HDL cholesterol. The doses used are: cholestyramine 0.6 g/kg per day or colestipol 10—20 g/day. For a resumé of lipid-lowering medications, *see Drug and Therapeutic Bulletin* (1987).

More complications, such as steatorrhoea, folate

Table 15.10 Cholesterol content of foods

Food	Cholesterol content (mg/100 g)
Cows' milk	14
Egg	484
Chicken	80
Beef	66
Liver	432
Sweetbreads	462
Prawns	149
Cheese	92
Butter	233
Vegetable margarine	0

Table 15.11 P : S ratio of vegetable oils

Oil	Polyunsaturates	Saturated fat	P : S
Coconut	0	86	—
Olive	7	11	0.36
Peanut	29	22	1.32
Soybean	59	15	3.93
Corn	54	10	5.40
Safflower	72	8	9.00

deficiency, vitamins A and E deficiency and inorganic phosphate deficiency have been associated with cholestyramine rather than colestipol. A more recently introduced drug, probucol, has been shown to cause the regression of xanthoma and produce a fall in serum cholesterol (Baker *et al.*, 1982).

Guar gum and other fibres have a hypocholesterolaemic effect in familial hypercholesterolaemia. Zavoral *et al.* (1983) recommend locust bean gum food products as a safe and useful method of lowering cholesterol in familial hypercholesterolaemia.

In the homozygous form of familial hypercholesterolaemia, diet and drug therapy may not be successful and procedures such as ileal or partial ileal bypass and portacaval shunt, as well as plasmaphoresis, have been attempted. A better technique than the latter is the specific removal of LDL by affinity chromatography. Chalstrey *et al.* (1982) advocate a combined surgical and medical approach. However, an innovative option is to stimulate LDL receptors with the hydroxymethylglutaryl CoA reductase inhibitor such as the now disgarded drug compactin (Yamamoto *et al.*, 1980), which was succeeded by the potent analogue mevinolin (Bilheimer *et al.*, 1983) and subsequently by lovastatin. Cholesterol synthesis depends upon β-hydroxy-β-methylglutaryl-CoA (HMG-CoA) reductase which is a rate limiting enzyme inhibited by the end-product cholesterol.

Familial hyperlipidaemia — type III

Dietary recommendations are similar to those for the type IIb disorder with particular emphasis on the maintenance of a normal weight. The fibric acid preparations (Anon, 1988) clofibrate, bezafibrate and gemfibrozil decrease serum triglycerides, may reduce LDL cholesterol and raise HDL cholesterol. These drugs are most effective in type III disorders.

Familial hypertriglyceridaemia — type IV

Hypertriglyceridaemia is not known to cause coronary heart disease, but it may prove to be an important independent risk factor. This condition in adults is often associated with a high intake of refined carbohydrate and obesity. Although the disorder is rarely manifested before puberty, children of affected parents should restrict their carbohydrate intake to unrefined sources as far as possible and avoid added sucrose. Dietary saturated fats should be restricted and polyunsaturated fats used in their place. Drug therapy is not usually required (Glueck, 1983).

Familial hyperlipidaemia — type V

In children the symptoms are similar to those of type I hyperlipidaemia with acute attacks of abdominal pain and pancreatitis. Dietary management is similar to that of the type I disorder; in addition, particular care is necessary to avoid high intakes of refined sugars and to maintain weight within the normal range. Marine oils rich in eicosapentaenoic and decosahexaenoic acids can decrease hypertriglyceridaemia. A concentrated fish oil preparation, Maxepa, may prove beneficial in type V hyperlipidaemia.

Nutrition and the prevention of coronary heart disease in the general paediatric population

By the age of 10 most children, even though of different geographical and ethnic origins, have fatty streaks deposited in their aorta, regardless of the composition of their diet and the incidence of coronary heart disease in their population.

However, levels of plasma cholesterol and LDLs are lower in children from less developed countries (Mendoza *et al.*, 1980). There is considerable controversy surrounding the role of diet in the prevention of atherosclerosis.

Dietary factors

Cholesterol

There is a positive correlation between serum particularly LDL cholesterol and atherosclerosis though there is no clear-cut association between dietary cholesterol intake and atherosclerosis. Studies have shown differing relationships between dietary intake and plasma levels in children (Laskarzewski *et al.*, 1979; Mellies and Glueck, 1983).

Much of the plasma cholesterol is of an endogenous source and intakes of less than 200 mg daily would be necessary to achieve a significant reduction. Such restriction is difficult to attain. Decreasing dietary cholesterol by approximately 50% led to a 15% fall in adolescents with plasma levels lower than 5.2 mmol/l (200 mg/100 ml). This effect was less marked in subjects with a lower initial value (McGandy *et al.*, 1972).

Fats

There appears to be a close correlation between the proportion of the energy in the diet which is derived from saturated fats and the development of atheroma although not between total dietary fat and atherosclerosis. The aetiology of the protective role of polyunsaturated fatty acids (PUFAs) in coronary heart disease is unclear but substitution of some of the saturated fat by PUFA might be advantageous. The reduction of the total fat content of the diet would seem to be the most beneficial dietary change that can be made. Despite this, there are disadvantages to both the reduction of total fat and the introduction of high levels of PUFA for the paediatric population. A high intake of PUFAs has been postulated in the aetiology of vitamin E deficiency and gallstones.

There is also evidence that increasing the intake of PUFAs reduces HDLs. A reduction in total fat in children and adults of normal weight means that the energy normally derived from fat must be substituted. Protein is expensive and there may be disadvantages to a high animal protein diet (*see below under* Protein). Replacement of refined carbohydrate for fat is nutritionally undesirable, because it provides few vitamins and trace elements and is associated with the development of dental caries. The use of unrefined carbohydrate would be beneficial in that it increases the fibre intake, but children under the age of 5 years with small appetites might achieve an inadequate intake from a diet with a low energy density.

Carbohydrates

High intakes of refined carbohydrate, particularly

sucrose, have been linked to elevated levels of LDLs and hypertriglyceridaemia. Also in one study a large amount of carbohydrate resulted in decreased plasma HDL cholesterol and raised triglycerides (Laskarzewski *et al.*, 1979), while others have found no correlation (Weidman *et al.*, 1978). A weak link was noted between total carbohydrate eaten, sucrose and plasma cholesterol levels in children (Mellies and Glueck, 1983), although no differentiation was made between refined and unrefined sources.

Fibre

Low quantities of dietary fibre will lead to high rates of reabsorption of bile acids in the ileum and a correspondingly diminished rate of excretion of cholesterol. A high fibre intake, particularly if consisting mainly of gums and pectins as found in vegetables and pulses, results in a lower plasma cholesterol level in adults.

Protein

Traditionally, the consumption of most animal proteins means the ingestion of large quantities of saturated fat. This might explain the correlation between coronary heart disease and dietary animal protein. Soy protein is associated with decreased plasma cholesterol levels. The protein intake, from whatever source, must meet the requirements of childhood and if a high animal protein intake is contraindicated then lower fat sources of protein should be sought (*see* Appendix IV.25)

Energy

Blood lipid levels have been shown to be higher in obese than lean children (Lauer, 1975), although obesity in adults *per se* is only a risk factor for coronary heart disease if it is complicated by other disorders, such as hypertension and diabetes mellitus. Because these diseases are frequently seen in obese adults, it would seem prudent to prevent excess weight in children and adolescents. Furthermore, there is some evidence that weight loss in obese children decreases plasma lipids.

Recommendations for the general paediatric population

Those with blood cholesterol levels between the 75th and the 90th percentile (4.4–4.8 mmol/l or 170–

185 mg/100 ml) require counselling about weight and diet and should be followed up. A reduction in dietary saturated fat to 10% of total energy, an increase in the P:S ratio (polyunsaturated fat: saturated fat) of the diet to 0.8 : 1.0 and a decrease in dietary cholesterol should reduce total and LDL cholesterol to below the 75th percentile (Glueck, 1986). Children with levels above the 90th percentile (> 4.8 mmol/l or 185 mg/100 ml) need more specific recommendations.

Advice from expert bodies for changes in national diets often overlooks guidelines for the paediatric population. However, the UK refers to children in its main report (DHSS, 1984); the Canadian report (Nutrition Committee of the Canadian Paediatric Society, 1981) and the USA (American Academy of Pediatrics, 1983) do make specific recommendations for children. A summary is given in Table 15.12.

Fat can be reduced by decreasing the amount fried foods and high fat snacks such as crisps, and by keeping to a minimum processed foods, e.g. burgers, sausages, biscuits and cakes, all of which contain large quantities of saturated fats. The white meats, chicken and turkey, are lower in total fat and cholesterol than red meats and eggs. The inclusion of white fish is advantageous because it is very low in fat and the consumption of fish oils found in the fatty fish may have a protective role against the development of atheroma. Low-fat yoghourt can be substituted for pouring cream in desserts, sauces and dressings, and home-made ice cream can be prepared from skimmed milk.

The benefits of substituting a PUFA margarine for butter are not clearly established; the use of any type of butter or margarine should be restricted to spreading on bread etc. and should not be added to vegetables or applied as a decoration. There is confusion over the amount of PUFAs in the various types of margarines. In the UK spreads containing a minimum of 40% of their total fat in the form of PUFAs can indicate on the packaging that a product is 'high' in PUFAs: soft margarines which do not make such a declaration generally have less than this amount.

Although fried foods should be kept to a minimum, when foods are prepared in this way an oil which is rich in polyunsaturates or which has a high P:S ratio would be preferable to one high in saturated fat. Confusion exists about the differences in P:S ratios between different types of vegetable fat; a list of P:S ratios is given in Table 15.11.

Infants

The previous feeding patterns of infants seems to have little influence on subsequent serum lipid profiles (Farris *et al.*, 1982). Breast-fed infants have

Table 15.12 Summary of recommendations for children not 'at risk'

Source	Fat	Cholesterol	Other recommendations
AHA	30% energy from fat <10% from PUF[a] 10% from MUF[b] 10% from SF[c]	100 mg/1000 kcal Maximum 300 mg/day	15% energy from protein 55% energy from carbohydrate primarily from complex sources Reduce sugar and salt
CMA	35% energy from fat Include a source of linoleic acid	No specific recommendations	Increase consumption of wholegrain cereals, fruit and vegetables Reduce refined sugar and salt
DHSS	35% energy from fat. <15% from SF P:S 0.45	No specific recommendations	Avoid obesity Increase consumption of wholegrain cereals Reduce refined sugar and salt

AHA : American Heart Association (1983).
CMA : Canadian Medical Association (Nutrition Committee of the Canadian Paediatric Society, 1981). For children over the age of 2 years.
DHSS: Department of Health and Social Security (1984). For children over the age of 5 years.
[a] Polyunsaturated fats; [b] monounsaturated fats; [c] saturated fats.

a higher plasma cholesterol level than those given formulae which include vegetable oils, but these differences disappear when solid foods are introduced and in older children there appears to be no correlation between breast or bottle feeding and cholesterol levels. Findings at birth are not predictive for infancy or childhood although after the age of one year plasma cholesterol is indicative of the probable subsequent percentile. Any future influences on plasma lipids should not be a consideration when selecting a feeding regimen for an infant. At weaning, very fatty foods are best avoided because infants often find difficulty in digesting them. They are also very energy dense and their use may cause satiety and deter consumption of other more beneficial foods. Low intakes of salt and sugar should be encouraged.

Infants and children up to the age of 5 years

After the age of 6 months cows' milk can be introduced. This should be a full fat milk because in infants and young children it is the major source of energy as well as of other nutrients. Beyond 2 years, should obesity appear, semi-skimmed or skimmed milk can be used, provided that vitamins A and D are given if the milk is unsupplemented, and if the overall diet is adequate. For pre-school children with a small appetite or who are finicky, it is advisable to continue with a full cream milk or

one in which vegetable oil has been substituted for butterfat. Wholly skimmed milk is not recommended for children less than 5 years (DHSS, 1987).

Children over the age of 5 years

With the proviso that the child can obtain an adequate energy intake the recommendations are as for adults.

Adolescents

This group may be reluctant to change its dietary customs. Unfortunately, many of the popular 'fast foods' are high both in total and saturated fat. Adolescents have a high energy requirement so will need to take in a fairly high-fat diet. For example, a requirement of 3000 kcal is not unusual for an active teenager and, if 35% of the energy is derived from fat, this will mean an intake of some 115 g fat daily. Hence the consumption of moderate quantities of fried foods is not unreasonable.

These recommendations are made because there is evidence to suggest that nutrition in childhood affects adult levels of plasma lipids and that an improved diet may slow the progress of later atherosclerosis. Dietary habits are formed in childhood, largely through home experience, and any changes should be adopted by the whole family if the future eating habits of the child are to be refashioned.

Section 3

NON-ENTERIC DISORDERS REQUIRING MODIFIED DIETS

16

Cardiac and Renal Disease

Congenital heart disease

Nutritional aspects

Children with congenital heart disease (CHD) may be growth retarded (Suoninen, 1971). This is particularly evident in those with cyanotic, as opposed to acyanotic, disease and, where the defect is accompanied by heart failure, growth is more markedly affected if the left-to-right shunt is large (Feldt *et al.*, 1969). In addition, infants with patent ductus arteriosus and pulmonary hypertension are more growth retarded than those with slight elevation of pulmonary artery pressure. Many factors could be implicated in the growth failure: these include hypoxia (although there is no linear relationship between the degree of hypoxia and growth retardation), altered haemodynamics, acidosis, repeated infections, genetic factors and poor nutrient intake.

Umansky and Hauck (1962) emphasize that prenatal factors and non-cardiac anomalies have a greater effect on post-operative growth than the severity of the congenital heart disease, although there is a suggestion that alterations to the haemodynamic state might have a long-term effect — even after surgical correction (Menaham, 1972). Most researchers are of the opinion that catch-up growth does occur after surgery (Naeye, 1965; Bayer and Robinson, 1969). It would appear that in the absence of a genetic abnormality contributing to growth failure (such as Down's syndrome), early corrective surgery will offer the best chance of a normal stature.

There will be little need for nutritional intervention for infants who receive early surgery, apart from maintenance of a moderate nutritional intake. For those where surgery is not available or must be delayed, then some modifications to the normal diet may be necessary to avoid stunting.

Energy

It remains unclear whether infants with congenital heart disease have increased requirements for their body mass or whether their growth failure is due entirely to a poor intake. They do, however, require an adequate energy intake for their age which may not be appropriate for their size. Appendix I.1 gives energy requirements for different ages and these recommendations should be followed in preference to those per kg body weight.

Protein

The protein intake should be generous for the infant's actual size rather than for age or expected weight because uraemia can be caused by an inappropriately high dietary protein intake. Intakes of 5–6 g protein/kg body weight per day may be tolerated and retained by infants provided a generous energy intake is achieved, but the blood urea should be monitored.

Fluid

Fluid intake is necessarily small in infants with congenital heart disease. This is because of the risk of exhaustion caused by sucking and, moreover, a high volume can result in abdominal distension and dyspnoea. In addition, there is the danger of circulatory overload. The maximum fluid intake that can be comfortably tolerated should be aimed for so that optimal nutrition is given.

Minerals and vitamins

The sodium intake should be kept to the minimum recommended for the infant's size (Appendix I.6). This is most easily met by using a dialysed whey milk (Appendix II.3). At 100 ml baby milk/kg body weight this will provide approximately 0.7 mmol sodium/kg body weight; this is less than the stated minimum requirement for an infant and care should be taken to ensure that hyponatraemia does not result. If the body sodium levels become very low, the absorption of nutrients from the gut is impaired and growth will cease. Usually (unless

a special low-sodium milk is used), if protein requirements are met from a milk source then
sodium needs are adequate. The low-fluid intake
may also mean that the daily requirements for
iron, calcium and trace elements will be insufficient
and supplements would be indicated. If diuretics
are given, the serum potassium level should be
observed and an appropriate preparation given if
indicated. A multivitamin supplement may become
necessary where a poor fluid intake continues and
this should contain vitamin K.

Feeding of infants with congenital heart disease

Infants with congenital heart disease are notoriously
poor feeders. In order to achieve a reasonable
intake it may be necessary to resort to a nasogastric
tube. Small frequent feeds will avoid the problem
of stomach distension and, if adequate supervision
is available, a continuous nasogastric infusion is
suggested. Nadas *et al.* (1981) describe a cyclic
phenomenon in which, when infants are well they
thrive nutritionally, but the resulting increase in
food intake provokes congestive cardiac failure
and, as a consequence, they undergo a period when
energy intake is suboptimal. It is important that
attention is paid to intake even when the infant
appears well so that overload is avoided.

The use of an appropriate volume of a dialysed
and adapted whey baby milk is recommended.
This may be supplemented by the addition of fat
and/or carbohydrate (Appendix III.9). If the infant
is breast fed, small quantities of a 15% solution of
glucose polymer in water, given by bottle or
spoon, will increase the energy content of the diet.
When the infant is weaned care should be taken
that the protein and energy intake does not fall;
enthusiastic encouragement of solids can mean that
milk intake is drastically reduced. If the milk is a
supplemented one this represents a large energy
deficit which is difficult to make up with weaning
foods. Solids should be introduced more slowly
than in normal infants; lumpy foods should be
introduced later than usual if the infant is a poor
feeder because there is a risk of choking. Weaning
foods should have a high protein and energy content
while being low in sodium. Items such as meat,
pulses and cereal are most suitable.

Older children

Very salty items, e.g. processed savoury items,
should be avoided in the diet and foods such as
meat, pulses and cereals encouraged (*see* Appendix
V.2). If a generous energy and protein intake is not
achieved then a high protein or high energy supplement, as described in Appendix III.12, can be
given as a drink with or between meals.

Dietary sodium and hypertension

It has been suggested that salted infant foods might
cause a predisposition to hypertension (Fries, 1976;
Guthrie, 1986). Indeed, since 1978 the commercial baby food industry in the UK has manufactured
only unsalted products. A prospective study by
Whitten and Stewart (1980) in black male infants
failed to reveal any influence of dietary sodium on
the infants' blood pressure, although a high-salt
diet caused a significant expansion of the extracellular fluid volume.

Hypertension

Sodium ought to be restricted to 1 mmol/kg per
day and occasionally to only 0.2 mmol/kg per day.
Details of the salt content of foods is given on
p. 286. Clinicians should remember that water
softening equipment can result in an increase in the
sodium load. Many medications contain sodium,
e.g. antacids, antibiotics, cough preparations, analgesics, laxatives and sedatives.

Renal disease

Acute and chronic renal failure

As renal function declines with a fall in glomerular
filtration rate (GFR), numerous metabolic, haematological, skeletal, endocrine, neurological, cardiovascular, nutritional and other sequelae arise as
attempts are made by the kidneys to maintain the
homeostasis of the internal milieu (Table 16.1).
Early dialysis, by whatever technique, and optimal
nutritional management to avoid catabolism will
stave off the onset of complications. Numerous
biochemical and multisystem disorders evolve jeop-
ardizing the well-being and ultimately the growth
of the child, unless close surveillance of the patient
is established.

Table 16.1 Summary of diet therapy in renal diseases

	Protein	Energy	Calcium and phosphorus	Sodium	Potassium	Others
GFR >50%	No restriction Adequate for age	Adequate for age	Decrease P when near GFR 50% Ca supplements if intake below recommendations	No restriction unless hypertension	No restriction	
GFR 25–50%	Normal for age Not excessive	Adequate/generous May need energy Supplement	Decrease P to requirement for height — age ? Ca supplement	No restriction unless hypertension	No restriction	Vitamin D therapy Phosphate binder
GFR 15–25%	WHO recommendations for height–age	Generous for height–age Energy supplement	Low P diet Ca supplement 1 g daily	May need 'no added salt' if NaHCO₃ used	Avoid high K foods	Vitamin D Phosphate binder Water-soluble vitamins
GFR <15%	Minimum requirements for height–age	Energy supplements	Low P diet Ca supplement	No added salt or low salt	Safe and adequate intake for height age. K/Ca resin	Vitamin D Phosphate binder Avoid excess Mg Full vitamin and trace element supplement
Haemodialysis	As tolerated At least WHO recommendations for height–age	Adequate May need energy supplement	Low P diet Ca supplement	No added salt or low salt	At least safe and adequate intake	Vitamin D Phosphate binder Full vitamin and trace element supplement
CAPD	150% WHO RDA for height–age	Normal for height–age	Low P diet Ca supplement	No added salt or normal for height–age	Normal for height–age	Vitamin D Phosphate binder Full vitamin and trace element supplement
Transplant	No restriction adequate for age	Not excessive for height–age	Normal	Normal	Normal	? vitamin D ? phosphate binder

Note: In Table 16.1, chemical formula should read $NaHCO_3$.

Dialysis

Most clinicians would agree that the following criteria justify dialysis:

1. Hyperkalaemia (K^+ > 6.5–7.0 mmol/l) unresponsive to ion-exchange resins.
2. Severe metabolic acidosis (plasma bicarbonate < 10 mmol/l) which cannot be treated with intravenous sodium bicarbonate because of the salt load.
3. Massive fluid overload.
4. Uraemic complications (e.g. neuropathy).

Complications of renal failure

Hyperkalaemia

With a fall in GFR total body potassium will rise. Most of the body's potassium is intracellular, therefore injury to tissues, e. g. acidosis, will cause a release of this electrolyte. End-stage renal failure combined with a high potassium intake in the diet will cause hyperkalaemia. Monitor blood K^+ frequently and note 'T' waves on the ECG as well as 'R' waves and the 'QRS' complex. Tall, 'tent-like' 'T' waves will indicate the presence of hyperkalaemia.

Treatment. Exchange resins where K^+ > 5.5 mmol/l. Sodium polystyrene sulphonate (Resonium A) 1 g/kg per day orally or rectally is effective where dietary control is not possible. This ion-exchange resin binds bowel K^+ and releases sodium. Where an additional sodium load is hazardous a calcium exchange resin might be preferable — calcium polystyrene sulphonate (Calcium Resonium) is such an alternative.

Rapid methods to correct hyperkalaemia include:

1. 10% calcium gluconate 1–3 ml/kg i.v. slowly under ECG control.
2. 3.75% sodium bicarbonate solution 1 or 2 ml/kg i.v. over 15 minutes.

3. Intravenous insulin and 10% glucose — 40 ml/kg of glucose followed by insulin 1 unit subcutaneously per 3 g of glucose.

With GFR <10 ml/min per 1.73 m^2 dietary K$^+$ should be less than 2 mmol/kg per day. Intravenous calcium antagonizes the influence of potassium on the myocardium.

With correction of the acidosis potassium will move into the cells thus lowering the serum level.

Hyponatraemia and hypernatraemia

Hyponatraemia in acute renal failure commonly occurs from excess fluid replacement whereas hypernatraemia might arise from a high solute load in the presence of enteritis which has caused acute renal failure. Dialysis might then be indicated to reduce the salt.

Hypertension and water retention

Hypertension in chronic renal failure is often due to sodium and water retention which cannot be handled by the diminishing number of functioning nephrons. Not infrequently, restriction of water and salt intake will control hypertension. Failing that, early dialysis to remove excess water might be indicated to control the elevated blood pressure. Anti-hypertensives such as hydralazine have a role: 0.1−0.2 mg/kg per dose i.m. or i.v. Diuretic therapy with frusemide 1−10 mg/kg per dose orally or parenterally is useful where fluid retention is suspected. If this drug is used the risk of ototoxicity, especially in the presence of very impaired renal function, needs to be considered.

Renal osteodystrophy (calcium, phosphorus and vitamin D metabolism)

A major aspect of optimal management of chronic renal failure is the early detection and prevention of skeletal or parathyroid complications.

Renal phosphate excretion is diminished in renal impairment leading to a raised plasma phosphorus and a decreased plasma ionized calcium. The parathyroid secretes parathormone in response to the hyperphosphataemia causing calcium and phosphate resorption from bone and an increased renal readsorption of calcium. Thus the calcium: phosphate ratio is normalized by this secondary hyperparathyroidism at the expense of bony tissue. The

situation is further complicated by poor gastrointestinal calcium absorption and a low drive to deposit calcium in bone due to the failing kidney's inability to hydroxylate cholecalciferol into 1,25-dihydroxycholecalciferol (1,25(OH)$_2$D$_3$). Treatment of potential bone disease should be one of the earliest therapeutic measures to be undertaken in chronic renal failure (Maschio *et al.*, 1980) and it should be started before there is a raised plasma phosphate. Treatment consists of the administration of 1,25-dihydroxycholecalciferol, but this should not be given before plasma phosphate is normalized. Aluminum hydroxide can be prescribed to bind phosphate in the gut. However, if such binders are used chronically, aluminum loading may cause toxic effects. Calcium, as calcium carbonate, should be given at a dose of 1−2 g daily. It is particularly important that any hypocalcaemia should be treated before acidosis as hypocalcaemic tetany can occur. The unpalatability of aluminum hydroxide can be disguised to some extent by baking it into sweet pastries and biscuits but non-compliance in the younger age group is a problem.

A low-phosphate diet should be followed from an early stage. A list of high- and low-phosphate foods appears in Appendix V.4. The recommended dietary allowance for phosphate appears in Appendix I.3 and the lower end of these figures should be aimed for. Milk and dairy foods are the main source of dietary phosphate in Western diets. The calcium: phosphate ratio varies in different milks (*see* Appendix II.8). Cows' milk is particularly high in phosphate and a useful method of keeping both the protein and the phosphorus content of the diet fairly low is to use a dialysed whey infant formula for older children.

Where dietary limitation of phosphate does not result in normophosphataemia, a phosphate-binding gel will help. A low phosphate diet should be followed from an early stage; this regimen has been shown to increase plasma calciferol levels, suppress hyperparathyroidism and improve growth velocity (McCrory *et al.*, 1987). The phosphate level must be monitored to ensure the gel has not induced too low a serum level.

With destruction of renal tissue, an essential active metabolite in the pathway of vitamin D synthesis is diminished (1,25-dihydroxycholecalciferol 1,25(OH)$_2$D$_3$. Hydroxylation of 25-hydroxycholecalciferol (25(OH)D$_3$) to 1,25(OH)$_2$D$_3$ does not take place thus causing rickets. Periodic radiographs of the hands and wrists will denote bone disease. 25 (OH)D$_3$ 25−50 µg/day or 1α(OH)D$_3$

4–6 µg/week might be necessary. The calcium must be monitored to avoid hypercalcaemia.

Anaemia

Depressed erythropoiesis, which is seen in chronic renal failure, causes a normochromic, normocytic anaemia. Failure of erythropoietin production and a low response to erythropoietin in uraemia leads to a decrease in red cell formation. In addition the erythrocyte has a shortened life and mobilization of red cells from body stores is below normal. Anorectic children have a low iron intake and there may be some iron loss from the gut. In addition, iron and blood are both lost during dialysis. Oral iron therapy of 2–3 mg elemental iron/kg actual body weight should correct deficiencies provided that there is no continuing loss of iron.

Blood transfusion is not commonly indicated. An excess load could provoke cardiac failure or, if blood has been stored under refrigeration, it might cause hyperkalaemia. Formerly, it was thought that transfusions jeopardized future transplantations because they stimulated circulating antibodies, but currently it is believed that some blood transfusions improve the likelihood of graft survival.

American clinical trials in 1987 with recombinant human erythropoietin have confirmed its effectiveness in stimulating erythropoiesis in adult dialysis patients. These cumulative research findings represent a major advance and will result in the improved management of anaemia and possibly anorexia too in chronic renal failure.

Hypercatabolism

Numerous complications and their sequelae are often seen in chronic renal failure including hypercatabolism (accentuated by any infection), seizures, peripheral neuropathies, encephalopathy, pericarditis, bleeding and hyperuricaemia.

A state of hypercatabolism is not uncommon in acute renal failure. This abnormal metabolic condition can be exacerbated by septicaemia or other infections.

Nutrition and chronic renal failure

Growth, energy and protein intake

Growth and body composition in children are profoundly affected by chronic renal failure (CRF) (Jones *et al.*, 1982). The failure in longitudinal growth is related to the duration of renal impairment with the most stunted children having congenital renal disorder, or having acquired the disease within the first 2 years of life. Changes in body composition in children with early acquired CRF resemble those seen in malnutrition with a low lean body mass (Jones *et al.*, 1982). These children with early CRF have a very limited capacity for catch-up growth. In order for permanent stunting to be avoided early attention should be paid to the child's nutritional status. Since height-for-age is generally low it is useful to consider the height–age of the child for determining an appropriate nutrient intake. The height–age is the age at which the measured height of the child lies on the 50th percentile of standard height charts (Wassner, 1982).

Various factors are thought to be involved in the growth failure of CRF. A deficient intake of nutrients, particularly energy, has been reported (Betts and Magrath, 1974). This may be due to anorexia or to the prescription of overly restricted diets. Children who consume less than 80% of the recommended intake for height–age or less than 60 kcal (248 kJ)/kg actual body weight fail to grow (Jones *et al.*, 1980). Experience of nocturnal nasogastric feeding in uraemic children has resulted in improve ponderal and linear growth velocity (Strife *et al.*, 1986). There is a correlation between the degree of stunting and renal impairment with a low growth velocity seen when the glomerular filtration rate falls below 25 ml/1.73 m^2.

The requirements for energy and protein for children with CRF are largely unknown. There is suggestion (Betts and Magrath, 1974) that uraemia increases the energy requirement for protein anabolism so that even children who are consuming their theoretical requirements may in fact have a deficient intake. An increased catabolic reaction to stress such as infection has been described (Chantler *et al.*, 1981) suggesting that a protein supplement, particularly of essential amino acids (EAAs) or ketoacid analogues (KAAs), might be advantageous during periods of intercurrent illness. Energy requirements can either be based on chronological age using a generous normal energy intake, or on height—age, when the intake should be 25% above the normal for height—age; when dietary protein is restricted an energy supplement should be given. Weight loss should be avoided because urea is released during tissue breakdown.

If the GFR is above 50% of normal, protein restriction has been considered to be unnecessary. It is essential that protein is not overly restricted in order that growth potential is maximized. Studies in adults have demonstrated the efficacy of a moderate protein restriction in slowing the decline of renal function. There is little evidence of the beneficial effect of early protein restriction in children (Berg *et al.*, 1987), but in any child with a reduced nephron mass, a high protein intake should be avoided (Brouhard, 1986). When the GFR falls by 25—50%, the protein intake should be based on the normal UK or USA recommendations for the child's height—age. This may mean a modest reduction in intake for some children. With a further decline in GFR, the protein intake should be based on WHO recommendations for height—age. When dietary intake of protein is restricted, it is important that requirements for EAAs are met and therefore care should be taken to ensure that high biological value protein forms the major part of the diet. For most children this means meat, fish, egg or milk protein; for vegetarian children milk should be the major source of protein with pulses or nuts contributing supplementary amounts.

It is often unnecessary formally to restrict protein because of the poor appetite shown by these children. Usually the child can be allowed to choose freely from preferred solid foods. There are several advantages to using a dialysed whey baby milk in place of cows' milk, even for older children, because not only does it contain a lower quantity of protein but probably a more advantageous balance of other nutrients. The recipe for a high-energy feed based on a milk of this type is shown in Appendix III.9.

In an unrestricted diet, protein usually contributes no more than 12—13% of the energy content of the diet, e.g. if protein intake is 20 g daily this provides 80 kcal (330 kJ). Total energy in the diet should therefore be in excess of 620 kcal (2560 kJ). When protein intake is restricted to minimal levels the protein may contribute as little as 6% of the total energy.

If protein does need to be restricted, then one method of achieving this is by using a protein-exchange system similar to the carbohydrate 'swopping' applied to diabetic diets. An example

of 6 g and 2 g exchanges used in the UK is given in Appendix V.1. A more complicated system involving food products exists in the USA; this uses food groups with variable amounts of protein.

The use of essential amino acids or ketoacid analogues of selected EAAs may decrease protein requirements; these may have advantages over EAAs in that there is evidence (Chantler *et al.*, 1980) that they stimulate protein synthesis. However, neither the minimum requirements, the optimum EAA pattern for children, the efficiency of conversion of KAAs into EAAs nor the long-term metabolic effects of their use are known.

Both EAA and KAA mixtures are available as relatively palatable drinks and the incorporation of these into the diet should present no great problem. Clinical trials have been disappointing because the construction of a palatable diet using minimal levels of natural protein is extremely difficult. Studies in infants have been more promising as the incorporation of a powder supplement into a low protein feed is less detectable.

Fat and carbohydrate

In the normal diet, energy is provided by protein, fat and carbohydrate. In renal disease the percentage energy from protein should not exceed 13%. Therefore fat and carbohydrate must be used to make up most of the energy intake. There are limitations to the use of both of these nutrients. High-carbohydrate feeding increases the hypertriglyceridaemia seen in CRF (Wassner, 1982), and insulin resistance is common. It would appear that fat is a preferable energy source, although hyperlipidaemia is a long-term problem. As much polyunsaturated fat should be used in the diet as is acceptable because the optimum P:S ratio to prevent atherogenesis is unknown. Examples of high-energy supplements are given in Appendices III.5 and IV.14.

Fibre

The amount of fibre to be included in a diet for children with CRF is difficult to quantify. Constipation should be avoided as it affects bladder emptying in young children. A high-fibre diet may impede the development of atheroma and, furthermore, it will have a low energy density. Fibre is high in phosphate, but most of this is bound in the form of phytate and is not absorbed. There are some data to suggest that certain fibre-rich diets are associated with marked malabsorption of zinc — this is particularly so in the Middle East (James, 1980). One explanation is that a high-fibre diet results in the greater ingestion of nutrients including phytate, which is known to strongly influence mineral absorption. Yet some fibres such as those rich in pectin have little effect on mineral absorption.

Sodium and potassium

Most children with CRF are able to maintain sodium balance, provided they receive a constant and moderate intake. Restriction of sodium in the diet is only necessary if hypertension, oedema or other signs of circulatory overload are present or if large quantities (up to 10 mmol/kg) of sodium bicarbonate are prescribed because of acidosis. Depletion of body sodium is more common than overload owing to the inability of the kidney to conserve sodium, diuretic therapy or the prescription of a low-sodium diet. The minimum requirements for the child's height–age should be adhered to, i.e. 25–50 mg or 1–2 mmol/kg actual body weight daily in infants and young children with a maximum of 2 g (90 mmol) daily total (including sodium prescribed as bicarbonate) in older children.

This can be achieved by a 'no added salt' diet which avoids very salty processed foods and also forbids salt added to food at the time of eating. If the dietary sodium is reduced further other problems arise: hyponatraemia, hypovolaemia and a worsening of renal function; in addition, a low-salt diet, where all food is cooked without the addition of salt, is unpalatable to children and is likely to increase the anorexia. A list of the sodium content of foods is given in Appendix V.2.

Generally potassium is the last nutrient to require dietary restriction as renal function fails. Avoidance of high potassium foods (Appendix V.3) is fairly easy but a low-potassium diet (10–20 mmol potassium daily) is unpalatable. Dialysed whey baby milks are considerably lower in potassium than cows' milk (Appendix II.4). Potassium exchange resins can be used.

Fluid intake

Fluid intake should only be restricted when signs of circulatory overload are present. Fluids present an excellent medium for increasing the energy intake by means of high-energy drinks. Children should be encouraged never to take plain water once any degree of dietary restriction has been introduced, as this has an energy value of zero. If fluids have to be restricted then it is usually necessary to restrict dietary sodium to avoid hypernatraemia.

Vitamins, minerals and trace elements

Any restriction of protein intake will result in a lowered intake of micronutrients and supplementation should be considered when protein restriction is introduced. Dialysed whey baby milks contain a useful amount of added micronutrients. A water-soluble vitamin supplement should be introduced if dietary potassium restriction is necessary and a complete vitamin and trace element supplement when dietary protein intake is down to WHO levels. Vitamin, mineral and trace element supplements are discussed in Appendix II.13.

Nutritional management of acute renal failure

The nutritional management of acute renal failure (ARF) is chiefly concerned with fluid and electrolyte intake. There is no evidence that restricting the protein intake, even if the blood urea is very high, affects the course of the disease. In practice, children with ARF are anorexic and rarely consume large quantities of protein. If a protein restriction is felt to be g desirable then an intake of 1–1.5 protein/kg body weight for children under the age of 2 years or 0.5–1.0 g protein/kg daily for older children would be suitable.

The energy intake should be as high as possible; ideally 25% above the recommendations for age should be taken to avoid catabolism and the release of nitrogen and potassium into the extracellular fluid (ECF). The energy can be boosted by giving concentrated drinks of glucose-based fluids or by clear sweets or candy.

The degree of salt restriction depends upon blood pressure and urine output; mild hypertension may require a 'no added salt' regimen if the child is taking solids, or a switch to a dialysed whey infant formula from cows' milk. For moderate and severe hypertension a low-salt diet of about 10 mmol daily along with a diuretic and a hypotensive agent may be necessary. Potassium may need to be restricted if the serum potassium is dangerously high. Soft and carbonated drinks offered to the child to boost energy intake may contain considerable amounts of sodium and/or potassium and brands should be checked for mineral content before they are offered. Most high-potassium foods should be avoided and there should be an intake of 10–20 mmol daily. A potassium/calcium exchange resin can also be used.

Fluid restriction depends upon urine output. The accepted minimal intake is 30 ml/kg body weight for infants, reducing to 10 ml/kg body weight for adolescents, plus the volume of urine passed during the previous 24 hours. If total fluid intake is less than half the normal requirement (Appendix II.6), then restriction of dietary sodium and potassium will be necessary.

For calculating intakes of fluid, nutrients and drugs, the child's normal pre-illness weight should be taken or, if this is not known, then a normal weight for the child's age can be used. The fluid and dietary restrictions described are used only for the duration of the anuria. Restrictions should be modified as soon as diuresis occurs.

Nephrotic syndrome

Dietary therapy for nephrotic syndrome involves manipulation of fluid, sodium and protein intakes to reduce oedema. In addition, obesity is a common problem in those receiving corticosteroids. Although the prescription of very low sodium diets is common there is no evidence that sodium restriction does reduce oedema. Very salty foods, however, do increase water retention and are best avoided. A 'no added salt' type of diet should be sufficient. The protein intake is determined by the degree of hypoalbuminaemia and if this does not exist then a normal protein intake for the child's age or pre-illness weight should be encouraged. If the serum albumin drops below 2 g/100 ml then a high-protein diet is indicated, and should be approximately 150% of the normal requirement. The protein needs to be of high biological value, ideally coming from fresh meat, fish and eggs. For vegetarian children or where animal foods are not available or liked by the child milk should provide at least 50% of the protein intake. A dialysed whey baby milk,

although containing less total protein, also has less sodium per gram of protein than does cows' milk.

In order to ensure that the protein in the diet is used for replacement of body stores and not for energy, an adequate non-protein energy intake must be ensured. Protein should provide no more than 14–15% of total dietary energy (Fomon, 1974). Restriction of fluid is not considered necessary unless renal failure occurs or there is hyponatraemia indicating excess fluid in relationship to sodium intake. Often children are thirsty and fluids are the best way of achieving an adequate protein and energy intake. A high-energy milk drink based on dialysed whey baby milk which would be suitable for children with nephrotic syndrome is shown in Appendix III.2. Various protein supplements with a low sodium content which can be added to milk drinks are described in Appendix IV.12.

Children with long-standing disease are likely to suffer from osteoporosis and extra calcium and vitamin D are advisable, as described under Nutrition and chronic renal failure. The serum lipid abnormalities seen in nephrotic syndrome often remain after clinical remission has occurred (Zilleruelo *et al.*, 1984) and frequent relapsers may be at risk of premature atherosclerosis. The dietary treatment for this is similar to the treatment of type IIa hyperlipidaemia and consists of reducing dietary saturated fat intake. Polyunsaturated fats can be used to improve the palatability and energy content of the diet (*see* Table 15.11).

Diet and renal replacement therapy

In general dietary restriction becomes much less important when any form of replacement therapy is started. There is a suggestion from some centres (Fennell *et al.*, 1984) that continuous ambulatory peritoneal dialysis (CAPD) results in a faster growth velocity than haemodialysis. Similarly there is a suggestion that renal osteodystrophy is improved in CAPD patients compared with haemodialysis. Calcium supplements, phosphate binders and vitamin D therapy are still used with all forms of renal replacement therapy at present.

Haemodialysis

The maximum protein intake possible which does not give rise to an unacceptable acidosis between dialyses should be aimed for. This sometimes means some degree of protein restriction although intakes should not fall below the WHO recommendations for height—age (Appendix I.2). Sodium restriction is usually of the 'no added salt' degree and high-potassium foods ought to be avoided in order to prevent hyperkalaemia. Sometimes a formal low-potassium diet is required in which case instructions should be given on appropriate food preparation methods to decrease the potassium content (Appendix V.3). The energy intake needs to be as high as can be practically managed in order that maximum growth occurs, but this is often difficult owing to the fluid restriction. At least average requirements for the child's height—age should be consumed. Water-soluble vitamins, particularly folic acid, and trace elements may be lost via the dialysate so adequate supplements for repletion should be given.

Continuous ambulatory peritoneal dialysis

Protein leaks through the peritoneum and up to 10 g amino acids and albumin daily can be lost to the body in this way. The dietary protein must be at a level which can compensate for these losses and should be of a high biological value. Protein intakes of up to 6 g protein/kg actual body weight may be required in young children; the individual requirement should be monitored by the serum albumin and, if possible, plasma amino acid levels. The protein intake in general should be approximately 50% greater than the WHO recommendations for height—age. The energy intake should be a generous one but need not necessarily be increased in line with the protein intake because glucose moves from the dialysate into the body fluids and provides an additional energy supply. Losses of water-soluble vitamins and trace elements occur and a full supplement should be prescribed.

Transplant

Once the transplanted kidney resumes full function most dietary restrictions can be lifted. However, children do show only a limited capacity for catch-up growth and care must be taken that these children do not become obese. Contributory factors to post-transplant obesity are a subnormal growth velocity, steroids and the consumption of an inappropriately high energy intake for the child's height—age.

17

Diabetes Mellitus

More numerous are the people that die at the cooking pot than are victims of starvation.

Julius Preuss

Insulin-dependent diabetes mellitus (IDDM) is one of the commonest disorders seen and affecting about 1 in 500 British children; in the USA alone there are 100 000 patients under the age of 20 years. In the last few years much progress has been made in the management of the disease such as the revolutionary recombinant DNA techniques used in the manufacture of highly purified 'human' insulin. However, the precise pathogenesis of this complex and widespread disorder is still ill understood. Secondary complications include blindness, renal failure, neuropathies and cardiovascular disease. In the UK, 1000 diabetics are added each year to the register of blind persons; in those between 30—49 years diabetes mellitus is the most common cause of blindness.

There is increasing but not conclusive evidence advocating a policy of 'tight control', i.e. not allowing the blood glucose range to deviate beyond the normal non-diabetic spectrum (Tamborlane and Sherwin, 1983; Leslie and Sperling, 1986). For succinct reviews on juvenile diabetes, *see* Castells (1984) and Travis (1987).

Prevalence and incidence

Diabetes in children is invariably of the insulin-dependent or type I variety. The prevalence ranges from 1.3 per 1000 for children under 17 years to an overall level of almost 2 per 1000 school-age children. The rates in the USA are very similar to those in England and Sweden. The two peaks in age are at 5 years and 11 years which are thought to be linked to the ages of junior or primary school entry and that of higher or secondary school admission. Seasonal analysis shows a fall in new cases during mid-summer and peaks in autumn and winter.

Aetiology

The cause of the clinical features is the diminished insulin secretion which ultimately, over a period of months or years, becomes exhausted. The major theories of aetiology include the hypotheses of genetic predisposition, infection and that of an autoimmune mechanism.

There is much animal experimental work, especially that involving an excellent model — the 'BB' wistar rat (Nakhooda *et al.*, 1976) — in addition to human observations that an environmental factor can provoke diabetes mellitus. The virus of foot and mouth disease in cattle has been linked with diabetes. Also a particular breed of mice can be made diabetic by Coxsackie B4 virus infection and epidemiologists have also associated IDDM in the human with Coxsackie B viruses (Gamble and Taylor, 1973; Hazra *et al.*, 1980). Furthermore, there may be a relationship between congenital rubella and diabetes. Specific viruses may be pancreatropic and initiate an autoimmune inflammatory reaction in the islets (insulinitis) resulting in insulin dependence.

There is a genetic susceptibility to diabetes mellitus in those with the HLA antigens HLA-B8, -DW3, -DW4 or -BW15. The HLA system which is located on chromosome-6 is the major histocompatibility complex and has an important role in immune responses.

Clinical features

The onset may be insidious but commonly it is present for less than one month. Major symptoms include: polyuria, polydipsia, weight loss and lethargy. In addition, monilial vaginitis may appear in adolescents. Only 10—20% present dramatically in a diabetic ketoacidotic state.

Insulin deficiency results in increased lipolysis

and elevated free fatty acids (FFAs). The FFAs are converted to the ketone bodies acetoacetate and hydroxybutyrate.

Diagnosis

The diagnosis can be established by an abnormal glucose tolerance test (GTT) but this is not considered essential (Wilkin *et al.*, 1987); however, a GTT will enable the renal threshold to be determined. The glucose load at 3 years of age is 2.5 g/kg decreasing to 1.75 g/kg (maximum 100 g) thereafter. Blood samples should be taken at 0, 30, 60, 90, 120 and 180 minutes. Different national and international authorities quote various values as indicating the abnormal 2-hour capillary or venous glucose level — WHO (1980, 1985) defined it as being above 7.8 mmol/l (140 mg/100 ml). Capillary samples give higher readings than venous specimens and the 2-hour glucose is probably the most reliable.

Management

The overall aim is for the child to have as near normal a lifestyle as is compatible with responsible management. The professional challenge is to bring the metabolic pathways into a state of near normality and to prevent hypoglycaemia, hyperglycaemia (Fig. 17.1) and increased lipolysis with elevated free fatty acids and ketosis. It would be a gross oversimplification to imagine that the goal of the paediatric diabetologist is solely to achieve normoglycaemia.

Proper management must include clinical surveillance of height and weight that has been recorded on centile charts. National organizations, such as the British Diabetic Association, have an educational and some an epidemiological role too. Support groups for parents and the patient are important and they should organize residential holidays with teaching seminars as well as school vacation diabetic camps.

Insulin (Fig. 17.2)

Insulins can be classified into three categories according to their duration of action:

1. Short-acting or soluble forms (approximately 1—2 hours), e.g. acid insulin and neutral insulin.
2. Intermediate acting (approximately 4—12 hours), e.g. isophane insulin and insulin zinc suspensions.
3. Long-acting (approximately 16—35 hours), e.g. ultratard.

In the UK, USA, Canada and elsewhere insulin is now dispensed in a standard strength of 100 units/ml (U 100). This policy will simplify management because formerly there were three concentrations of insulin. Furthermore, special disposable syringes for use with U 100 insulin facilitates the daily regimen. Fountain-pen style non-disposable syringes will ease management for pre-adolescents (e.g. Fig. 17.3). For some years highly purified insulins have been available in the form of short-acting (soluble), lente, ultralente and isophane types. Also there are premixed combinations of soluble and isophane insulins in a 50:50 or 30:70 proportion. An average daily dosage is 0.5—1.0 units/kg. Most diabetics, particularly prepubertal children, will need two injections a day but some during times of remission ('honeymoon period') can be satisfactorily managed on a single dose of a medium acting

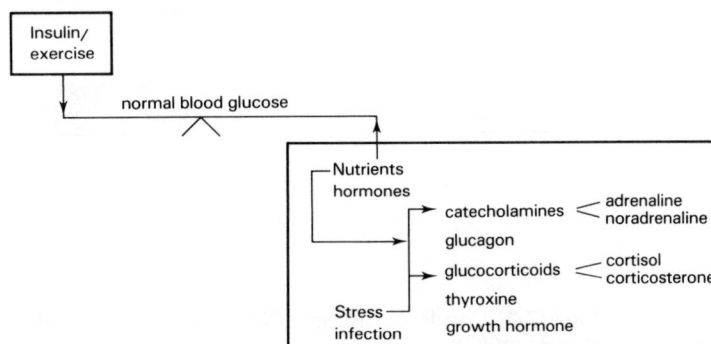

Fig. 17.1 The balance in the metabolic states of hypoglycaemia, normality and hyperglycaemia.

Preparation	Manu-facturer	Origin	Onset, peak activity and duration of action (approximate) Hours 2 6 10 14 18 22 26 30 34
NEUTRAL INSULIN INJECTION BP (INSULIN INJECTION, SOLUBLE INSULIN)			
Human Actrapid (monocomponent)	Novo	Human (emp)	
Human Velosulin (highly purified)	Nordisk/Wellcome	Human (emp)	
Humulin S	Eli Lilly	Human (prb)	
Velosulin (highly purified)	Nordisk/Wellcome	Pork	
Neutral	Evans	Beef	
Hypurin Neutral (highly purified)	C. P. Pharm	Beef	
Quicksol	Boots	Beef	
Neusulin (purified)	Wellcome	Beef	
ACID INSULIN INJECTION BP (ACID INSULIN)			
Acid Insulin (purified)	Wellcome	Beef	
Hypurin Soluble (highly purified)	C. P. Pharm	Beef	
PROTAMINE ZINC INSULIN BP			
Hypurin Protamine Zinc (highly purified)	C. P. Pharm	Beef	
ISOPHANE INSULIN INJECTION BP (ISOPHANE PROTAMINE INSULIN)			
Human Insulatard (highly purified)	Nordisk/Wellcome	Human (emp)	
Human Protaphane (monocomponent)	Novo	Human (emp)	
Humulin I	Eli Lilly	Human (prb)	
Insulatard (highly purified)	Nordisk/Wellcome	Pork	
Isophane	Evans	Beef	
Hypurin Isophane (highly purified)	C. P. Pharm	Beef	
Monophane	Boots	Beef	
Neuphane (purified)	Wellcome	Beef	
INSULIN ZINC SUSPENSION BP (AMORPHOUS)			
Semitard MC (monocomponent)	Novo	Pork	

Fig. 17.2 Available insulins. (With permission of ML Rogers (1987).)

Preparation	Manufacturer	Origin	Onset, peak activity and duration of action (approximate) — Hours (2 6 10 14 18 22 26 30 34)
INSULIN ZINC SUSPENSION BP (MIXED)			
Human Monotard (monocomponent)	Novo	Human (emp)	
Humulin Lente	Eli Lilly	Human (prb)	
Lentard MC (monocomponent)	Novo	Pork / Beef	
Lente	Evans	Beef	
Hypurin Lente (highly purified)	C. P. Pharm	Beef	
Tempulin	Boots	Beef	
Neulente (purified)	Wellcome	Beef	
INSULIN ZINC SUSPENSION BP (CRYSTALLINE)			
Humulin Zn	Eli Lilly	Human (prb)	
Human Ultratard (monocomponent)	Novo	Human (emp)	
BIPHASIC INSULIN BP			
Rapitard MC (monocomponent)	Novo	Pork / Beef	
PRE-MIXED NEUTRAL + ISOPHANE INSULINS			
Human Actraphane (monocomponent)	Novo	Human (emp)	
Human Initard 50/50 (highly purified)	Nordisk/Wellcome	Human (emp)	
Human Mixtard 30/70 (highly purified)	Nordisk/Wellcome	Human (emp)	
Humulin M1	Eli Lilly	Human (prb)	
Humulin M2	Eli Lilly	Human (prb)	
Humulin M3	Eli Lilly	Human (prb)	
Humulin M4	Eli Lilly	Human (prb)	
Initard 50/50 (highly purified)	Nordisk/Wellcome	Pork	
Mixtard 30/70 (highly purified)	Nordisk/Wellcome	Pork	

Dispensing of Insulin Preparations

Monocomponent, Human and Purified Insulins are not interchangeable with each other or with conventional insulins.

Insulins of porcine origin and human origin have a slightly shorter onset and duration of action than equivalent bovine insulins.

Human Insulins are named (emp) or (prb) according to whether they have been enzymatically prepared (semisynthetic emp) or are chain recombinant DNA bacterial (biosynthetic prb) products. The prb insulins were formerly called crb insulins; the starting point for their manufacturing process has changed.

Mixing of Insulins

Patients may be allergic to a particular species or preservative.

1. The shorter acting insulin should be drawn into the syringe first to prevent contamination of the vial by the longer acting preparation.
2. It is advisable to inject any mixture immediately.
3. Acid Insulin (pH 3.0-3.5) should not be mixed with any Insulin with neutral pH.
4. Neutral Insulin may be mixed with Isophane and Biphasic Insulins. There is some evidence of a rapid reduction in amount of Neutral Insulin when mixed with Insulin Zinc Suspensions. This seems to be greatest with pork and least with beef insulins.
5. When Neutral Insulin is mixed with Protamine Zinc Insulin there is a variable diminution of immediate effect due to reaction with excess Protamine. The combination is therefore not recommended.
6. Insulin Zinc Suspensions may be mixed with each other but not with Protamine Zinc or Isophane (because buffering media differ).

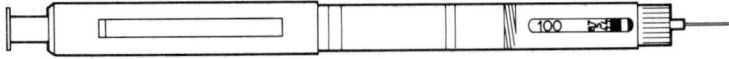

Fig. 17.3 An insulin syringe in the form of a fountain pen. The push button activates the plunger to deliver the required dose of rapid-acting insulin.

insulin. Many diabetics following the initial stabilization require less than 0.5−1.0 units/kg per day because of the influence of the residual β cells of the pancreas. The phase commonly lasts several weeks or months and rarely 1−2 years.

Some, in an endeavour to achieve very tight control, recommend three injections a day on a long-term basis but this places a considerable burden on the patient. Following an acute admission, it is an unrealistic aim to expect optimal stability on the basis of the findings in a hospital setting. The sooner the child is returned to his normal environment the better. Activity, stress, diet at school and home are quite different to an acute clinical ward and only in a more typical environment is it possible to assess the child's dietary and insulin requirements.

Insulin pumps

For optimal glucose control patients can be switched, where it is appropriate, to a subcutaneous pump delivering 1.5 units/kg per day of insulin. Such a pump offers rapid acting insulin continuously by means of a battery powered external infusion system carried by the patient. The pump is programmed to deliver low volumes of insulin but by manual means additional aliquots can be infused 15−30 minutes before a meal. A 27-gauge needle is inserted into the subcutaneous tissues of the anterior abdominal wall. Of the normal total daily dose 30−50% is given as the basal infusion and the remainder used before each meal with the largest supplemental bolus being delivered at breakfast time. Adjustments to insulin dosage should be made on the basis of frequent blood glucose samples. Although some studies have reported both improved short- and long-term control of glycaemia, the use of pumps is not without problems, including infection at the infusion site, increased risk of nocturnal hypoglycaemia and the possibility of ketoacidosis due to unnoticed cessation of the infusion (Leslie and Sperling, 1986).

Insulin source

Previously the two main sources of animal insulin were beef (bovine) and pork (porcine). The amino acid discrepancy is given in Table 17.1. From this it can be seen that porcine insulin is more closely allied to human insulin in its amino acid composition than is bovine, because it differs in only one amino acid position rather than three. The more recent highly purified insulins produced by recombinant DNA technology are thought to be less immunogenic than earlier preparations and this is probably a desirable quality, although spontaneous autoantibodies have been detected in about 38% of type I diabetics before insulin therapy has begun (Anon, 1986). Of the animal insulins, bovine is regarded as the most antigenic. Commercial insulin preparations contain a number of impurities. These are known as the:

1. 'a' fraction — non-insulin proteins.
2. 'b' fraction — proinsulin and insulin dimers.
3. 'c' fraction — monomeric insulin, insulin esters, desamido insulin and arginine insulin.

Purification is now carried out by anion exchange chromatography which removes most of these impurities and produces the so-called 'single peak' insulin.

Insulin with the exact amino acid sequence of the human hormone is now available. Novo (Copenhagen) have regular B30-alanine or porcine insulin (*see* Fig. 17.2), with a threonine residue added to the porcine insulin by an enzymatic technique, so mimicking exactly the human insulin structure.

Eli Lilly (Indianapolis) produce human insulin from proinsulin synthesized by bacteria using recombinant DNA technology (prb); this is also known as 'biosynthetic insulin'. Nordisk and Wellcome manufacture highly purified porcine insulin. Semi-synthetic insulins are labelled as 'emp'

Table 17.1 Amino acid discrepancies in porcine and bovine insulins

Position	A8	A10	B30
Human	Threonine	Isoleucine	Threonine
Porcine	Threonine	Isoleucine	Alanine
Bovine	Alanine	Valine	Alanine

(enzymatic modification of porcine insulin). Novo make both beef and porcine insulins including some that are altered to the human configuration (*see* Fig. 17.2.)

Monitoring

A written record must be kept of selective daily postprandial blood glucose readings, preinsulin levels, hypoglycaemic episodes, extra physical stress, illnesses, daily insulin dosage and urine glucose and ketone test results where indicated. In the early phase of the disease the blood glucose should be checked frequently — perhaps 2 hours after each main meal and late at night to prevent nocturnal hypoglycaemia too, as well as prior to the insulin injection(s). When the glycosylated haemoglobin and other parameters such as weight are satisfactory, the capillary sampling can be reduced to alternate days. If hypoglycaemia or the Somogyi effect is suspected, the times of peak insulin activity and the blood glucose level should be checked. If weight is falling, yet the daily record depicts normoglycaemia and the HbA$_1$ (or fructosamine) is raised, the credibility of the observations must be questioned.

Early independence in management has its advantages, but if the child is pressurized to achieve self-reliance too rapidly psychological consequences may arise.

The 24-hour fractional urine test

A random one-off urine glucose specimen is of very limited value. If the Clinitest reagent is used to test urine, the two-drop method is preferable to the standard five-drop method. Using two drops of urine and 10 drops of water the scale of urine sugars obtained after adding the Clinitest tablet is 0—5% rather than 0—2%. The appropriate colour charts can be obtained from Ames Division, Miles Laboratories. This two-drop method is now widely used in UK diabetic clinics. Diabur-Test 5000 sticks (MCP Pharmaceuticals) are more convenient than Clinitest tablets and preferable to Diastix because they read up to 5% and their colour formation is not inhibited by ketones (Kinmonth, 1987).

Clearly, a total 24-hour collection made up of different timed samples (08.00—12.00, 12.00—16.00, 16.00—20.00 and 20.00—08.00 hours) gives valuable and very relevant information (Craig, 1981). A urine glucose concentration of 0—25 g/24 hours represents good control whereas a level > 100 g/24 hours is unsatisfactory.

Self-monitoring of blood glucose at home

Self-monitoring reflects the influence of physical and emotional stresses on blood sugar levels and will detect cases of unrecognized nocturnal hypoglycaemia (Baumer *et al.*, 1982). Samples taken at a hospital clinic do not truly reflect what is happening on a normal (non-hospital) day. Parents and patients should be taught to obtain blood from a skin prick using spring-fired lances (e.g. Glucolet, Ames; Autolet, Owen Mumford). These are not painless but are usually acceptable. Topical application of an analgesic (e.g. lignocaine) prior to capillary sampling can help. There are a variety of test sticks and reflectance meters for determining blood glucose, e.g. Dextrostix, a glucose oxidase reagent (Miles Laboratories), the BM test — Glycemie (Boehringer Corporation), Glucometer II (Ames & Co.) and Reflolux II (Boehringer). Reflectance meters are designed to interpret the reading on the blood reagent preparation (Brooks *et al.*, 1986); however, the need for these expensive meters is not essential (Earis *et al.*, 1980).

Glycosylated haemoglobin (HbA$_1$)

Persistent hyperglycaemia alters the haemoglobin fraction. Unlike blood glucose specimens which constantly vary HbA$_{1c}$ specimens ('c' is the largest of the fractions a, b and c) give information about the blood glucose over the previous 4 weeks. The technique of measuring HbA$_1$ is promising and will help to achieve better monitoring particularly where there is poor clinic attendance or suboptimal management.

Unfortunately, difficulties with methodology and reliability are such that the measurement of glycosylated haemoglobin concentration is unsatisfactory as a routine laboratory technique. However, fructosamine, which is a measure of glycosylated proteins, may be preferable as an index of blood glucose control over a period of 1—3 weeks because estimation can be fully automated. There is a statistically significant correlation between fructosamine concentrations and fasting plasma glucose (Baker *et al.*, 1983).

Children and especially adolescents often have dietary whims and ignore advice from the hospital nutritionist. Diet must not be allowed to become a territory for a perennial battleground. It is known that certain types of dietary fibre (unabsorbable plant polysaccharides) will allow reduction of insulin. Guar crispbread has been shown to reduce the urinary glucose excretion by 38% (Jenkins *et al.*, 1978) and may be useful as an adjunct to treatment.

Prevention of diabetes and complications

Some features of type I IDDM suggest a genetic predisposition, detected by the HLA system, which may ultimately lead to a method of prevention. The DR4 locus is an important susceptibility factor (Schober *et al.*, 1981). Moreover, the triad of HLA identity, pancreatic islet cell antibodies and reduced insulin secretion can identify siblings at high risk of developing IDDM (Ginsberg-Fellner *et al.*, 1985). The 'honeymoon period' — during which there is still viable endocrine pancreatic tissue — could be an opportunity for treatment to prevent further damage to the islet cells with subsequent insulin dependence. Methods of immunosuppression or immunization against the viruses linked to the cause of IDDM may have a role in the treatment of those who are genetically vulnerable, although to date newly diagnosed diabetics have not benefited from treatment with interferon, azathioprine, steroids, antilymphocytic globulin or plasmaphoresis.

Varying incidence of complications has been reported in childhood onset type I diabetes. An early paper describing children with one daily insulin injection and an unmeasured diet found that after 10 years of diabetes, 52% of the patients had evidence of retinopathy and 10% were blind. There were signs of neuropathy and retinopathy in 35% and death from renal failure had occurred in 10% of the patients, all of whom were in their twenties and thirties (Knowles *et al.*, 1961). There is growing evidence that the degree of metabolic control is linked with the incidence of complications in some diabetics, although genetic susceptibility also appears to play a part. Dornan *et al.* (1982) have suggested that retinopathy is more common in patients with HLA-DR4 than in those without. Certainly, some diabetics appear to remain free of complications despite poor control, while a number with good control do develop vascular changes. Frequent monitoring of blood glucose, use of the HbA$_1$, or fructosamine assay, urine sugar fractionation and appropriate changes in insulin regimen and diet are important. The use of fluorescein angiography, though not without risk, might become a useful diagnostic tool in the early assessment of retinal changes.

Methods of treatment should be continuously reviewed; for example Kinmonth and Baum (1980) demonstrated that the timing of the morning injection of insulin was important, because it influenced the level of postprandial hyperglycaemia. If hyperglycaemia is undesirable, should the 'open-loop' subcutaneous infusion system of insulin be used (Pickup *et al.*, 1979; Watkins, 1980)?

Hypoglycaemia

Hypoglycaemia can be manifested by sweating, confusion, irritability, headache, hunger, abdominal pain, weakness or bizarre behaviour. In young children anger or a change in the behavioural pattern may be the earliest clue. The polypeptide glucagon (1 mg i.m.) can be administered if oral treatment is unsuccessful. This is usually effective and parents can be trained to use this hormone in an emergency.

The most likely causes of hypoglycaemia are incorrectly measured insulin, dietary omissions and/or strenuous exercise. If parents and children are taught the causes of hypoglycaemia then they are able to predict the predetermining factors such as physical activity or a delayed meal. During a hypoglycaemic attack a rapidly absorbed form of refined sugar is indicated — 10 g glucose as a tablet or a drink should be administered immediately, then a further 10 g of a longer acting, less readily absorbed carbohydrate should also be given if the next meal is not due within 30 minutes of the episode. A concentrated glucose gel which is absorbed through the mucous membrane of the mouth has recently become available in the UK for the treatment of hypoglycaemia. Hypoglycaemia at night is usually a source of anxiety to parents and reassurance should be given that children invariably awake when symptoms occur. Tablets of glucose or a sweet drink should be placed within easy reach at night.

Ketoacidosis

Many diabetic children present initially in a ketoacidotic condition which is an extreme medical emergency. Features include drowsiness, vomiting, dehydration, hyperglycaemia, ketosis, metabolic acidosis, glycosuria and ketonuria. With progression coma may ensue. Air hunger is manifest when Kussmaul breathing is observed. This deep rapid respiration is a compensatory measure to remove excess carbon dioxide and thus correct the metabolic acidosis.

Ketoacidosis is a serious and potentially fatal condition which requires expert care and above all an awareness of cerebral oedema. The principles of management involve accurate assessment of the dehydration and acidosis and then the use of physiological saline. The fluid loss should be repleted over 3 hours and isotonic sodium bicarbonate infused if the pH is less than 7.2.

However, it must be emphasized that inappropriate use of sodium bicarbonate can accentuate the cerebral acidosis (Craig, 1981; Castells, 1984). We have witnessed potentially lethal situations because of medical complacency and lack of expertise during the recovery phase. Meticulous and regular acid–base status and electrolyte monitoring is essential until the acidosis has resolved and also the patient is alert and able to tolerate oral nutrition. For an authoritative review of the biochemistry and physiology of diabetic ketoacidosis, *see* Krane (1987).

The future

Future research developments with great promise include the implantation of embryonic islet cells ('cytograft') into diabetics (Peterson *et al.*, 1988) or once a year injections by the use of an encapsulation system (*Diabetes Bulletin*, 1985). It is now almost two decades since the first transplants of the pancreas were carried out at the University of Minnesota but modern biotechnology might supersede surgical options (Anon, 1987).

Dietary management

The diabetic associations of several Western countries have published similar recommendations for dietary management (American Diabetes Association, 1979; Canadian Diabetes Association, 1981; British Diabetic Association, 1982) and,

although these recommendations are not specifically for children, they serve as guidelines.

Nutritional requirements

Energy

The energy intake should meet individual requirements and allow for growth; in a newly diagnosed diabetic child who is not overweight, the best guide is the child's pre-illness energy intake. This should be determined by means of a detailed diet history or the recommended daily allowances (Appendices I.1 and I.2) can be used as an indicator. The energy intake must not be excessive because there is a tendency towards obesity, especially after puberty.

Carbohydrate and fibre

The proportion of the energy intake as carbohydrate should ideally constitute about 50%. Not only is the quantity of carbohydrate important but also the type has an effect on maintenance of normal blood sugar levels. Some types of fibre such as pectin and guar depress the postprandial rise in blood glucose (Jenkins *et al.*, 1981). Peas, beans and lentils are particularly effective; cereal fibre does not appear to have the same influence. Good control in children is more closely related to the total amount of dietary fibre rather than to the carbohydrate content of the diet (Hackett *et al.*, 1986). Fibre, particularly guar in the form of granules added to food or liquid, has been investigated and does appear to delay glucose absorption provided the product is adequately mixed with food. Another development is that the enzyme inhibitors such as α-glucosidase which blocks intestinal sucrase and maltase and the luminal hydrolysis of starch (Jenkins, 1982). Both of these methods of delaying or blocking glucose absorption from the gut have yet to be widely tested in children.

It is customary to recommend that isolated or concentrated sources of mono- and disaccharides (refined sugars) such as household sugar, sweets, sweet biscuits and cakes are avoided and unrefined high fibre foods are consumed in their place, especially legumes. This means that a diet providing 50% energy from carbohydrate is a bulky one; children may find difficulty in consuming an adequate energy intake and it is often necessary to decrease the percentage of carbohydrate in the diet to 40% of total energy.

The carbohydrate should be distributed throughout the day to coincide with peak insulin activity. It is important that insulin-dependent children are instructed about the need for eating at predetermined times. Because the blood sugar pattern is less abnormal if carbohydrate is ingested in small regular quantities, the carbohydrate should be proportioned with the three meals and three snacks during the day. A method of distributing carbohydrate throughout the day is suggested in Appendix VI.6.

In most countries an exchange system for carbohydrate has been devised to allow greater flexibility with the diet. Any quantity of food containing a known amount of carbohydrate (10 g or 15 g) is known as an 'exchange' and can be substituted for any other exchange portion. A list of exchanges used by the British and American Diabetic Associations is given in Appendices VI.4—VI.5. In some centres a 'free' system is used where diabetics are advised to eat approximately the same amount of carbohydrate each day at the same time. Advice is given about the type of carbohydrate that is most beneficial, but foods or exchanges are not measured.

Fats

Due to the acknowledged risk of vascular disorders in diabetes and hypercholesterolaemia associated with cardiovascular disease, most authorities recommend that total fat should be restricted to 30—35% of the energy intake, with polyunsaturated fats replacing saturated ones where practical (*see* p. 163). Strict control of dietary cholesterol is probably unrealistic for a meat-eating diabetic and moderate restriction of this source has little effect on serum cholesterol levels. However, excessive consumption of high cholesterol foods (Appendix IV.26) should be discouraged. Diabetics should avoid fried and fatty foods and children over the age of 5 years ought to be encouraged to take low-fat skimmed milk. Under the age of 5 years it may be difficult to achieve an adequate energy intake if skimmed milk is used.

Protein

The protein requirement in diabetes is the same as for a non-diabetic child of the same size. Protein will usually contribute about 15% of the total energy intake. With the exception of skimmed milk which contains carbohydrate, it should be remembered that most sources of animal protein contain significant quantities of animal fat and the consumption of these carbohydrate-free foods, such as cheese, on a regular basis outside mealtimes should be avoided. If the child is hungry then this indicates that the energy content of the diet needs to be increased.

Minerals and vitamins

It is recommended that a low or moderate salt intake is consumed by the diabetic because of the risk of hypertension and cardiovascular disease. Children should be encouraged to add no salt to their food at the table and to avoid highly salted processed foods (Appendix V.2). Other minerals should not give cause for concern because the diabetic diet is in essence a normal one. If a low-fat unfortified milk is taken to reduce the total fat intake then a supplement of fat-soluble vitamins may be advantageous.

Special dietary foods

Special diet foods fall into three main categories and use depends upon their composition. In the first group a product such as sucrose is replaced by a low-energy artificial sweetener and these products include sugar substitutes and sugar-free drinks. The major low-energy artificial sweeteners are saccharin, aspartame and acesulphamine. Although doubts have been expressed about the safety of saccharin, the FAO/WHO Committe on Food Additives consider that an intake of 2.5 mg/kg daily is acceptable for adults. However, children should be strongly discouraged from using sugar substitutes. After a short time children become accustomed to the unsweetened taste of foods and are less likely to crave sweet foods. The use of low-energy soft drinks should be in alignment with the family policy — if the child were allowed to take this type of confectionary freely prior to the onset of diabetes then there is no real reason for its exclusion.

A second type of diabetic food has the sucrose replaced by a metabolizable sugar substitute, usually sorbitol (glucose alcohol) or fructose. Both of these have the same energy value as sucrose although their ingestion does not greatly influence blood glucose levels. This type of product often contains fat and the energy value is at least as great as its normal counterpart. Because energy is now considered to be the most important consideration in the diabetic diet there can be little place for this type of product which includes some sugar substitutes, biscuits, cakes, desserts, sweets and candies. Other disadvantages include the high price of such products, the laxative effect of sorbitol which can cause abdominal cramp and diarrhoea in young children and the hyperlipidaemic response to large quantities of this type of sweetener. If the family feels that sweet foods cannot be entirely omitted, then a small quantity of ordinary confectionary can be included at the end of a meal containing protein, fat and fibre because the absorption of sucrose will be slower under these conditions.

A further type of special diet product is that developed primarily for reducing diets. Some of these, mainly drinks, chocolate and biscuits, are designed as meal replacements and are unsuitable for diabetics. Certain types of foods such as jams, jellies and canned fruits have a reduced quantity of added sucrose and can be included in small quantities.

Diet and exercise

Exercise and/or an appropriate sport is particularly advantageous for diabetics. They should be encouraged to take regular daily exercise and to participate in games. Parents who are overprotective should be advised that obesity and poor control are commoner in sedentary children. If extra carbohydrate is not given prior to exercise then there is a risk of hypoglycaemia. It is recommended that an extra 10–20 g carbohydrate is given before a period of physical activity. In prolonged strenuous exercise small quantities of refined carbohydrate in the form of glucose tablets or drinks will help maintain a normal blood glucose profile.

Management of illness in diabetes

The principles of management of a diabetic with an intercurrent infection are still the maintenance of a normal blood glucose and avoidance of ketosis. Even if a child is not eating, insulin is essential to avoid ketoacidosis. A change to a soluble or rapid-acting insulin administered three times daily will improve control. Frequent checks should be made on the blood glucose levels and carbohydrate administered accordingly. Usually at least a half to two-thirds of the child's normal carbohydrate intake needs to be given. If the child is anorexic then carbohydrates can be given as small frequent drinks containing sucrose or glucose sipped throughout the day until the appetite improves.

General aspects of dietary treatment

Although the diet is basically a normal one, the fact that some foods — usually those attractive to children — are excluded or restricted and that foods containing carbohydrate need to be consumed at set times are likely to make the diabetic different from his peers and indeed alienate him. It is most important that the insulin regimen and the diet is tailored to the lifestyle of the child and his family. Where possible, the whole family should follow the diabetic diet to reduce feelings of isolation. The reason for the withdrawal of sweets and candies should be explained and realistic substitutes such as peanuts or sugar-free chewing gum offered. It is not uncommon for young children to believe that the injections and withdrawal of sweet foods represent punishment. Although the consumption of snacks is essential, care should be taken to design a regimen which minimizes the necessity for a diabetic child to transport and eat food at times dissimilar to that of his schoolfriends. Lack of motivation over diet has been identified as contributing to poor control in adolescents (Käär *et al.*, 1984) and it is vital that the paediatrician and dietitian continue to discuss nutritional recommendations in a non-authoritarian style with teenagers. The pre-school child represents another age group in which careful monitoring of blood glucose and considerable flexibility in diet and management is required (Golden *et al.*, 1985).

18

Psychonutritional Disorders

Obesity is harmful to the body and makes it sluggish, disturbs its functions and hinders its movements.
The Medical Aphorisms of Moses Maimonides (1135–1204)

Obesity

It takes a wise doctor to know when not to prescribe.
Gracián: *The Art of Wordly Wisdom*, 1647

Obesity — which is the presence of excessive body fat — is the commonest nutritional problem in the industrialized world. Although as many as 50% of some schoolgirl populations diet (Nylander, 1971) and despite the fact that there is much awareness of the hazards of overeating, many aspects of obesity are still controversial. Even such basic questions regarding the influences of genetic and environmental factors are disputed. The fundamental 'fat cell number and size' hypothesis, expounded more than a decade ago, is now rejected and we seem to have returned to the 'burn it off' theory (Hull, 1980). Maybe the only straightforward facet of the subject is that if the observer suspects increased body fat then indeed this is likely to be confirmed when the skinfold measurements are recorded. The clinical estimate of body fat by skinfold thickness correlates well with physicochemical techniques.

Obese children need help since much teasing and unhappiness is an invariable experience at school. Even though an adverse social and psychological background can produce overeating and subsequently obesity, it is not unreasonable while establishing therapy or support to start the child on a diet. It is undeniable that unhappiness can cause obesity and obesity unhappiness. In addition, obesity in adulthood is no longer believed to be inevitable after a childhood problem with weight; furthermore, most obese babies are not obese by the age of 4 years.

Assessment of body fatness

Clinical examination needs to include an assessment of pubertal development and anthropometry which must be carefully evaluated. Body fatness can be assessed with a skinfold caliper (e.g. Holtain) (Fig. 18.1), a tapemeasure, a stadiometer and weighing equipment. Centile charts for triceps skinfold thickness in boys and girls are available (Fig. 18.2). Where values exceed the 97th centile there is obesity (Tanner and Whitehouse, 1975). Weight in itself is a poor way to assess body fatness (Brook, 1980). Centile standards for height, weight, age and sex enable a diagnosis of obesity to be made; one criterion defines obesity as a weight exceeding the height-related weight by two times the standard deviation or more.

In adults one indicator of obesity is Quetelet's index which determines the body mass (weight/height^2 = body mass), but in children it is less useful because of a variation with age. However, body mass can be related to a theoretical child with height and weight upon the 50th centile and the measure then given a percentage value:

90% = underweight
90 – 110% = normal weight
110 – 120% = overweight
> 120% = obese (Poskitt, 1987).

Prevalence of obesity in childhood

Estimates indicate that as many as one-third of the population of the developed countries are overweight. As different definitions are used internationally to diagnose obesity, comparable comparisons are difficult: in Finnish schoolchildren it is 3% for girls and 3.5% for boys, whereas it is

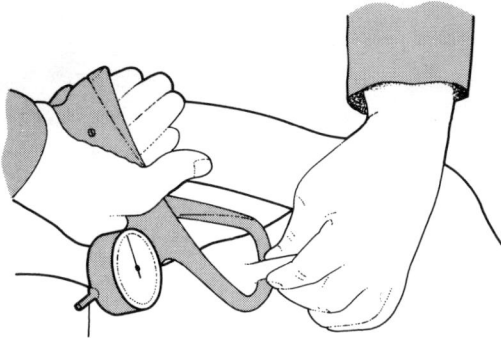

Fig. 18.1 Measuring skinfold thickness with calipers.

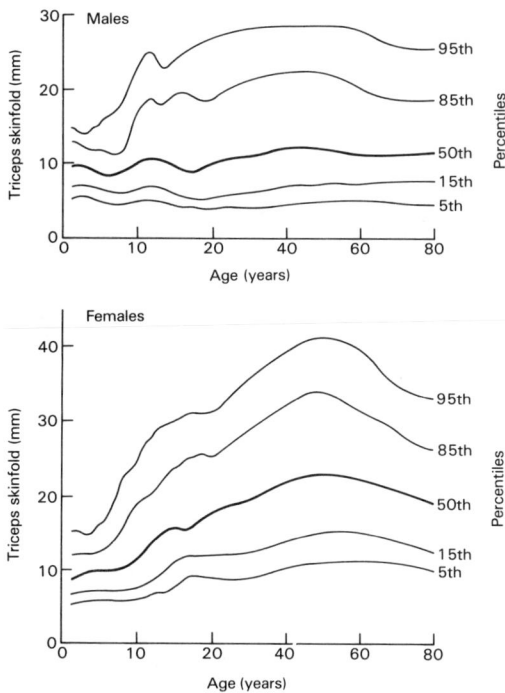

Fig. 18.2 Centiles for thickness of triceps skinfolds in white Americans based on the Ten-State Nutrition Survey of 1968–70.

0–6% in Sweden (Sveger *et al.*, 1975) and 14–35% in English infants.

Aetiology of childhood obesity

Children uncommonly have obesity secondary to a pathological disease but if present this must be identified (e.g. Prader–Willi or Laurence–Moon–

Biedl syndrome). Obesity develops only if there is a positive energy balance. Adipose tissue is formed in childhood with only a small positive energy balance. During the first years of life the average rate of energy store in fat is 37 kcal/day (155 kJ/day) which falls to 13 kcal/day (54 kJ/day). The 'adipose-cell hypothesis' arose from overfeeding or underfeeding rats during the first 3 weeks of life to produce a long-term change in adiposity. The overfed rat had more and larger adipocytes than the underfed or control animals (Knittle and Hirsch, 1968). Rats wih an increased number of fat cells later become obese. However, current evidence rejects this hypothesis in man.

Contrary to some professional subjective opinions, not all obese children eat excessively. Overweight children are less active than their leaner counterparts and this pattern of reduced physical activity is more important than overeating (Stefanik *et al.*, 1959). Observations in animals and adult men have shown that with reduced activity a corresponding decrease in food intake does not happen (Mayer *et al.*, 1954a,b). Many factors are involved in the aetiology of obesity including behavioural problems, feeding patterns within the family, nature of feeding in the newborn period, attitude of parents and siblings to obesity and physical activity.

A huge investigation into the genetic aspects of human obesity was the Ten-State Nutrition Survey (1968–1970 in USA) (*see* Fig. 18.2). Obesity was found to be significantly more common in children of fat parents and in the parents of fat children. However, a genetic explanation may not be the answer because Mason (1970) demonstrated that overweight dogs are more likely to have obese than slim owners. The implication is that people differ in the level of obesity they find acceptable both in their families as well as their pets.

The most important determinants of obesity at 2 years old have been found to be: birth weight (large babies tend to remain large) and maternal weight; breast feeding seems to protect against the development of obesity (Kramer *et al.*, 1985).

Management

Specialized obesity clinics have many advantages particularly if they are located in schools. After the initial assessment by an experienced clinician it is not essential that such a service be maintained at consultant or equivalent level.

All but a few paediatricians advocate dietary

restriction as the mainstay of treatment. Compliance can be so poor that the child and parent(s) must be highly motivated in initiating a programme of nutritional re-education to justify the enterprise (Poskitt, 1987).

In the Prader—Willi syndrome, the voracious appetite can result in gross and unsightly obesity (Fig. 18.3) unless early attempts are made to curtail excessive eating.

Methods of management

Energy restriction. Whatever the cause(s) of obesity there must be a reduction in the caloric intake. Serial measurements of height, weight and skinfold thickness need to be recorded. An integrated school-based programme of behaviour modifications, nutritional education and physical education over 10 weeks resulted in 60 (95%) of the 63 children losing weight compared with three (21%) of the 14 controls. The average loss in this very successful study was 4.4 kg (Brownell and Kaye 1982). Similarly a school-based behavioural weight-reduction programme in New York on junior highschool attenders resulted in 51% losing weight compared with 16% of the controls (Botvin *et al.*, 1979). A slow weight loss is more beneficial in the long term if deceleration of linear growth and rapid regain is not to occur. Total fasting ('zero calories regimen') is not recommended in growing individuals.

Physical exercise. Clinical studies have shown that regular exercise results in weight loss but, not surprisingly, when combined with dieting is even more effective in achieving weight reduction (Epstein *et al.*, 1985).

Behaviour therapy. This has produced promising results and should form part of a comprehensive therapeutic and educational programme of management (Brownell and Stunkard, 1978).

Anorectic drugs. These are effective but not indicated. Lorber (1966) used amphetamines and his 22 patients achieved a weight loss of 3.4 kg in the first month but later follow-up revealed most were still obese.

Surgery. Grossly obese adults have had bypass surgery which induces malabsorption to cause weight loss. Patients also reduce their food intake to avoid diarrhoea. This procedure is not without undesirable sequelae and children should not have bypass procedures carried out.

Joint management. A multidisciplinary approach

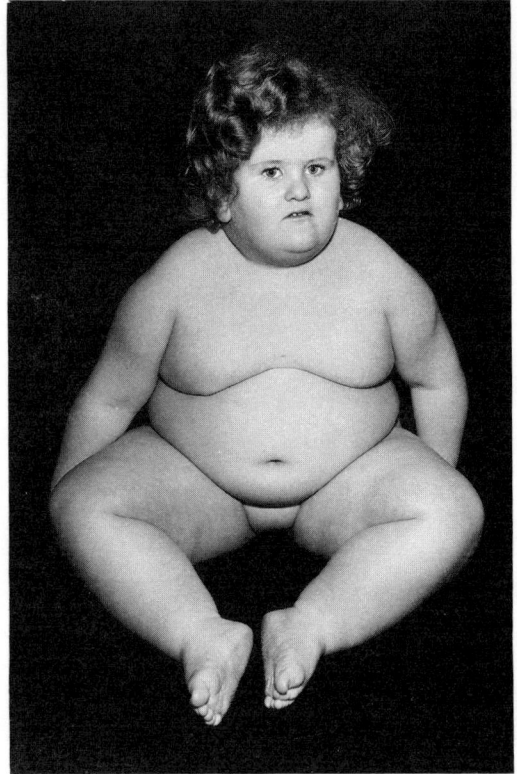

Fig. 18.3 The Prader—Willi syndrome. (Courtesy of Professor V Dubowitz.)

involving the support of parents, peers, nutritionist, paediatrician and behavioural therapist or clinical psychologist is the most advisable method of joint management (Blackburn and Greenberg, 1980). Without eliciting an attitude of high motivation most endeavours will fail. A change in lifestyle is recommended in the useful and comprehensive guidelines issued by the Office of Health Information and Health Promotion (OHIHP — USA) in a publication entitled *Matrix for Action.*

Dietary treatment

Dietary history. The child and parents should be interviewed separately in an endeavour to determine the cause of previous failures, if any, of dieting. The child's age, degree of obesity, motivation and parental support are important factors in selecting the dietary regimen to be recommended. Details of ethnic background, family structure, typical daily schedules, activities and interests provide useful information of the family lifestyle.

Food-purchasing habits, methods of preparation, availability of money and frequency of eating outside the home enable the child's meal pattern to be ascertained. A 24-hour recall, combined with frequency of consumption of individual items can be a useful guide. The dietician ought to be aware of bizarre habits such as night feasting.

Principles of dietary treatment

The nutritional adequacy of any diet is of prime importance if growth is not to be jeopardized. Furthermore, treatment can provoke antagonistic psychological responses.

Both parents and child need to be jointly involved in planning the dietary regimen. Such shared management encourages motivation and participation. Ideally, a target weight should be agreed at an early stage.

Parents should be told that fad and crash diets are potentially dangerous and must be avoided. The aim of the treatment is to correct faulty eating habits. In mild or moderate obesity it is recommended that the intake be modified to keep weight stable and allow for catch-up growth (Lole-Harris *et al.*, 1983), whereas in severe obesity the purpose is to induce a negative energy balance and slow loss of body weight. Very low energy diets need careful supervision.

Infants. Dietary restriction is not recommended for infants under 18 months old. Excessive weight gain can be controlled by correcting inappropriate feeding practices. For example, bottle-fed infants may be force-fed the residual volume of a feed to fulfil the parent's desire for an empty bottle (McWilliams, 1980). A smaller feed may be all the infant requires. Food is frequently used as a reward and also the infant's cries may be misinterpreted as hunger.

The use of low-fat milks is not recommended until the child reaches an age when he/she is receiving most of their calories from non-milk sources (Merritt and Batrus, 1980). Parents of fat infants may be in the habit of unnecessarily encouraging the child to empty the bowl or jar. If physical activity is confined to chair or playpen and the child force-fed in any way the self-regulating mechanism for weight control is over-ruled (McWilliams, 1980).

Childhood. Parents of children under 5 years old need general advice to avoid a high intake of fat and sugar. This includes removal of visible fat, use of butter or margarine in moderation and substitution of frying with other methods of cooking. A policy to limit crisps, chips (French fries), sweets and chocolate needs to be carefully planned to avoid feelings of deprivation and isolation from peers. Parents need to be aware that eating patterns established during the formative years lay the foundation for later life.

Children over 5 years can increasingly participate in the management of their eating habits. Foods taken in excess must be identified. It is unrealistic to expect total avoidance and both parents and child need to learn how to include these foods occasionally. Smaller portions, no second helpings and low-calorie brands of items such as sugar-free drinks may be sufficient to control weight gain. Any modification must ensure variety and satiety and be based on the existing family diet.

In cases of moderate obesity, the child needs to grow into his present weight whereas in more severe cases the aim is to achieve a slow loss avoiding harmful fluctuations. As one pound of excess body weight represents 3500 kcal (14.7 MJ), a daily reduction of 500 kcal (2 MJ) is needed to lose one pound (450 g) of weight per week. An average weight loss over a month shows a realistic trend. Weighing easily becomes an obsessive habit and when no weight loss is observed disappointment, if not negativism and disinterest, ensue.

A reducing diet must provide 60% of the energy requirements for the child's age. An intake of between 800–1200 kcal (3.4–5.1 MJ) is generally advised and most children lose weight on 1000 kcal (4.2 MJ) (Brooke and Abernethy, 1985). If the nutritional adequacy of the diet is in doubt supplements may be needed. Parents need to know of the unrestricted foods and of items to use with caution as well as the interchangeable isocaloric portions (Appendices VI.1 and VI.2). The skilled help of a dietitian is invaluable in aiding parents to use this information to develop an acceptable eating pattern. Once initial weight has levelled out increased exercise is recommended to balance the lowered metabolic rate (Taitz, 1983).

Adolescents. A long-standing history of childhood obesity and associated psychological difficulties is not uncommon. It is important not to pressurize this group to lose weight particularly in early adolescence when motivation is less evident (Merritt and Batrus, 1980). Emphasizing the child's failure to lose weight can result in poor self-esteem. Psychological support and behavioural modification techniques may be valuable.

At each consultation there should be an opportunity to discuss feelings and experiences and plan coping strategies for dealing with identifiable problems. A food diary can provide useful insights into eating behaviour and associated emotions. Non-diet-related asignments given between visits encourage participation (Merritt and Batrus, 1980) and help to keep the issue of food and weight in perspective. Planned activities and an exercise programme should be encouraged. Endeavours to counteract boredom should be emphasized, particularly during the school holidays, because long periods of unstructured time provide ample opportunities for eating and inactivity.

In cases of severe obesity, a protein-sparing modified fast may be useful as part of a supervised programme. However, there is the risk of inducing eating disorders such as 'bingeing' when advocating strict dietary measures.

In-patient treatment is used as a last resort to show both child and parent that weight loss can be achieved. However, facilities for intensive education are rarely available and weight is often regained after discharge from hospital. Group therapy is not as widely used with children as with adults. Successful treatment of obesity requires a prolonged commitment by the whole family. Compliance consists of implementing dietary knowledge over considerable time and long-term positive support is essential in maintaining motivation. There is a need for programmes that encourage positive attitudes and awareness of self-image and an easier relationship with food and body weight. In addition, health professionals must understand more of the psychological dynamics of food choice, eating behaviour, self-image and weight control.

Anorexia nervosa

Whosoever fasts for the sake of self-affliction is termed a sinner.
      Talmud, Ta'anit 11a The Babylonian Mar Samuel
                                    (circa 165–257)

Anorexia nervosa is a very serious disorder which is seen predominantly in young girls. It was first described in 1873 in the French medical literature by Ernest C. Laségue under the title 'anorexia hysterique' and in the same year Sir William Gull in England used the term 'anorexia nervosa' (Fig. 18.4). However, prior to 1873, sporadic case reports of what was known as 'apepsia hysterica'

appeared in publications such as the *British Medical Journal* (Anon, 1870). The disease is characterized by profound anorexia, marked weight loss and a distorted self-image with a bizarre attitude to both food and eating. In essence the diagnosis implies a terror of weight gain in a starving teenager (Crisp, 1983). Those who have reached reproductive age frequently have amenorrhoea. Cases may present as young as 7 years of age. The female to male ratio is 10:1. The morbid fear of obesity is such that the mean weight loss, when calculated on the norm for height and age, can be as high as 32% (Casper *et al.*, 1981). In the UK, there are about 100 000

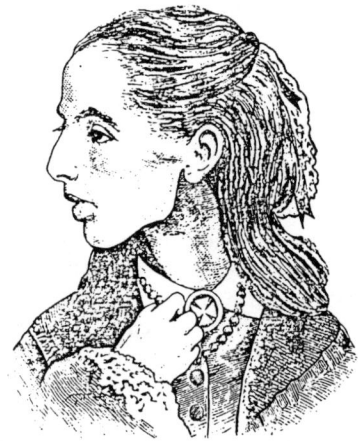

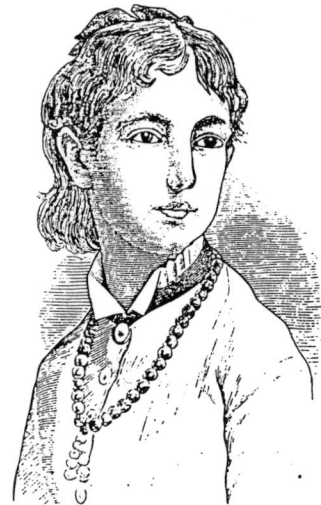

Fig. 18.4 (a) Anorexia nervosa in a 15-year-old girl (Miss C., 1873). (b) The same girl fully recovered one year later. (Woodcuts form the original paper of Gull (1874).)

cases and the average length of illness is 4 years. In one small study over a 7-year period, a poor prognosis was associated with an early age of onset (11 years) (Bryant-Waugh *et al.*, 1988). An early onset is associated with a better outcome.

Many of the girls have been described as 'over-achievers' (Warren and Wiele, 1973). Numerous endocrine and hypothalamic anomalies accompany anorexia nervosa, including abnormal thyroid function. Some may be adaptive phenomena secondary to the malnutrition. Many investigators have reported abnormal gonadotrophins and there is also a delayed response to thyrotrophin-releasing hormone. Basal plasma cortisol level can be elevated and a loss of the diurnal variation occurs.

The diagnosis is readily suspected. Any young girl, especially if from a middle-class family, with drastic weight loss from starvation and self-induced vomiting and/or diarrhoea and obsessed with food needs to be regarded as a case of anorexia nervosa. Crohn's disease can coexist with anorexia nervosa and indeed at times be mistaken for this psychopathological disorder (Jenkins *et al.*, 1988). Both of these diseases are increasing in frequency. Restlessness and insomnia with early wakening may result in the erroneous label of 'severe depression'.

Management

The essential need is to save the patient's life and correct the malnutrition. Pancreatic insufficiency and lactose intolerance may arise from the long-term inadequacies of nutrition. The mortality rate is as high as 10% in some series of hospitalized patients. Suicide is a common cause of death. Williams (1958) reported, in a retrospective analysis, that 10 out of 53 patients had died, eight solely from malnutrition. If untreated, half the patients will be severely crippled psychologically and physically compared with a quarter when given intensive therapy (Crisp, 1983). Some psychiatrists have commented that feeding helps the emotional state (Crisp, 1965). Currently it is thought that tube feeding and intravenous nutrition are rarely indicated because of the benefits of drug therapy (e.g. phenothiazines, benzodiazepines), behaviour modification, encouragement, individual and family psychotherapy or a combination of these options. Those with a weight loss below 75% of the ideal weight for height need hospital admission and those with drastic weight loss (35—40% below their usual weight), cardiac arrhythmias or under

metabolic stress justify enteric infusions of nutrients (Drossman *et al.*, 1979). This technique may achieve an impressive response (Fig. 18.5). If admitted into hospital, close surveillance is essential so as to deter illicit physical activity and the disposal of food. Out-manoeuvring of the nursing and medical staff is common and patients often undertake brisk walks through the wards until confined to bed.

Nutritional management

Enteral and parenteral feeding

Enteral or parenteral infusions are only justifiable as a life-saving measure (Fig. 18.5). Raised liver enzymes have been described in two anorectics fed intravenously with greater than 80 kcal/kg body weight daily (336 kJ/kg) (Croner *et al.*, 1985). Any regimen should have as its main aim the correction of fluid and electrolyte disturbances; the replacement of body tissue is a long-term objective best met by voluntary feeding.

In any state of chronic malnutrition a deficiency of sodium and potassium exists. The deficits should be repleted over 48 hours. If correction is too rapid then severe metabolic consequences will result. When protein deficiency is marked, an infusion of plasma may be used as a short-term replacement. Whatever enteral preparation is chosen it should be introduced slowly, giving no more than half strength and half the estimated volume requirements in the first 24 hours. An 'adult' preparation is usually suitable (*see* Appendix III.1).

Continuous infusion is likely to cause less distress than bolus feeding; the introduction of enteral feeds can induce nausea and a 'bloated' feeling. Supervision by nursing staff is vital at all times, because infusions can be disconnected and enteral fluids disposed of by the anorectic.

Oral feeding

When planning a scheme for nutritional rehabilitation it is essential that all members of the team — psychiatrist, paediatrician, nursing staff and dietician — are fully involved. Adolescents with anorexia are notoriously manipulative and quickly perceive which staff are unsure about procedures. The full nutritional requirements, taking height and age into consideration, should be calculated and a realistic 'target weight' set. The complete energy intake may not be achieved immediately but with a

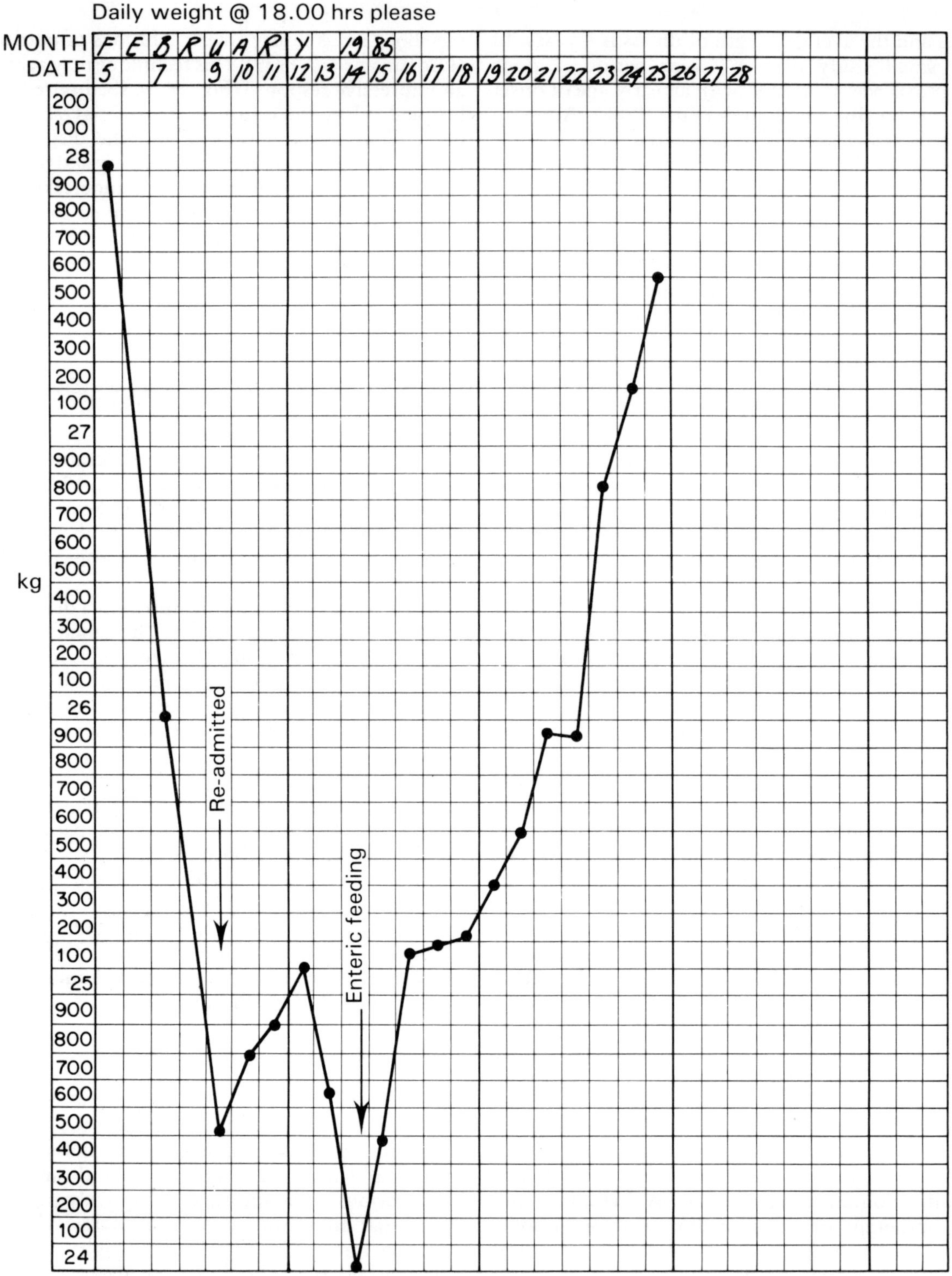

Daily weight @ 18.00 hrs please

Fig. 18.5 Daily weight chart of a 16-year-old girl with anorexia nervosa on an enteric feeding regimen.

planned series of increments should be reached over a period of 5—7 days.

The regimen should be based on normal meals that are appropriate for age. Too much choice is to be avoided, because this facilitates manipulation. A long list of 'dislikes' must be discouraged, as such items will always include bread and potato which are regarded as 'fattening'. Ideally all portions should be weighed to avoid conflict about daily variations of quantity. If this is not possible, then portion sizes should be clearly stated in handy measures such as tablespoons, slices, number of biscuits etc. and displayed so that food service staff and patients can see them. Rules about mealtimes and exactly what may be uneaten must be established at an early stage. If the patient is very underweight, then a fortified milk shake (Appendix III.3) or fruit juice supplemented with a glucose polymer (Appendix III.5) may provide extra supplements. Unfortunately, a dogmatic, inflexible attitude is justified in view of the bleak outlook. A schedule that is acceptable to the patient needs to be negotiated and it may be useful to draw up a 'contract' specifying what has been agreed upon about eating and levels of physical activity. This protocol can be signed by the patient and care staff. A punitive rather Victorian punishment and reward system is used in some centres. Pleasurable activities, for example watching television or being allowed outside the ward area, are used to encourage good behaviour and bed rest or restriction of visitors is imposed if compliance is poor. All members of the caring team must be fully conversant and in agreement regarding decisions and procedures to be followed in any circumstance.

Bulimia nervosa or the bulimic syndrome

Bulimia means 'ox-hunger' and is also known as 'binge-eating'. It was described by Russell (1979) as an 'ominous variant of anorexia nervosa'. This psychiatric disorder is characterized by episodic overeating which is followed by self-induced vomiting, purgation or periodic starvation in an endeavour to avoid weight gain. In common with anorexia nervosa, to which it is related, the patients are mainly young women who have a fear of obesity — indeed a history of obesity and anorexia is seen in almost 50% of cases. There may be a switch from bulimia nervosa to anorexia nervosa

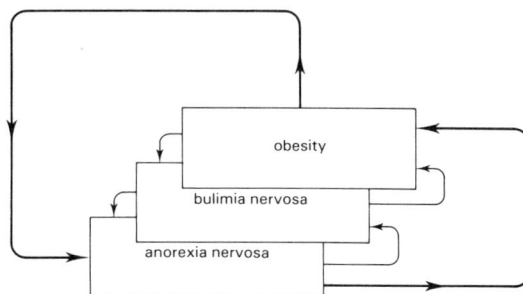

Fig. 18.6   Interrelationship between anorexia nervosa, bulimia nervosa and obesity.

or the features of both might coexist (Fig. 18.6).

Depression, suicidal ideas, shop-lifting, alcoholism and drug abuse are some of the characteristics of this psychological disease. Bulimic episodes are associated with distress and anger. Diagnostic criteria have been defined by Russell (1979) and the American Psychiatric Association (1980).

Management

Since the main characteristics of this condition are 'binge-eating' coupled with a desire to lose weight, the nutritional management is aimed at normalizing eating habits initially, followed by advice on moderate calorie restriction later.

In a similar way to that described for the treatment of anorexia nervosa (p. 193), firm rules must be laid down. A meal plan, with times that foods must be eaten, is drawn up and the bulimic encouraged to consume foods at set times, whether she is hungry or not. The meals should still be consumed even if there has been a recent incident of hyperphagia. All meals should include carbohydrate, usually 50—60 g, because a low intake appears to be one of the triggers for binge-eating. Once the patient has achieved some measure of control over her eating pattern, then a planned programme of gradual weight loss can be instituted. Psychotherapeutic support and behavioural therapy may also have a role (Lacey, 1983; Freeman *et al.*, 1988).

Drug treatment has relied on antidepressants and other thymoleptic agents. It has been suggested that an abnormal regulation of endogenous opioid peptides is the cause of this disorder. Jonas and Gold (1986), using the opioid antagonist, naltrexone, support the theory that opioids may have a role in the pathophysiology of bulimia.

Appendix I: Nutrient requirements and height/weight data

I.1 Recommendations for energy intake

Age	FAO[a]	Age	Energy (kcal/day) UK[b]	Age	USA[c]
		0−3/12	kg × 115	0−6/12	kg × 115
3−6/12	kg × 100	3−6/12	kg × 100		
6−9/12	kg × 95	6−9/12	kg × 100		
9−12/12	kg × 100	9−12/12	kg × 100	6−12/12	kg × 105
		Boys			
1−2 years	kg × 105	1 year	1200	1−3 years	1300
2−3	kg × 100	2	1400		
3−5	kg × 95	3−4	1560	4−6	1700
		Girls			
		1 year	1100		
		2	1300		
		3−4	1500		
Boys		Boys			
5−7	kg × 90	5−6	1740		
7−10	kg × 78	7−8	1980	7−10	2400
		9−11	2280		
Girls		Girls			
5−7	kg × 85	5−6	1680		
7−10	kg × 67	7−8	1900		
		9−11	2050		
Boys		Boys		Boys	
10−12	2200				
12−14	2400	12−14	2640	11−14	2700
14−16	2650				
16−18	2850	15−17	2880	15−18	2800
Girls		Girls		Girls	
10−12	1950				
12−14	2100	12−14	2150	11−14	2200
14−16	2150				
16−18	2150	15−17	2150	15−18	2100

[a] Energy and Protein Requirements: Report of Joint FAO/WHO/UNU Expert Committee (FAO, 1985).
[b] Recommended daily amounts of food energy and nutrients for groups of people in the United Kingdom (DHSS, 1979).
[c] Food and nutrition board recommended dietary allowances (Natl Acad. Sci., 1980).

I.2 Recommendations for protein intake

Age	FAO[a]	Age	Protein (g per day) UK[b]	Age	USA[c]
0–3/12	kg × 2.40	0–3/12	kg × 2.80	0–6/12	kg × 2.20
3–6/12	kg × 1.85	3–6/12	kg × 2.50		
6–9/12	kg × 1.65	6–9/12	kg × 2.50		
9–12/12	kg × 1.50	9–12/12	kg × 2.50	6–12/12	kg × 2.00
		Boys			
1–2 years	kg × 1.20	1 year	30	1–3 years	23
2–3	kg × 1.50	2	35		
3–5	kg × 1.10	3–4	39	4–6	30
		Girls			
		1 year	27		
		2	32		
		3–4	37		
		Boys			
5–7	kg × 1.00	5–6	43	7–10	34
		7–8	49		
7–10	kg × 1.00	9–11	57		
		Girls			
		5–6	42		
		7–8	47		
		9–11	51		
Boys		Boys		Boys	
10–12	kg × 1.00				
12–14	kg × 1.00	12–14	66	11–14	45
14–16	kg × 0.95				
16–18	kg × 0.90	15–17	72	15–18	56
Girls		Girls		Girls	
10–12	kg × 1.00				
12–14	kg × 0.95	12–14	53	11–14	46
14–16	kg × 0.90				
16–18	kg × 0.80	15–17	57	15–18	46

[a] Energy and Protein Requirements: Report of Joint FAO/WHO/UNU Expert Committee (FAO, 1985).
[b] Recommended amounts of food energy and nutrients for groups of people in the United Kingdom (DHSS, 1979).
[c] Food and nutrition board recommended dietary allowances (Natl Acad. Sci., 1980).

I.3 Recommendations for intakes of minerals

Age	Calcium (mg)			Phosphorus (mg)	Magnesium (mg)	Iron (mg)			Zinc (mg)	Iodide (µg)
	FAO[c]	UK[a]	USA[b]	USA[b]	USA[b]	FAO[c]	UK[a]	USA[b]	USA[b]	USA[b]
0−6/12	500−600	600	360	240	50	5−10	6	10	3	40
6−12/12	500−600	600	540	360	70	5−10	6	15	5	50
1−3 years	400−500	600	800	800	150	5−10	7−10	15	10	70
4−6	400−500	600	800	800	200	5−10	10	10	10	90
Boys										
7−9	400−500	600	800	800	250	5−10	10	10	10	120
10−12	600−700	700	800	800	350	5−10	12	10	10	150
13−15	600−700	700	1200	1200	350	9−18	12	18	15	150
16−19	500−600	600	1200	1200	400	5−9	12	18	15	150
Girls										
7−9	400−500	600	800	800	250	5−10	7−10	10	10	120
10−12	600−700	700	800	1200	300	5−10	12	18	10	150
13−15	600−700	700	1200	1200	300	12−24	12	18	15	150
16−18	400−500	600	1200	1200	300	14−28	12	18	15	150

[a] Recommended amounts of food energy and nutrients for groups of people in the United Kingdom (DHSS, 1980).
[b] Food and nutrition board recommended dietary allowances (Natl Acad. Sci., 1980).
[c] Handbook on Human Nutritional requirements (WHO, 1974).
FAO and UK — no recommendations for phosphorus, magnesium, zinc and iodide.

I.4 Recommendations for intakes of B vitamins

Age	Thiamine (mg)			Riboflavin (mg)			Niacin (mg NE[a])			Pyridoxine (mg)	Folate (µg)			Vitamin B$_{12}$ (µg)	
	FAO[d]	UK[b]	USA[c]	FAO	UK[b]	USA[c]	FAO[d]	UK[b]	USA[c]	USA[c]	FAO[d]	UK[b]	USA[c]	FAO[d]	USA[c]
0−6/12	0.3	0.3	0.3	0.5	0.4	0.4	5.4	5	6	0.3	60	50	30	0.3	0.5
6−12/12	0.3	0.3	0.5	0.5	0.4	0.6	5.4	5	8	0.6	60	50	45	0.3	1.5
1−3 years	0.5	0.6	0.7	0.8	0.5−0.8	0.8	9	7−9	9	0.9	100	100	100	0.9	2
4−6	0.7	0.7	0.9	1.1	0.9	1	12.1	10	11	1.3	100	200	200	1.5	2.5
Boys															
7−9	0.9	0.8	1.2	1.3	1	1.4	14.5	11	16	1.6	100	200	300	1.5	3
10−12	1	0.9	1.4	1.6	1.2	1.4	17.2	14	18	1.8	100	200	300	2	3
13−15	1.2	1.1	1.4	1.7	1.4	1.7	19.1	16	18	1.8	200	300	400	2	3
16−18	1.2	1.2	1.4	1.8	1.7	1.7	20.3	19	18	2.0	200	300	400	2	3
Girls															
7−9	0.9	0.8	1.2	1.3	1	1.4	14.5	11	16	1.6	100	200	300	1.5	3
10−12	0.9	0.8	1.1	1.4	1.2	1.3	15.5	14	15	1.8	100	200	300	2	3
13−15	1	0.9	1.1	1.5	1.4	1.3	16.4	16	14	1.8	200	300	400	2	3
16−18	0.9	0.9	1.1	1.4	1.7	1.3	15.2	19	14	2	200	300	400	2	3

[a] mg nicotinic acid equivalents.
[b] Recommended amounts of food energy and nutrients for groups of people in the United Kingdom (DHSS, 1980).
[c] Food and nutrition board recommended dietary allowances (Natl Acad. Sci., 1980).
[d] *Handbook on Human Nutritional Requirements* (WHO, 1974).
FAO and UK — no recommendation for pyridoxine.
UK — no recommendation for vitamin B$_{12}$.

I.5 Recommendations for intakes of fat-soluble vitamins and vitamin C

Age	Vitamin A (µg RE)			Vitamin D (µg)			Vitamin E (mg)	Vitamin C (mg)		
	FAO[c]	UK[a]	USA[b]	FAO[c]	UK[a]	USA[b]	USA[b]	FAO[c]	UK[a]	USA[b]
0−6/12	300	450	420	10	7.5	10	3	20	20	35
6−12/12	300	450	400	10	7.5	10	4	20	20	35
1−3 years	250	300	400	10	10	10	5	20	20	45
4−6	300	300	500	10	10	10	6	20	20	45
Boys										
7−9	400	400	700	2.5	(10[d])	10	7	20	20	45
10−12	575	575	1000	2.5	(10[d])	10	8	20	25	50
13−15	725	725	1000	2.5	(10[d])	10	8	30	25	50
16−18	750	750	1000	2.5	(10[d])	10	10	30	30	60
Girls										
7−9	400	400	700	2.5	(10[d])	10	7	20	20	45
10−12	575	575	800	2.5	(10[d])	10	8	20	25	50
13−15	725	725	800	2.5	(10[d])	10	8	30	25	50
16−18	750	750	800	2.5	(10[d])	10	8	30	30	60

[a] Recommended amounts of food energy and nutrients for groups of people in the United Kingdom (DHSS, 1980).
[b] Food and nutrition board recommended dietary allowances (Natl Acad. Sci., 1980).
[c] *Handbook on Human Nutritional Requirements* (WHO, 1974).
[d] 10 µg vitamin D recommended daily in winter for children and adolescents; no recommendation for summer months if exposed to sunlight.
FAO and UK — no recommendation for vitamin E.
RE = retinol equivalent.

I.6 Recommendations for intakes of fluids and electrolytes

Age	Fluid (ml/kg)	Sodium (mmol/kg)	USA[a] (mmol/day)	Potassium (mmol/kg)	USA[a] (mmol/day)	Chloride (mmol/kg)	USA[a] (mmol/day)
0−3/12	150	2.5−3.8	5.0−15.2	2.8−4.0	9.0−23.7	2.5−3.8	7.7−19.7
3−6/12	130	2.0−3.8		2.5−3.8		2.0−3.8	
6−9/12	120	1.5−3.6	10.8−32.6	2.3−3.6	11.0−32.6	1.5−3.6	11.2−33.8
9−12/12	110	1.2−3.6		2.0−3.4		1.2−3.6	
1−3 years	95	1.0−3.3	14.1−16.3	1.1−3.3	14.1−42.3	1.0−3.3	14.1−42.2
4−6	85	0.9−3.0	19.5−58.6	1.0−3.0	19.8−59.6	0.9−3.0	19.7−59.1
7−10	75	0.8−2.8	26.0−78.2	0.9−2.8	25.6−77.9	0.8−2.8	26.0−78.2
11−14	55	0.8−2.4	39.1−117.4	0.8−2.4	39.1−117.3	0.8−2.4	39.4−118.3
15+	50	0.7−2.0	39.1−117.4	0.7−2.0	39.1−117.3	0.7−2.0	39.4−118.3

[a] Estimated safe and adequate dietary intakes (Natl Acad. Sci., 1980).

I.7 Estimated safe and adequate dietary intakes of additional nutrients[a]

Age	Vitamin (μg)	Biotin (μg)	Pantothenic acid (mg)	Copper (mg)	Manganese (mg)	Fluoride (mg)	Chromium (mg)	Selenium (mg)	Molybdenum (mg)
0–6/12	12	35	2	0.5–0.7	0.5–0.7	0.1–0.5	0.01–0.04	0.01–0.04	0.03–0.06
6–12/12	10–20	50	3	0.7–1.0	0.7–1.0	0.2–1.0	0.02–0.06	0.02–0.06	0.04–0.08
1–3 years	15–30	65	3	1.0–1.5	1.0–1.5	0.5–1.5	0.02–0.08	0.02–0.03	0.05–0.10
4–6	20–40	85	3–4	1.5–2.0	1.5–2.0	1.0–2.5	0.03–0.12	0.03–0.12	0.06–0.15
7–10	30–60	120	4–5	2.0–2.5	2.0–3.0	1.5–2.5	0.05–0.20	0.05–0.20	0.10–0.30
11+	50–100	100–200	4–7	2.0–3.0	2.5–5.0	1.5–2.5	0.05–0.20	0.05–0.20	0.15–0.50

[a] Estimated safe and adequate dietary intakes (Natl Acad. Sci., 1980).

I.8 Length (cm) by age of boys aged 0–36 months

Age (months)	Centiles		
	3rd	50th	97th
0	46.2	50.5	54.8
1	49.9	54.6	59.2
2	53.2	58.1	62.9
3	56.1	61.1	66.1
4	58.6	63.7	68.7
5	60.8	65.9	71.0
6	62.8	67.8	72.9
7	64.5	69.5	74.5
8	66.0	71.0	76.0
9	67.4	72.3	77.3
10	68.7	73.6	78.6
11	69.9	74.9	79.9
12	71.0	76.1	81.2
13	72.1	77.2	82.4
14	73.1	78.3	83.6
15	74.1	79.4	84.8
16	75.0	80.4	85.9
17	75.9	81.4	87.0
18	76.7	82.4	88.1
19	77.5	83.3	89.2
20	78.3	84.2	90.2
21	79.1	85.1	92.2
22	79.8	86.0	91.2
23	80.6	86.8	93.1
24	81.3	87.6	94.0
25	82.1	88.5	94.8
26	82.8	89.2	95.7
27	83.6	90.0	96.5
28	84.4	90.8	97.2
29	85.1	91.6	98.0
30	85.8	92.3	98.7
31	86.6	93.0	99.5
32	87.3	93.7	100.2
33	88.0	94.5	100.9
34	88.6	95.2	101.7
35	89.3	95.8	102.4
36	89.9	96.5	103.2

Length = recumbent body length.
These data were intended for use within the USA.
United States Public Health Service,
Health Resources Administration.
NCHS Growth Charts,
Rockville, MD, 1976 (HRA 76-1120, 25, 3).

I.9 Length (cm) by age of girls aged 0–36 months

Age (months)	Centiles		
	3rd	50th	97th
0	45.8	49.9	53.9
1	49.2	53.5	57.9
2	52.2	56.8	61.3
3	54.9	59.5	64.2
4	57.2	62.0	66.8
5	59.2	64.1	69.0
6	61.0	65.9	70.9
7	62.5	67.6	72.6
8	64.0	69.1	74.2
9	65.3	70.4	75.6
10	66.6	71.8	77.0
11	67.8	73.1	78.3
12	69.0	74.3	79.6
13	70.1	75.5	80.9
14	71.2	76.7	82.1
15	72.2	77.8	83.3
16	73.2	78.9	84.5
17	74.2	79.9	85.6
18	75.1	80.9	86.7
19	76.1	81.9	87.8
20	77.0	82.9	88.8
21	77.8	83.8	89.8
22	78.7	84.7	90.8
23	79.5	85.6	91.7
24	80.3	86.5	92.6
25	81.1	87.3	93.5
26	81.9	88.2	94.4
27	82.7	89.0	95.3
28	83.4	89.8	96.1
29	84.2	90.6	96.9
30	84.9	91.3	97.7
31	85.6	92.1	98.5
32	86.3	92.8	99.3
33	87.0	93.5	100.1
34	87.6	94.2	100.8
35	88.2	94.9	101.6
36	88.8	95.6	102.3

Length = recumbent body length.
These data were intended for use within the USA.
United States Public Health Service,
Health Resources Administration.
NCHS Growth Charts,
Rockville, MD, 1976 (HRA 76-1120, 25, 3).

I.10 Stature (cm) by age of boys aged 2–18 years

Age (years)	(months)	Centiles		
		3rd	50th	97th
2	0	79.6	85.6	91.6
2	6	83.8	90.4	97.1
3	0	87.8	94.9	102.1
3	6	91.5	99.1	106.7
4	0	94.9	102.9	111.0
4	6	98.2	106.6	114.9
5	0	101.3	109.9	118.6
5	6	104.2	113.1	122.0
6	0	107.0	116.1	125.2
6	6	109.6	119.0	128.3
7	0	112.1	121.7	131.3
7	6	114.5	124.4	134.2
8	0	116.9	127.0	137.0
8	6	119.2	129.6	139.9
9	0	121.5	132.2	142.8
9	6	123.7	134.8	145.9
10	0	126.0	137.5	149.0
10	6	128.3	140.3	152.3
11	0	130.6	143.3	155.9
11	6	133.0	146.4	159.7
12	0	135.5	149.7	163.8
12	6	138.1	153.0	167.9
13	0	140.9	156.5	172.0
13	6	143.8	159.9	175.9
14	0	147.0	163.1	179.2
14	6	150.4	166.2	182.0
15	0	153.8	169.0	184.2
15	6	157.1	171.5	185.8
16	0	160.0	173.5	187.1
16	6	162.3	175.2	188.0
17	0	163.9	176.2	188.6
17	6	164.5	176.7	189.0
18	0	164.4	176.8	189.2

Stature = standing height.
These data were intended for use within the USA.
United States Public Health Service,
Health Resources Administration.
NCHS Growth Charts,
Rockville, MD, 1976 (HRA 76-1120, 25, 3).

I.11 Stature (cm) by age of girls aged 2–18 years

Age (years)	(months)	Centiles		
		3rd	50th	97th
2	0	78.5	84.5	90.5
2	6	82.9	89.5	96.0
3	0	86.9	93.9	100.9
3	6	90.6	97.9	105.3
4	0	94.0	101.6	109.2
4	6	97.2	105.1	113.0
5	0	100.1	108.4	116.7
5	6	102.8	111.6	120.3
6	0	105.4	114.6	123.9
6	6	107.9	117.6	127.4
7	0	110.3	120.6	130.9
7	6	112.6	123.5	134.3
8	0	115.0	126.4	137.7
8	6	117.5	129.3	141.1
9	0	120.0	132.2	144.5
9	6	122.6	135.2	147.8
10	0	125.4	138.3	151.2
10	6	128.5	141.5	154.5
11	0	131.7	144.8	157.8
11	6	135.2	148.2	161.2
12	0	138.7	151.5	164.4
12	6	141.9	154.6	167.2
13	0	144.6	157.1	169.7
13	6	146.5	159.0	171.6
14	0	147.8	160.4	172.9
14	6	148.6	161.2	173.9
15	0	149.1	161.8	174.5
15	6	149.5	162.1	174.8
16	0	149.9	162.4	175.0
16	6	150.4	162.7	175.0
17	0	151.1	163.1	175.0
17	6	151.8	163.4	174.9
18	0	152.5	163.7	174.9

Stature = standing height.
These data were intended for use within the USA.
United States Public Health Service,
Health Resources Administration.
NCHS Growth Charts,
Rockville, MD, 1976 (HRA 76-1120, 25, 3).

I.12 Weight (kg) by age of boys aged 0–36 months

Age (months)	Centiles		
	3rd	50th	97th
0	2.5	3.3	4.2
1	3.0	4.3	5.6
2	3.6	5.2	6.7
3	4.2	6.0	7.6
4	4.8	6.7	8.4
5	5.4	7.3	9.1
6	6.0	7.8	9.7
7	6.5	8.3	10.2
8	7.0	8.8	10.7
9	7.4	9.2	11.1
10	7.7	9.5	11.5
11	8.0	9.9	11.9
12	8.2	10.2	12.2
13	8.5	10.4	12.5
14	8.7	10.7	12.8
15	8.8	10.9	13.1
16	9.0	11.1	13.3
17	9.1	11.3	13.6
18	9.3	11.5	13.8
19	9.4	11.7	14.0
20	9.5	11.8	14.2
21	9.7	12.0	14.4
22	9.8	12.2	14.6
23	9.9	12.4	14.8
24	10.1	12.6	15.0
25	10.2	12.8	15.2
26	10.4	13.0	15.4
27	10.5	13.1	15.6
28	10.6	13.3	15.8
29	10.8	13.5	16.0
30	10.9	13.7	16.2
31	11.1	13.8	16.4
32	11.2	14.0	16.6
33	11.3	14.2	16.8
34	11.5	14.4	17.0
35	11.6	14.5	17.3
36	11.8	14.7	17.5

These data were intended for use within the USA.
United States Public Health Service,
Health Resources Administration.
NCHS Growth Charts,
Rockville, MD, 1976 (HRA 76-1120, 25, 3).

I.13 Weight (kg) by age of girls aged 0−36 months

Age (months)	Centiles		
	3rd	50th	97th
0	2.3	3.2	3.9
1	2.9	4.0	5.0
2	3.4	4.7	6.0
3	4.0	5.4	6.9
4	4.6	6.0	7.6
5	5.1	6.7	8.3
6	5.6	7.2	8.9
7	6.0	7.7	9.5
8	6.4	8.2	10.0
9	6.7	8.6	10.4
10	7.0	8.9	10.8
11	7.3	9.2	11.2
12	7.6	9.5	11.5
13	7.8	9.8	11.8
14	8.0	10.0	12.0
15	8.1	10.2	12.3
16	8.3	10.4	12.5
17	8.5	10.6	12.7
18	8.6	10.8	13.0
19	8.8	11.0	13.2
20	8.9	11.2	13.4
21	9.1	11.4	13.6
22	9.3	11.5	13.9
23	9.4	11.7	14.1
24	9.6	11.9	14.3
25	9.7	12.1	14.6
26	9.9	12.3	14.8
27	10.1	12.4	15.0
28	10.2	12.6	15.2
29	10.4	12.8	15.5
30	10.5	12.9	15.7
31	10.6	13.1	15.9
32	10.8	13.3	16.1
33	10.9	13.4	16.3
34	11.0	13.6	16.6
35	11.2	13.8	16.8
36	11.3	13.9	17.0

These data were intended for use within the USA.
United States Public Health Service,
Health Resources Administration.
NCHS Growth Charts,
Rockville, MD, 1976 (HRA 76-1120, 25, 3).

I.14 Weight (kg) by age of boys aged 2–18 years

Age		Centiles		
(years)	(months)	3rd	50th	97th
2	0	10.2	12.3	15.5
2	6	10.9	13.5	16.8
3	0	11.6	14.6	18.0
3	6	12.4	15.7	19.3
4	0	13.1	16.7	20.5
4	6	13.9	17.7	21.8
5	0	14.7	18.7	23.2
5	6	15.5	19.7	24.7
6	0	16.3	20.7	26.2
6	6	17.1	21.7	27.9
7	0	17.9	22.9	29.8
7	6	18.7	24.0	31.8
8	0	19.5	25.3	34.1
8	6	20.2	26.7	36.5
9	0	21.0	28.1	39.2
9	6	21.8	29.7	42.1
10	0	22.7	31.4	45.2
10	6	23.7	33.3	48.4
11	0	24.8	35.3	51.7
11	6	26.1	37.5	55.1
12	0	27.6	39.8	58.7
12	6	29.3	42.3	62.3
13	0	31.2	45.0	65.9
13	6	33.4	47.8	69.5
14	0	35.9	50.8	73.2
14	6	38.4	53.8	76.7
15	0	40.9	56.7	80.1
15	6	43.4	59.5	83.4
16	0	45.7	62.1	86.4
16	6	47.8	64.4	89.2
17	0	49.6	66.3	91.6
17	6	51.0	67.8	93.7
18	0	52.0	68.9	95.3

These data were intended for use within the USA.
United States Public Health Service,
Health Resources Administration.
NCHS Growth Charts,
Rockville, MD, 1976 (HRA 76-1120, 25, 3).

I.15 Weight (kg) by age of girls aged 2—18 years

Age (years)	(months)	Centiles		
		3rd	50th	97th
2	0	9.6	11.8	14.4
2	6	10.5	13.0	16.2
3	0	11.3	14.1	17.8
3	6	12.1	15.1	19.1
4	0	12.8	16.0	20.4
4	6	13.4	16.8	21.6
5	0	14.0	17.7	22.9
5	6	14.6	18.6	24.3
6	0	15.3	19.5	25.8
6	6	15.9	20.6	27.6
7	0	16.7	21.8	29.7
7	6	17.4	23.3	32.2
8	0	18.3	24.8	35.0
8	6	19.2	26.6	38.0
9	0	20.2	28.5	41.3
9	6	21.3	30.5	44.7
10	0	22.5	32.5	48.2
10	6	23.8	34.7	51.8
11	0	25.2	37.0	55.3
11	6	26.7	39.2	58.7
12	0	28.3	41.5	62.0
12	6	30.0	43.8	65.1
13	0	31.7	46.1	68.0
13	6	33.5	48.3	70.7
14	0	35.2	50.3	73.0
14	6	36.8	52.1	75.1
15	0	38.3	53.7	76.8
15	6	39.7	55.0	78.2
16	0	40.8	55.9	79.1
16	6	41.6	56.4	79.7
17	0	42.3	56.7	80.0
17	6	42.7	56.7	80.0
18	0	42.9	56.6	79.9

These data were intended for use within the USA.
United States Public Health Service,
Health Resources Administration.
NCHS Growth Charts,
Rockville, MD, 1976 (HRA 76-1120, 25, 3).

I.16. Weight (kg) by length of boys and girls 49—54 cm in height

Length (cm)	Centiles		
	3rd	50th	97th
Boys			
49	2.5	3.1	4.1
50	2.6	3.3	4.3
51	2.7	3.5	4.5
52	2.8	3.7	4.7
53	3.0	3.9	5.0
54	3.1	4.1	5.2
Girls			
49	2.6	3.3	3.9
50	2.7	3.4	4.1
51	2.8	3.5	4.4
52	2.9	3.7	4.6
53	3.0	3.9	4.9
54	3.2	4.1	5.1

Length = recumbent body length.
These data were intended for use within the USA.
United States Public Health Service, Health Resources Administration.
NCHS Growth Charts, Rockville, MD, 1976 (HRA 76-1120, 25, 3).

I.17. Weight (kg) by stature of boys 55—145 cm in height

Length (cm)	Centiles		
	3rd	50th	97th
55	2.9	4.3	6.6
56	3.2	4.7	6.9
57	3.5	5.0	7.3
58	3.8	5.4	7.6
59	4.1	5.7	7.9
60	4.4	6.0	8.3
61	4.6	6.3	8.6
62	4.9	6.6	8.9
63	5.2	6.9	9.2
64	5.4	7.2	9.5
65	5.7	7.5	9.8
66	5.9	7.7	10.1
67	6.2	8.0	10.4
68	6.4	8.3	10.7
69	6.7	8.5	10.9
70	6.9	8.8	11.2
71	7.1	9.0	11.5
72	7.4	9.2	11.7
73	7.6	9.5	12.0
74	7.8	9.7	12.2
75	8.0	9.9	12.5
76	8.2	10.1	12.7
77	8.4	10.4	13.0
78	8.7	10.6	13.2

I.17. *(Contd)*

Length (cm)	Centiles		
	3rd	50th	97th
79	8.9	10.8	13.5
80	9.1	11.0	13.7
81	9.3	11.2	13.9
82	9.5	11.5	14.2
83	9.7	11.7	14.4
84	9.9	11.9	14.6
85	10.1	12.1	14.9
86	10.3	12.3	15.1
87	10.5	12.6	15.3
88	10.7	12.8	15.5
89	10.9	13.0	15.8
90	11.1	13.3	16.0
91	11.3	13.5	16.2
92	11.5	13.7	16.5
93	11.7	14.0	16.7
94	11.9	14.2	17.0
95	12.1	14.5	17.2
96	12.3	14.7	17.5
97	12.5	15.0	17.8
98	12.7	15.2	18.0
99	12.9	15.5	18.3
100	13.2	15.7	18.6
101	13.4	16.0	18.9
102	13.6	16.3	19.2
103	13.9	16.6	19.5
104	14.1	16.9	19.8
105	14.3	17.1	20.2
106	14.6	17.4	20.5
107	14.8	17.7	20.9
108	15.1	18.0	21.2
109	15.4	18.3	21.6
110	15.6	18.7	22.0
111	15.9	19.0	22.4
112	16.2	19.3	22.8
113	16.5	19.6	23.3
114	16.8	20.0	23.7
115	17.1	20.3	24.2
116	17.4	20.7	24.7
117	17.7	21.1	25.2
118	18.1	21.4	25.7
119	18.4	21.8	26.2
120	18.8	22.2	26.8
121	19.1	22.6	27.3
122	19.5	23.0	27.9
123	19.8	23.4	28.6
124	20.2	23.9	29.2
125	20.6	24.3	29.8
126	21.0	24.8	30.5
127	21.4	25.2	31.2
128	21.8	25.7	31.9
129	22.2	26.2	32.7
130	22.6	26.8	33.5

I.17. *(Contd)*

Length (cm)	Centiles		
	3rd	50th	97th
131	23.0	27.3	34.3
132	23.4	27.8	35.1
133	23.8	28.4	35.9
134	24.3	29.0	36.8
135	24.7	29.6	37.7
136	25.2	30.2	38.7
137	25.6	30.9	39.6
138	26.0	31.6	40.6
139	26.5	32.3	41.6
140	27.0	33.0	42.7
141	27.4	33.7	43.8
142	27.9	34.5	44.9
143	28.3	35.2	46.1
144	28.8	36.1	47.2
145	29.3	36.9	48.5

Stature = standing height.
These data were intended for use within the USA.
United States Public Health Service, Health Resources Administration.
NCHS Growth Charts, Rockville, MD, 1976 (HRA 76-1120, 25, 3).

I.18. Weight (kg) by stature of girls 55–137 cm in height

Length (cm)	Centiles		
	3rd	50th	97th
55	3.0	4.3	6.6
56	3.3	4.7	6.9
57	3.6	5.0	7.3
58	3.8	5.3	7.6
59	4.1	5.7	7.9
60	4.4	6.0	8.3
61	4.6	6.3	8.6
62	4.9	6.6	8.9
63	5.1	6.9	9.2
64	5.4	7.1	9.4
65	5.6	7.4	9.7
66	5.8	7.7	10.0
67	6.1	7.9	10.2
68	6.3	8.2	10.5
69	6.5	8.4	10.7
70	6.7	8.6	11.0
71	7.0	8.9	11.2
72	7.2	9.1	11.4
73	7.4	9.3	11.7
74	7.6	9.5	11.9
75	7.8	9.7	12.1
76	8.0	10.0	12.4
77	8.2	10.2	12.6
78	8.4	10.4	12.8

I.18. *(Contd)*

Length (cm)	Centiles		
	3rd	50th	97th
79	8.6	10.6	13.0
80	8.8	10.8	13.3
81	9.0	11.0	13.5
82	9.2	11.2	13.7
83	9.4	11.4	13.9
84	9.6	11.6	14.2
85	9.8	11.8	14.4
86	10.0	12.0	14.6
87	10.2	12.3	14.9
88	10.4	12.5	15.1
89	10.6	12.7	15.4
90	10.8	12.9	15.6
91	11.0	13.2	15.9
92	11.2	13.4	16.2
93	11.4	13.6	16.4
94	11.6	13.9	16.7
95	11.8	14.1	17.0
96	12.0	14.3	17.3
97	12.2	14.6	17.6
98	12.4	14.9	17.9
99	12.6	15.1	18.2
100	12.8	15.4	18.5
101	13.0	15.6	18.8
102	13.3	15.9	19.1
103	13.5	16.2	19.4
104	13.7	16.5	19.8
105	14.0	16.7	20.1
106	14.2	17.0	20.5
107	14.4	17.3	20.8
108	14.7	17.6	21.2
109	15.0	17.9	21.5
110	15.2	18.2	21.9
111	15.5	18.6	22.3
112	15.8	18.9	22.7
113	16.1	19.2	23.1
114	16.4	19.5	23.6
115	16.7	19.9	24.0
116	17.0	20.3	24.5
117	17.3	20.6	25.0
118	17.6	21.0	25.5
119	18.0	21.4	26.1
120	18.3	21.8	26.7
121	18.6	22.2	27.3
122	19.0	22.7	27.9
123	19.4	23.1	28.6
124	19.7	23.6	29.3
125	20.1	24.1	30.1
126	20.5	24.6	30.9
127	20.9	25.1	31.8
128	21.3	25.7	32.6
129	21.7	26.2	33.6

I.18. *(Contd)*

Length (cm)	Centiles		
	3rd	50th	97th
130	22.1	26.8	34.6
131	22.6	27.4	35.6
132	23.0	28.0	36.7
133	23.5	28.7	37.8
134	23.9	29.4	39.0
135	24.4	30.1	40.3
136	24.9	30.8	41.6
137	25.3	31.5	43.0

Stature = standing height.
These data were intended for use within the USA.
United States Public Health Service, Health Resources Administration.
NCHS Growth Charts, Rockville, MD, 1976 (HRA 76-1120, 25, 3).

I.19. Nomogram for determination of surface area

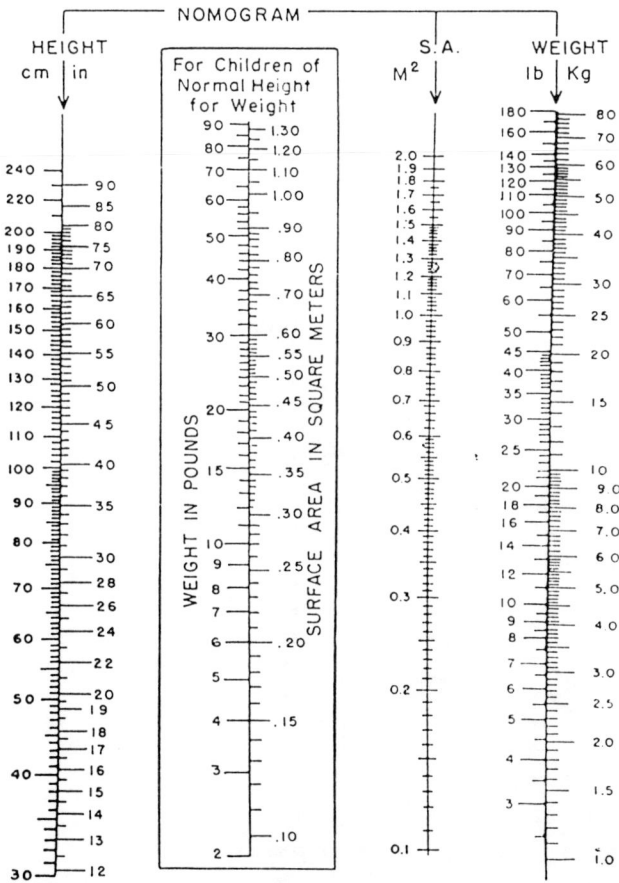

Weight range (kg)	Approximate SA (m²)
1–5	$m^2 = 0.05 \times W^* + 0.05$
6–10	$m^2 = 0.04 \times W + 0.10$
11–20	$m^2 = 0.03 \times W + 0.20$
21–70	$m^2 = 0.02 \times W + 0.40$

* W = weight (kg)

The surface area is indicated where a straight line connecting the height and weight intersects the surface area (SA) column or, if the patient is roughly of normal proportions, from the weight alone (enclosed area). (From Shirkey HC (1975) *Pediatric Therapy*, 5th edn, p. 26, CV Mosby, St Louis)

I.20. Growth and development chart. © Creaseys of Hertford Limited. Reprinted with kind permission.

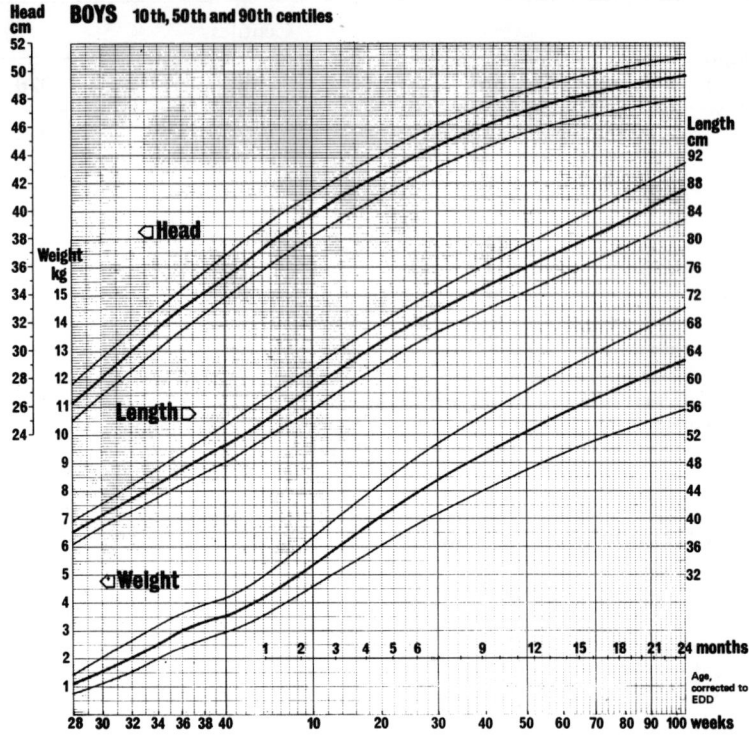

BOYS 10th, 50th and 90th centiles

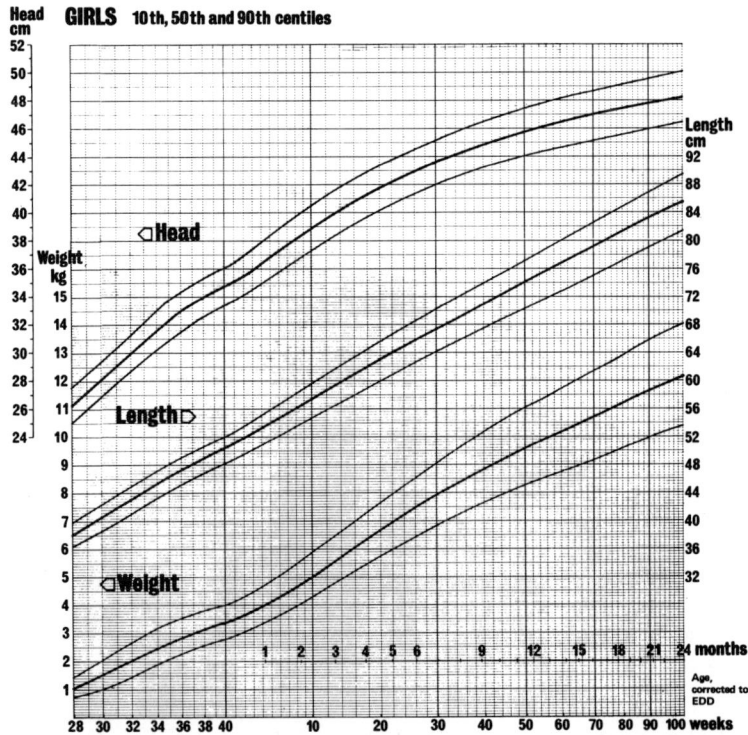

GIRLS 10th, 50th and 90th centiles

Appendix II: Preparations for normal and premature infants, oral and intravenous fluids and vitamin/mineral supplements

II.1 Recommendations for composition of infant formulae: macronutrient and vitamin content per 100 available kilocalories

	WHO[a]	UK[b]	USA[c]
Protein (g)	1.8−4.0	Unmodified cow's milk protein 2.1−2.9 Casein: whey ratio similar to human milk 1.7−2.9	1.8−4.5
Fat (g)	3.3−6.0	No recommendation	3.3−6.0
Linoleic acid (mg)	≥300	No recommendation	≥300
Carbohydrate (g)	No recommendation	Lactose 3.6−11.4 Total 6.8−14.3	No recommendation
Vitamin A (μg retinol equivalent)	75−150	57−214	75−225
Vitamin D (μg)	1−2	1−1.9	1−2
Vitamin E (mg)	≥0.7 or 0.7 mg/g linoleic acid	≥0.4 or 0.4 mg Vit. E: 1.02 g PUFA	≥3 or 0.7 mg/g linoleic acid
Vitamin K (μg)	≥4	≥2.1	No recommendation
Vitamin C (mg)	≥8	≥4	≥8
Thiamine (μg)	≥40	≥18.5	≥40
Riboflavin (μg)	≥60	≥43	≥60
Niacin (μg)	≥250	≥328	≥250
Pyridoxine (μg)	≥35 min. 15 μg/g protein	≥7	≥35 min. 15 μg/g protein
Folate (μg)	≥4	≥4	≥4
Vitamin B_{12} (μg)	≥0.15	≥0.14	≥0.15
Biotin (μg)	≥1.5	≥0.7	≥1.5
Pantothenic acid (μg)	≥300	≥285	≥300
Choline (mg)	≥7	No recommendation	≥7
Inositol (mg)	No recommendation	No recommendation	≥4

[a] FAO/WHO recommended international standards for foods for infants and children (Joint FAO/WHO Food Standards Programmes Codex Alimentarius Comission, 1976, Rome, FAO).

[b] Artificial feeds for the young infant (DHSS Report on Health and Social Subjects No. 18 (1980) *Artificial Feeds for the Young Infant*, London, HMSO).

[c] Commentary on breast feeding and infant formulae, including proposed standards for formulae (Committee on Nutrition of the American Academy of Pediatrics (1976) Commentary on breast-feeding and infant formulas, including proposed standards for formulas. *Pediatrics*, **57**, 278−285).

II.2 Recommendations for composition of infant formulae: mineral content per 100 available kilocalories

	WHO[a]	UK[b]	USA[c]
Sodium (mg)	20−60	21−50	20−60
Potassium (mg)	80−200	71−143	80−200
Chloride (mg)	55−150	57−114	55−150
Calcium (mg)	≥50	43−171	≥50
Phosphorus (mg)	≥25	21−86	≥50
	Ca:P ratio ≥1.2 and ≤2	Ca:P ratio ≥1.2 and ≤2.2	Ca:P ratio ≥1.1 and ≤2
Magnesium (mg)	≥6	4−17	≥6
Iron (mg)	≥0.15 if not labelled as 'fortified' ≥1 if iron fortified	1−10	≥0.15
Zinc (mg)	≥0.5	No recommendation	≥0.5
Iodide (μg)	≥5	No recommendation	≥5
Copper (μg)	≥60	No recommendation	≥60
Manganese (μg)	≥5	No recommendation	≥5

[a] FAO/WHO recommended international standards for foods for infants and children (*see* Appendix II.1).
[b] Artificial feeds for the young infant (*see* Appendix II.1).
[c] Commentary on breast feeding and infant formulae, including proposed standards for formulae (*see* Appendix II.1).

II.3 Normal infant formulae

Most normal infant formulae are based on heat treated cows' milk, with the addition of fats, carbohydrates, vitamins and trace elements to provide a composition similar to that of mature human breast milk. Dried milk powders based on whole or skimmed milk and fresh cow or goat milk are not suitable under the age of 6 months because the protein and renal solute load is undesirably high. Such milks can be used for infants if there is no alternative, but the product must be diluted. Appendix II.6 gives suggestions for modification of such milks.

Formulae which have a composition similar to that of human milk are known as modified milks and are considered to be suitable for the feeding of infants from birth onwards if the mother is not breast feeding. In the USA, the UK and countries where legislation exists to prevent the marketing of unmodified formulae, it can be assumed that all milks on sale to the general public will conform to the guidelines for that country or to the FAO/WHO recommendations (p. 218). However, many of the less developed countries do not have such legislation and it is common for milks to be sold indicating that they are designed for infants, when they are in fact unmodified milk powders. The composition of all formulae should be checked against the guidelines before it is recommended to mothers.

Two main types of modified infant formulae exist: those based on whole milk protein, with a whey:casein ratio of 18:82 and those based on dialysed whey protein with a whey:casein ratio of 60:40, similar to that found in human milk. Provided the protein content of the formula is not higher than the levels recommended, there appears to be little advantage of one type of formula over another. If an infant is receiving a low protein diet and the protein intake is close to the minimum, the amino acid pattern found in the whey-based preparations might be more beneficial. This type of formula is usually lower in electrolytes than the non-whey formulae.

The carbohydrate in human milks and the majority of infant formulae is lactose. Some modified formulae contain other carbohydrates which partially replace lactose; this type of formula may be useful for infants after surgery or where a partial intolerance to lactose is suspected. The fat of human milk is more readily digested and absorbed than that of whole cows' milk. For this reason most modified infant formulae have wholly or partially replaced the butterfat with a mixture of other animal fats or vegetable oils. Formulae which contain animal fat other than butterfat are not suitable for use for infants of Moslem, Jewish or Hindu faith.

The standard energy density of feeds is 65–75 kcal per 100 ml (270–315 kJ per 100 ml). Some manufacturers also produce dilute (half strength) formulae which should only be used for short periods when grading infants onto full strength feeds. Formulae with a higher energy concentration than that recommended are also available, and these should be used with caution since they have a high osmolality and can cause an osmotic diarrhoea.

'Follow on' formulae have been designed for use for infants over the age of 6 months. They are usually higher in protein content than modified formulae and contain a higher quantity of minerals including sodium. Vitamins are added to these milks. The use of such formulae is not particularly beneficial for infants who receive a good weaning diet, because unmodified cows' milk is considered by most authorities to be suitable for infants over the age of 6 months. However, for infants who are reluctant with solids, who fail to gain weight, or who are considered to need additional vitamins, and in areas where fresh pasteurized cows' milk is not available, this type of formula will be useful.

Infant milks are available in the form of dried milk powder for reconstitution with water, and as ready-to-feed products in pre-measured sterile disposable bottles. These have the advantage of accuracy and hygiene but are extremely expensive compared with the powder product. Care must be taken to ensure that the mother or person preparing the formula is able to prepare it correctly. Most modified baby milks enclose a scoop or spoon with the package and the milk is reconstituted using one scoop to either 1 or 2 fluid ounces (30 ml or 60 ml) water. If the mother changes to a different formula she should be aware that the recipe for making up the feed may differ between formulae.

The availability of clean water is important in the less developed countries. Every effort must be made to continue breast feeding if there is any doubt about the quality of the local water. Bottled potable or mineral water is expensive and may be too high in sodium and calcium for use in the preparation of infant feeds, and this should be checked before its use is recommended.

II.4 Composition of normal infant formulae

Product	Manufacturer	Protein (g/100 ml)	Fat		Carbohydrate		Energy (kcal/100ml)
			Source	(g/100 ml)	type	(g/100 ml)	
Whey-based starter formulae (reconstituted or ready-to-feed)							
SMA — Gold Cap	Wyeth	1.5	Animal and vegetable	3.6	Lactose	7.2	65
Enfamil	Mead-Johnson	1.5	Vegetable	3.8	Lactose	6.9	65
NAN	Nestlé	1.6	Vegetable	3.4	Lactose	7.3	66
Almiron	Nutricia	1.5	Vegetable	3.5	Lactose	7.5	67
Premium	Cow & Gate	1.5	Vegetable	3.8	Lactose	7.2	66
Non-whey-based starter formulae							
SMA	Wyeth	1.5	Animal and vegetable	3.6	Lactose	7.2	65
Similac	Ross	1.7	Vegetable	3.7	Lactose	7.1	65
Milumil	Milupa	1.9	Butterfat	3.1	Lactose Amylose Maltodextrin	8.4	68
Babymilk Plus	Cow & Gate	1.9	Butterfat and vegetable	3.4	Lactose	7.3	66
Lactogen	Nestlé	2.1	Butterfat and vegetable	3.1	Lactose	6.9	64
Follow-on formulae							
Progress	Wyeth	2.9	Vegetable	2.6	Lactose Maltodextrin	8.0	65
Modar	Wander	2.2	Butterfat and vegetable	3.1	Lactose Maltodextrin	7.9	70

II.5 Formulae designed for premature and low-birth-weight infants

Product	Manufacturer	Protein (g/100 ml)	Fat		Carbohydrate		Energy
			Type	(g/100 ml)	Type	(g/100 ml)	(kcal/100ml)
Prematalac	Cow & Gate	2.4	Butterfat and vegetable	5.0	Lactose	6.6	79
SMA — LBW formula	Wyeth	2.0	Animal Vegetable MCTs	4.4	Lactose Maltodextrin	8.6	80
Preaptamil	Milupa	2.1	Vegetable and butterfat	3.6	Lactose	8.7	76
Osterprem	Farleys	2.0	Vegetable and butterfat	4.9	Lactose Maltodextrin	7.0	80
Enfamil — Prem formula	Mead-Johnson	2.0	Vegetable and MCTs	3.4	Glucose polymer Lactose	7.4	68
Nenatal	Nutricia	1.8	Vegetable and MCTs	4.5	Maltodextrin Glucose Lactose	7.5	76
Alprem	Nestlé		Butterfat MCTs Vegetable	3.4	Lactose Glucose polymer	8.0	70
Vita-Nova	United Dairymen	2.2	Butterfat MCTs	4.6	Maltodextrin Lactose	7.4	79

All premature and low-birth-weight formulae are only available in 'ready-to-feed' format, except Vita-Nova which is only available in powder form.
MCTs = medium chain triglycerides

II.6 Milks not adapted as infant formulae

Manufacturers of infant formulae have generally designed the milk so as to meet the requirements of the small infant. Where possible a normal or a specialized milk should be used. However, in situations where such formulae are not available through economic or geographical reasons, other milks can be used to provide adequate nutrition.

Cows' milk

This must be pasteurized or boiled before it is fed to an infant. Undiluted cows' milk is not recommended for infants of less than 6 months of age because of its high protein and sodium content. For infants of less than 6 months of age, a diluted formula is suitable.

Preparation of diluted formula To each 70 ml boiled cows' milk add 30 ml boiled water. In addition carbohydrate (glucose, glucose polymer, maltodextrin or sucrose) should be added at 5 g/100 ml diluted feed.

This adapted formula falls within the FAO guidelines for the major nutrients (*see* p. 224), but is deficient in iron, retinol, cholecalciferol, ascorbic acid and nicotinic acid and these should be supplemented if cows' milk is to be fed for a period of longer than a few days.

Canned evaporated whole milk

The composition of evaporated whole milk is subject to the regulations in force in the country where it is marketed. The figures given in Appendix II.7 are for milks available in the UK. In North America evaporated milk contains more water, and the content of all nutrients is about 1% lower than the figures in the table. Other regulations may affect the nutrient content of evaporated milk: in some countries iron and/or cholecalciferol may be added. For small infants, where whole milk is not available or where the quality of the milk is in doubt, a diluted formula can be prepared.

Preparation of diluted formula To each 25 ml evaporated milk add 75 ml boiled water. In addition carbohydrate (glucose, glucose polymer, maltodextrin or sucrose) should be added at 5 g/100 ml diluted feed.

This adapted formula falls within the FAO guidelines with the same exceptions as for whole cows' milk (*see* p. 224). Care should be taken to ascertain if iron of cholecalciferol have already been added to the product. The total intake of cholecalciferol should not exceed 2 µg per 100 kcal.

Canned, condensed, skimmed or sweetened cows' milk

This type of product is generally not suitable for adaptation into a feed for infants.

Goats' milk

This should always be boiled or pasteurized before it is fed to an infant. Undiluted goats' milk is not recommended for feeding to infants of less than 6 months of age, but where there is no suitable alternative, a dilute formula can be devised.

Preparation of dilute formula To each 70 ml boiled goats' milk add 30 ml boiled water. In addition carbohydrate (glucose, glucose polymer, maltodextrin or sucrose) at 4 g/100 ml diluted feed should be added.

The nutrient content of this adapted formula will fall within the FAO guidelines for the major nutrients (*see* p. 224). However, the vitamin and mineral content of domestic goats' milk, particularly where goats are reared in less than ideal surroundings, is not well known. It would seem advisable to give a complete vitamin and mineral supplement under these circumstances. The folic acid content of goat milk is known to be particularly low, and a vitamin supplement should always include this vitamin.

II.7 Composition of non-adapted milks (per 100 ml)

Milk	Protein (g)	Fat (g)	Carbohydrate (g)	Energy (kJ)	Sodium (mmol)
Cows' milk	3.3	3.8	4.7	272	2.17
diluted formula, as in text	2.3	2.6	8.3	275	1.52
Canned evaporated milk	8.6	9.0	11.3	660	7.8
diluted formula, as in text	2.1	2.2	7.8	165	1.95
Goats' milk	3.3	4.5	4.6	296	1.8
diluted formula, as in text	2.3	3.1	7.2	275	1.26

II.8 Nutrient and renal solute content of milks

	Renal solute load (msmol/l)	Protein (g/100 ml)	Energy (kcal/100 ml)	Calcium (mg/100 ml)	Phosphorus (mg/100 ml)	Sodium (mmol/100 ml)	Potassium (mmol/100 ml)
Cows' milk	225	3.4	67	124	98	2.26	4.10
Canned evaporated milk	590	7.8	155	290	254	7.00	12.87
Modified baby milk	127	1.8	65	70	50	1.30	2.28
Dialysed whey baby milk	95	1.5	68	40	30	0.78	1.54
Mature human milk	90	1.4	70	35	15	0.65	1.74

II.9 Composition of normal, concentrated and premature milks

		per 100 ml formula		
		Normal formula 12% dilution[a]	Normal formula 20% dilution[a]	Premature formula[b]
Energy	(kJ)	284	473	330
	(kcal)	68	113	79
Protein	(g)	1.5	2.5	2.4
Sodium	(mmol)	0.78	1.3	2.6
Calcium	(mmol)	1.0	1.67	1.67
	(mg)	40	67	67
Phosphorus	(mmol)	0.87	1.45	1.71
	(mg)	27	45	53
Ca:P ratio		1.48	1.48	1.26
Iron	(mmol)	0.012	0.02	0.012
	(mg)	0.65	1.08	0.65
Zinc	(mmol)	0.005	0.008	0.006
	(mg)	0.34	0.57	0.4
Vitamin D	(mg)	0.0011	0.0018	0.0011
Vitamin E	(mg)	1.0	1.67	1.0
Vitamin C	(mg)	5.5	9.2	6.5
Vitamin B_6	(mg)	0.08	0.13	0.08
Folic acid	(mg)	0.0035	0.0058	0.0035
Vitamin K	(mg)	0.0028	0.0047	0.0032

[a] Cow & Gate Premium Babymilk.
[b] Cow & Gate Prematalac Formula.

II.10 Copper concentration and copper:zinc ratio of milks

	Copper (µmol/100 ml)	Copper:zinc ratio
Mature human milk	0.6	0.14
Standard formulae		
SMA/Wysoy	0.79	0.14
Premium	0.6	0.1
Ostermilk 2	0.25	0.08
Baby milk Plus	0.25	0.05
Milumil	0.2	0.06
Preterm formulae		
Osterprem	1.89	0.12
Nenatal	1.26	0.1
SMA LBW	1.10	0.14
Prematalac	0.79	0.13
Preaptamil	0.16	0.1

From Sutton *et al.* (1985) *Archives of Disease in Childhood*, Vol. 60, pp. 644–651.

II.11 Oral rehydration mixtures

Name	Manufacturer	Form
Dioralyte	Armour Pharmaceuticals	Sachet: 1 sachet + 200 ml water
Infalyte	Penwalt Corporation	Sachet: 1 sachet + 960 ml water
Oral electrolyte solution	Wyeth	Ready-to-feed (bottles)
Pedialyte	Abbott	Ready-to-feed (bottles)
Dextrolyte	Cow & Gate	Ready-to-feed (bottles)
Lytren	Mead Johnson	Ready-to-feed (bottles) Powder (cans)
Oral rehydration salts I and II	Nutricia	Ready-to-feed (bottles) Sachet: 1 sachet + 1000 ml water
Rehidrat	Searle Pharmaceuticals	Sachet: 1 sachet + 250 ml water
Resol	Wyeth	Ready-to-feed (cartons)

II.12 Composition of oral rehydration fluids per litre (powdered products reconstituted as directed on package)

Name	Osmolality (mosmol/kg water)	Carbohydrate (g)	Energy (kJ)	Sodium (mmol)	Potassium (mmol)	Chloride (mmol)	Base anion	(mmol)
Dioralyte	310	40	669	35	20	37	Bicarbonate	18
Infalyte	251	23	384	50	20	40	Bicarbonate	30
Oral electrolyte solution	393	75	1325	30	20	30	Citrate	23
Pedialyte	300	50	840	30	20	30	Citrate	28
Dextrolyte	297	36	565	35	13	30	Lactate	18
Lytren	290	79	1397	30	25	25	Citrate	36
Oral rehydration salts I	285	30	504	35	25	35	Bicarbonate	25
II	330	20	336	90	25	90	Bicarbonate	25
Rehidrat		48	800	50	20	50	Bicarbonate Citrate	29
Resol	269	20	336	50	20	50	Citrate	34

II.13 Vitamin and mineral supplements

Preparations available in the UK

Oral preparations
1. Abidec drops (Parke-Davis)
   0.6 ml contains:
   - vitamin A, 120 μg
   - thiamine hydrochloride, 1 mg
   - riboflavin, 400 μg
   - nicotinamide, 5 mg
   - pyridoxine hydrochloride, 500 μg
   - ascorbic acid, 50 mg
   - ergocalciferol, 10 μg
2. Orovite elixir (Bencard)
   5 ml contains:
   - thiamine hydrochloride, 20 mg
   - riboflavin, 2 mg
   - nicotinamide, 80 mg
   - pyridoxine hydrochloride, 2 mg
   - ascorbic acid, 40 mg
   Diluent: syrup. Life of diluted elixir: 14 days.
3. Ketovite tablets (Paines & Byrne)
   Per tablet:
   - ascorbic acid, 16.6 mg
   - riboflavin, 1 mg
   - thiamine hydrochloride, 1 mg
   - pyridoxine hydrochloride, 330 μg
   - nicotinamide, 3.3 mg
   - calcium pantothenate, 1.16 mg
   - α-tocopheryl acetate, 5 mg
   - inositol, 50 mg
   - biotin, 170 μg
   - folic acid 250 μg
   - acetomenaphthone, 500 μg
   (Supplement) liquid:
   - vitamin A, 750 μg
   - vitamin D, 10 μg
   - choline chloride, 150 mg
   - cyanocobalamin, 12.5 μg
   Diluent: purified water, freshly boiled and cooled.
   Life of diluted liquid: 7 days
4. Juvel tablets and elixir (Bencard)
   Per tablet:
   - vitamin A, 150 μg
   - thiamine hydrochloride, 2.5 mg
   - riboflavin, 2.5 mg
   - nicotinamide, 50 mg
   - vitamin D, 12.5 μg
   - pyridoxine hydrochloride, 2.5 mg
   - ascorbic acid, 50 mg
   5 ml elixir:
   - vitamin A, 1200 μg

thiamine hydrochloride, 2 mg
riboflavin, 2 mg
nicotinamide, 40 mg
vitamin D, 10 μg
pyridoxine hydrochloride, 2 mg
ascorbic acid, 40 mg
Diluent: syrup. Life of diluted elixir: 14 days
5. Multivitamins tablets (Evans)
Per tablet:
vitamin A, 750 μg
thiamine hydrochloride, 1 mg
riboflavin, 500 μg
nicotinamide, 7.5 mg
ascorbic acid, 15 mg
vitamin D, 7.5 μg

Injectable preparations

1. Multibionta — for addition to infusion fluids (Merck)
10 ml contains:
ascorbic acid, 500 mg
dexpanthenol, 25 mg
nicotinamide, 100 mg
pyridoxine hydrochloride, 15 mg
riboflavin sodium phosphate, 19 mg
thiamine hydrochloride, 50 mg
tocopheryl acetate, 5 mg
vitamin A, 3 mg
2. Solivito — powder for reconstitution (KabiVitrum)
Each vial contains:
biotin, 300 μg
cyanocobalamin, 2 μg
folic acid, 200 μg
glycine, 100 mg
nicotinamide, 10 mg
pyridoxine hydrochloride, 2.43 mg
riboflavin (as sodium phosphate), 1.8 mg
sodium ascorbate, 34 mg
sodium pantothenate, 11 mg
thiamine mononitrate, 1.24 mg
3. Parentrovite (Bencard)
IMM injection, vitamins B and C — weak for intramuscular use
IMHP injection, vitamins B and C — strong for intramuscular use
IVHP injection, vitamins B and C — strong for intravenous use

Preparations available in the USA

Oral preparations

1. Vitamins A, C and D liquid
1 ml contains: vitamin A, 2.5 mg

              vitamin C, 83.3 mg
              vitamin D, 41.7 µg

2. Cod Liver Oil (USP)
   Each gram contains:
      vitamin D, not less than 2.125 µg (85 units)
      vitamin A, 1.2 mg

3. Hexavitamin capsules, tablets and liquid
   per capsule/tablet:
      vitamin A, 1500 µg
      vitamin D, 10 µg
      thiamine hydrochloride (or mononitrate), 2 mg
      riboflavin, 3 mg
      nicotinamide, 20 mg
      ascorbic acid, 75 mg

4. Decavitamin capsules (USP)
   per capsule:
      vitamin A, 1.5 mg
      vitamin D, 10 µg
      ascorbic acid, 75 mg
      thiamine hydrochloride (or mononitrate), 2 mg
      riboflavin, 3 mg
      nicotinamide, 20 mg
      pyridoxine hydrochloride, 2 mg
      calcium pantothenate, 5 mg
      folic acid, 0.25 mg
      cyanocobalamin, 2 µg

Injectable preparations

Vitamin B complex with ascorbic acid
Each vial contains:
   ascorbic acid, 150 mg
   thiamine HCl (or mononitrate), 2.5 mg
   riboflavin, 2.5 mg
   nicotinamide, 50 mg
   pyridoxine hydrochloride, 1 mg
   calcium pantothenate, 10 mg
   folic acid, 0.75 mg
   cyanocobalamin, 0.5 µg

Iron preparations

Preparations available in the UK

Oral preparations

1. Fersamal syrup (Duncan-Flockhart)
   5 ml contains: ferrous fumarate 140 mg (45 mg iron)
   Diluent: syrup. Life of diluted mixture: 14 days

2. Plesmet syrup (Napp)
   5 ml contains: ferrous glycine sulphate 141 mg (25 mg iron)

3. Ferrous sulphate mixture, paediatric BP
   5 ml contains: ferrous sulphate 60 mg (12 mg iron)
   To be taken well diluted with water

4. Sytron Elixir (Parke-Davis)
   5 ml contains: sodium iron edetate (equivalent to 27.5 mg iron)
   Diluent: water for preparations. Life of diluted elixir: 14 days

Injectable preparations

1. Jectofer (Astra)
   Iron sorbitol injection 5% (50 mg/ml) of iron
2. Imferon (Fisons)
   Iron dextran injection 5% (50 mg/ml) of iron

Preparations available in the USA

Oral preparations

1. Vitron C — chewable tablets
   Each tablet contains:
       ferrous fumarate, 200 mg
       ascorbic acid, 125 mg
2. Fer-in-Sol syrup (USP)
   5 ml contains: ferrous sulphate 90 mg

Injectable preparations

As for the UK

Potassium preparations

Preparations available in the UK

Oral preparations

1. Potassium tablets — effervescent
   Each tablet contains:
       potassium bicarbonate, 500 mg
       potassium acid tartrate, 300 mg
   (each tablet provides 6.5 mmol of K^+)
2. Slow-K (Ciba) — slow release tablets
   Each tablet contains: potassium chloride 600 mg
   (each tablet provides 8 mmol of K^+)
3. Sando-K tablets (Sandoz) — effervescent
   Each tablet contains:
       potassium bicarbonate, 400 mg
       potassium chloride, 600 mg
   (each tablet provides 12 mmol K^+ and 8 mmol Cl^-)
4. Kay-Cee-L syrup (Geistlich) — sugar-free potassium chloride
   1 mmol/ml
   Do not dilute
5. Potassium citrate mixture for infants (BPC 1959):
       potassium citrate, 731.2 mg
       citric acid monohydrate, 146.4 mg
       benzoic acid solution, 0.083 ml
       amaranth solution, 0.033 ml
       syrup, 1.33 ml

chloroform water to 4 ml
Dose: 4—8 ml, well-diluted with water

Injectable preparations

1. Strong potassium chloride solution (BP 1973)
   10 ml contains: A sterile 15% solution of potassium chloride in
   water for injection pH 5—7. Contains approx. 20 mmol (20
   mequiv.) of potassium and of chloride and must be diluted
   before use with not less than 50 time its volume of sodium
   chloride 0.9% injection or other suitable diluent.
2. Potassium chloride, sodium chloride and glucose intravenous
   infusion BP: A sterile solution of potassium chloride 0.17—
   0.19% and sodium chloride 0.17—0.19%. Anhydrous
   glucose 3.8—4.2% in water for injection.

Preparations available in the USA

Oral preparations

1. Potassium chloride elixir (USP)
   (Rum-K) 10 mequiv. K^+ and Cl^- per 5 ml (sugar free)
   (Cena K) 13.3 mequiv. K^+ and Cl^- per 5 ml (sugar free)
2. Potassium gluconate elixir (Kaon)
   Elixir NF, 6.7 mequiv. K^+ and $C_6H_{11}O_7^-$ per 5 ml with
   alcohol up to 5% (sugar free)

Injectable preparations

1. Potassium chloride injection (USP)
   A sterile solution in water for injections pH 4—8. To be diluted
   before use.
2. Potassium phosphate injection (USP)
   4.4 mmol of K^+
   3 mmol of HPO_4^{2-} (provided by potassium phosphate dibasic
   236 mg and potassium phosphate monobasic 224 mg/ml)

Calcium preparations

Preparations available in the UK

Oral preparations

1. Sandocal effervescent tablets (Sandoz)
   Each tablet contains:
   3.08 g calcium lactate gluconate (equivalent to 400 mg calcium)
   (10 mmol:20 mequiv. Ca^{2+})
   137 mg sodium (6 mmol:6 mequiv. Na^+)
   176 mg potassium (4.5 mmol:4.5 mequiv. K^+)
   1.1 g anhydrous citric acid (1.08 g citrate ion)
2. Calcium-Sandoz (R) syrup (Sandoz)
   15 ml contains:
   calcium glubionate, 3.27 g
   calcium lactobionate, 2.17 g

(325 mg calcium or 8.1 mmol Ca^{2+}/15 ml)
Diluent: syrup. Life of diluted elixir: 14 days
3. Calcimax Syrup (Wallace Mfg)
   5 ml contains:
   thiamine hydrochloride, 500 µg
   riboflavin, 125 µg
   nicotinamide, 2 mg
   pyridoxine hydrochloride, 125 µg
   cyanocobalamin, 125 µg
   ascorbic acid, 5 mg
   ergocalciferol, 400 units
   calcium glycine hydrochloride, 500 mg
   calcium pantothenate, 125 µg

Injectable preparations

1. Calcium chloride injection BP
   (13.4% w/v $CaCl_2$) $2H_2O$
   1.34 g in 10 ml
   9.12 mmol Ca^{2+} ⎫
   18.23 mmol Cl^- ⎬ in 10 ml
2. Calcium gluconate BP
   calcium gluconate 10% (5 and 10 ml ampoules)
   2.25 mmol Ca^{2+} in 10 ml

Preparations available in the USA

Oral preparations

Calcium gluconate tablets (USP)
Tablets containing anhydrous calcium gluconate.

Injectable preparations

1. Calcium gluconate injection (USP)
   A sterile solution of anhydrous calcium gluconate in water for
   injections. It may contain small amounts of calcium saccharate
   or other suitable calcium salts as stabilizers; sodium hydroxide
   may be added to adjust the pH to 6–8.2.
2. Calcium Gluceptate Injection (USP)
   A sterile solution of calcium gluceptate in water for injections.
   It contains the equivalent of 17–19 mg Ca^{2+} in each millilitre,
   pH 5.6–7.

Magnesium salts

Preparations available in the UK

Injectable preparations

1. Magnesium sulphate 20% (BP)
   10 ml contains: 8.14 mmol Mg^{2+}
2. Magnesium sulphate 50% (BP)
   10 ml contains: 20.4 mmol Mg^{2+}

Preparations available in the USA

Oral preparations

Magnesium gluconate tablets (USP)
GYN (Amfre-Grant)
Each gram represents approximately 2.2 mmol (4.4 mequiv.) of magnesium

Injectable preparations

Magnesium sulphate (USP)
A sterile solution of magnesium sulphate in water for injections. pH of 5% solution 5.5—7.

Trace elements

Preparations available in the UK

Injection/solution

1. Addamel (KabiVitrum)
    Electrolytes and trace elements for addition to Vamin infusion solution.
    10 ml contains:
    Ca^{2+} 5 mmol
    Mg^{2+} 1.5 mmol
    Cl^- 13.3 mmol
    Traces of Fe^{2+}, Zn^{2+}, Mn^{2+}, Cu^{2+}, F^-, I^-
    For adult use.
2. Ped-El, sterile solution (KabiVitrum)
    For addition to Vamin infusion solutions
    1 ml contains:
    Ca^{2+} 0.15 mmol
    Mg^{2+} 25 μmol
    Fe^{3+} 0.5 μmol
    Zn^{2+} 0.15 μmol
    Mn^{2+} 0.25 μmol
    Cu^{2+} 0.075 μmol
    F^- 0.75 μmol
    I^- 0.01 μmol
    P   75 μmol
    Cl^- 0.35 mmol
    For paediatric use.

Mineral supplements

Aminogran Mineral Mixture
Allen & Hanbury

Mineral		per 100 g powder	per 2.7 g scoop	per 8 g (recommended dose)
Potassium	(mmol)	210	5.7	16.8
Calcium	(mg)	8100	218	650
Phosphorus	(mg)	6000	162	480
Sodium	(mmol)	170	4.6	13.6
Magnesium	(mmol)	40	1.1	3.2
Iron	(mg)	63	1.7	5.0
Zinc	(mg)	48	1.3	3.8
Copper	(mg)	13	0.3	1.0
Manganese	(mg)	4	0.1	0.4
Iodine		Trace		
Aluminium		Trace		
Cobalt		Trace		
Molybdenum		Trace		

Metabolic Mineral Mixture
Scientific Hospital Supplies

Mineral		per 100 g	per 8 g (recommended daily dose for > 5.5 kg body weight; infants < 5.5 kg, dosage 1.5 g/kg)
Calcium*	(mg)	8200	656
Potassium	(mmol)	212	17.0
Sodium	(mmol)	172	13.8
Magnesium	(mg)	970	77.6
Chloride	(mmol)	51	4.1
Phosphorus	(mg)	5960	477
Iron	(mg)	63	5.0
Copper	(mg)	13	0.1
Zinc	(mg)	48	0.38
Manganese	(mg)	5.7	0.046
Iodine	(µg)	760	60.8
Molybdenum	(µg)	150	12.0
Aluminium	(µg)	20	1.6

* Calcium-free product also available.

Vitamin supplements

Supplementary vitamin tablets for infants   Cow & Gate

	per tablet	per 12 tablets (recommended dose)
Ascorbic acid (mg)	10.0	120
Thiamine hydrochloride (mg)	0.25	3.0
Riboflavin (mg)	0.25	3.0
Pyridoxine hydrochloride (mg)	0.083	1.0
Nicotinamine (mg)	0.83	10.0
Biotin (mg)	0.008	0.1
Calcium pantothenate (mg)	0.5	6.0
Folic acid (mg)	0.063	0.8
Cyanocobalamin (mg)	0.001	0.012
Acetomenaphthone (mg)	0.125	1.5
d-α-Tocopherol acetate (mg)	1.24	14.9
Iron (as sulphate) (mg)	0.85	10.2
Zinc (as sulphate) (mg)	0.62	7.4
Manganese (as sulphate) (mg)	0.005	0.06
Copper (as sulphate) (mg)	0.034	0.41
Molybdenum (as NH_4^+ salt) (mg)	0.006	0.07
Iodine (as K^+ salt) (mg)	0.012	0.14

Multivite, pellets   Duncan Flockhart

	per tablet (recommended dose)
Vitamin A (μg)	750
Thiamine (mg)	0.5
Vitamin C (mg)	12.5
Vitamin D (μg)	6.25

Mineral and vitamin supplements

Poly-Vi-Flor (0.5 mg) Tablets   Mead Johnson

		Regular	With iron per tablet (recommended dose)
Vitamin A	(μg)	750	750
Vitamin D	(μg)	10	10
Vitamin E	(mg)	15	15
Vitamin C	(mg)	60	60
Folic acid	(mg)	0.3	0.3
Thiamine	(mg)	1.05	1.05
Riboflavin	(mg)	1.2	1.2
Niacin	(mg)	13.5	13.5
Vitamin B_6	(mg)	1.06	1.06
Vitamin B_{12}	(μg)	2.0	—
Iron	(mg)	—	10.0
Fluoride	(mg)	0.5	0.5

Poly-Vi-Flor (1.0 mg) Tablets — Mead Johnson

		Regular	With iron per tablet (recommended dose)
Vitamin A	(µg)	750	750
Vitamin D	(µg)	10	10
Vitamin E	(mg)	15	15
Vitamin C	(mg)	60	60
Folic acid	(mg)	0.3	0.3
Thiamine	(mg)	1.05	1.05
Riboflavin	(mg)	1.2	1.2
Niacin	(mg)	13.5	13.5
Vitamin B_6	(mg)	1.05	1.05
Vitamin B_{12}	(µg)	4.5	4.5
Iron	(mg)	—	12.0
Copper	(mg)	—	1.0
Zinc	(mg)	—	10.0
Fluoride	(mg)	1.0*	1.0*

* 0.5 mg fluoride per tablet in Poly-Vi-Flor (0.5 mg) Tablets.

Poly-Vi-Flor (0.25 mg) Drops — Mead Johnson

		Regular	With iron per ml (recommended dose)
Vitamin A	(µg)	450	450
Vitamin D	(µg)	10	10
Vitamin E	(mg)	5	5
Vitamin C	(mg)	35	35
Thiamine	(mg)	0.5	0.5
Riboflavin	(mg)	0.6	0.6
Niacin	(mg)	8.0	8.0
Vitamin B_6	(mg)	0.4	0.4
Vitamin B_{12}	(µg)	2.0	—
Iron	(mg)	—	10.0
Fluoride	(mg)	0.25*	0.25*

* 0.5 mg/ml in Poly-Vi-Flor (0.5 mg) Drops

Tri-Vi-Flor (0.25 mg) Drops — Mead Johnson

		Regular	With iron per ml (recommended dose)
Vitamin A	(µg)	450	450
Vitamin D	(µg)	10	10
Vitamin C	(mg)	35	35
Iron	(mg)	—	10
Fluoride	(mg)	0.25*	0.25*

* 0.5 mg fluoride in Tri-Vi-Flor (0.5 mg) Drops

Tri-Vi-Flor Tablets		Mead Johnson
		per tablet (recommended dose)
Vitamin A	(µg)	750
Vitamin D	(µg)	10
Vitamin C	(mg)	60
Fluoride	(mg)	1

Paediatric Seravit Powder				Scientific Hospital Supplies
		per 100 g	per 8 g (recommended dose 0−6/12)	per 12 g (recommended dose 6/12−1 year)
Calcium	(mg)	4500	360	540
Phosphorus	(mg)	3000	240	360
Magnesium	(mg)	625	50	75
Iron	(mg)	103	8.25	12.4
Copper	(mg)	7.5	0.6	0.9
Zinc	(mg)	72.2	5.8	8.65
Iodine	(µg)	750	60	90
Manganese	(mg)	7.2	0.58	0.87
Molybdenum	(µg)	469	37.5	56.3
Selenium	(µg)	281	22.5	33.7
Chromium	(µg)	281	22.5	33.7
Vitamin A	(mg)	8.33	0.67	1.0
Vitamin D	(µg)	118	9.4	47.0
Vitamin E	(mg)	77.3	6.19	9.3
Vitamin K	(µg)	700	56.0	84.0
Vitamin C	(mg)	640	51.2	76.9
Thiamine	(mg)	6.25	0.5	0.75
Riboflavin	(mg)	9.38	0.75	1.1
Pyridoxine	(mg)	5.38	0.43	0.64
Nicotinamide	(mg)	70.2	5.62	8.43
Vitamin B_{12}	(µg)	15	1.2	1.8
Folic acid	(µg)	600	48.0	72.0
Biotin	(µg)	400	32.0	48.0
Pantothenic acid	(mg)	27.3	2.19	3.28
Inositol	(mg)	1562	125	187
Choline	(mg)	1015	81	122

Seravit Powder   Scientific Hospital Supplies

		per 100 g	per 5 g (one scoop)	per 25 g (adult dose)
Magnesium	(mg)	1250	62.5	312
Iron	(mg)	83.2	4.16	20.8
Zinc	(mg)	83.2	4.16	20.8
Iodine	(µg)	666	33.3	166
Manganese	(mg)	12.4	0.62	3.1
Copper	(mg)	8.2	0.41	2.0
Aluminium	(µg)	8.6	0.43	2.1
Molybdenum	(µg)	666	33.3	166
Chromium	(µg)	90	4.5	22.5
Phosphorus	(mg)	1600	80	400
Vitamin A	(mg)	6.5	0.32	1.6
Vitamin D	(µg)	38	1.9	9.5
Vitamin E	(mg)	166	8.3	41.5
Vitamin C	(mg)	566	28.3	141.5
Vitamin K	(mg)	3.9	0.20	0.98
Thiamine	(mg)	11.6	0.58	2.9
Riboflavin	(mg)	11.6	0.58	2.9
Vitamin B_6	(mg)	15.0	0.75	3.7
Vitamin B_{12}	(µg)	36.0	1.8	9.0
Nicotinamide	(mg)	83.2	4.2	20.8
Folic acid	(mg)	1.66	0.08	0.5
Biotin	(µg)	1.16	0.06	0.3
Inositol	(mg)	184	9.2	46.0
Choline	(mg)	1832	91.6	458
Pantothenic acid	(mg)	40	2.0	10.0

II.14 Thickening agents for milk feeds

Nestargel   *Nestlé*

Powder derived from carob seed flour. Low in protein, gluten free, milk protein and lactose free.
Dosage 0.5–1.0 g (0.5–1 scoop) Nestargel powder to each 100 ml liquid.

Carobel   *Cow & Gate*

Powder derived from carob bean endosperm. Low in protein, gluten free, milk protein and lactose free.
Dosage 0.5–1.0 g (1 scoop to each 60 ml liquid) Carobel powder to each 100 ml liquid.

Infant Gaviscon   *Reckitt & Colman*

Powder. Ingredients: alginic acid; magnesium trisilicate; aluminium hydroxide gel; sodium bicarbonate. Free of protein, gluten and lactose.
Dosage: infants up to 2 months, half a sachet; infants over 2 months half to one sachet mixed with made-up feed.
NB Contains 4.0 mmol sodium per 2 g sachet.

II.15 Composition of some preparations and solutions for intravenous infusion

Name	Electrolyte content (mmol/l)					Osmolality (mosmol/kg)	Energy (kcal/l)
	Na^+	K^+	Cl^-	HCO_3^- (or equivalent)	Ca^{2+}		
0.9% saline (physiological saline)	150	—	150			300	0
Dextrose 5% in 0.9% saline	150	—	150			586	200
Hartmann's solution (= lactate Ringer)	131	5	111	29 (lactate)	2	278	0
Ringer's solution	147	4	155	—	2	308	0
Human plasma protein fraction (HPPF 5%)	130–160	≯1		≯15 (citrate)		300	0
Human plasma protein fraction (HPPF 20%) — salt poor	≯130	≯1		≯15 (citrate)		1200	0
Dextran 70 in 5% dextrose (mol. wt 70 000)	None					315	200
70 in 0.9% saline (mol. wt 70 000)	150	—	150			300–310	0
Plasma	132–151	3.4–5.2	101–111		2.02–2.6	285–300	0

Appendix II.16 Realimentation formulae

These formulae have been designed to act as an intermediate stage between clear oral fluids and full milk feeds or normal solid diet during diarrhoea or protein−energy malnutrition. They are usually lower in lactose and higher in electrolytes than normal infant formulae. Although these products can be useful in the above-mentioned condition, the products are expensive and are unlikely to be available to infants and children who would derive the most benefit from them.

HN 25 *Milupa*

Casein based, low in lactose and fat; carbohydrates derived from banana, apple, corn and rice. Gluten free. Complete feed, no supplements recommended; meets FAO criteria. Manufacturers recommend a maximum of 7−10 days use as sole source of nutrients.
Preparation: 3 scoops (14 g) HN 25 powder added to 85 ml water.

Composition of Realimentation Formulae

	Protein (g)	Fat (g)	Carbohydrate Total (g)	Lactose (g)	Energy (kcal)	Sodium (mmol)	Potassium (mmol)
HN 25							
100 g powder	17.5	8.4	67.6	0.6	416	12.2	17.7
100 ml feed	2.5	1.2	9.5	0.1	58	1.7	2.5

Appendix III: Enteral feeding and feeds with increased protein/energy density

III.1 Products used for enteral feeding

Several types of commercially produced products are available for enteral feeding. The diet or whole meal replacement should contain the recommended daily intake of all macro- and micronutrients within a stated volume which is consumed over a 24-hour period (usually 1500—2500 ml). Products designed as supplements to the diet may not contain the whole range of essential minerals, trace elements and vitamins. They are generally taken in smaller quantities than a complete feed by patients with increased nutrient requirements or a poor appetite.

Complete feeds may be recommended as an oral or a tube feed; it is important to determine whether a feed of this type is palatable before recommending it to be taken orally. The products described as supplementary feeds are usually palatable as they are intended to be taken orally.

Products may be in the form of a powder which is reconstituted with water or milk. These have the advantages of economy and ease of transport and storage, but if they are to be reconstituted by untrained personnel there is a danger of contamination due to poor hygiene practices and to inaccuracies occurring. Ready-to-feed products are normally marketed in sterile cans and require no reconstitution. Although these feeds are expensive and are difficult to transport and store they have the advantage of accuracy and ease of use.

Few enteral feeding products are designed specifically for children. The products described in this section are all intended for adult use. Adaptation of enteral products for use in infants and children is described in the chapter on enteral and parenteral feeding on p. 31.

Complete feeds

Isocal   *Mead Johnson*

Ready to feed; 250 ml cans. Adult RDA contained in 2000 ml. Unflavoured. Soy and milk protein; vegetable oil and MCTs (20% of total fat); glucose syrup; lactose free. Osmolality: 350 mosmol/kg.

Clinifeed Iso   *Roussel*

Ready to feed; 375 ml cans. Adult RDA contained in 1875 ml. Vanilla flavour. Milk protein; vegetable oil and butterfat; maltodextrin and lactose. Osmolality: 270 mosmol/l.

Fortison Standard   *Cow & Gate*

Ready to feed; 500 ml bottles. Adult RDA contained in 2000 ml. Vanilla flavour. Milk protein; vegetable oil; maltodextrin; minimal lactose. Osmolality: 300 mosmol/kg.

Fortison is also available as a high energy formula, low sodium formula and soy formula.

Ensure RTF   *Abbott*

Ready to feed; 250 ml cans; adult RDA in 1900 ml. Flavoured. Milk and soy protein; vegetable oil; hydrolysed cornstarch and sucrose; lactose free. Osmolarity: 380 mosmol/l.

Ensure Powder   *Abbott*

Powder; 400 g cans; reconstitute with water. Adult RDA contained in 1900 ml. Vanilla flavour. Ingredients as for RTF formula.

Enteral 400   *Scientific Hospital Supplies*

Powder; 86 g pack; reconstitute with water. Adult RDA in 2000 ml. Flavoured. Milk protein; vegetable oil and MCTs (25% total fat as MCTs); maltodextrin; minimal lactose. Osmolarity 330 mosmol/l.

Compleat   *Doyle*

Ready to feed; 250 ml bottles and cans. Adult RDA in 1500 ml. Beef; cereals; vegetables; milk; vegetable oil; maltodextrin; fruit. Contains gluten and lactose.

Compleat Modified Formula   *Doyle*

As for Compleat, except lactose and milk protein free.

Supplementary feeds

Supplement   *Wyeth*

Ready to feed; 200 ml cartons. Milk protein; vegetable oils; lactose and maltodextrin.

Fortisip   *Cow & Gate*

Ready to feed; 200 ml bottles. Milk protein; vegetable oils; maltodextrin; lactose free.

Build up   *Carnation*

Powder; 38 g sachets reconstituted with 250 ml whole or skimmed
milk. Milk protein; low fat; lactose and maltodextrin.

Energy supplements

Where an energy rather than a protein supplement is required, or
where a child dislikes milk, a fruit-flavoured, protein-free supplement is a useful addition to the diet. These can be prepared using a
carbohydrate module such as a glucose polymer as described in
Appendix III.2, or commercially prepared products are available.
These usually contain glucose polymers, colourings and flavourings to improve palatability. In addition most are low in sodium
and potassium and are suitable for use in diets restricted in these
nutrients. It should be noted, however, that such supplements are
usually extremely high in carbohydrate (approximately 60% w/v)
and consequently have a high osmolality (up 9 to 900 mosmol/kg).
They should be introduced slowly and should be diluted with at
least an equal volume of water to reduce the risk of an osmotic
diarrhoea developing. Alternatively they can be diluted with Cola
or fizzy drinks in the ratio 30% supplement : 70% fizzy drink.
Such products are generally not suitable for use in children under
the age of 3–4 years.

III.2 Composition of enteral feeds

Product	Nutrient composition			
	Protein (g)	Fat (g)	Carbohydrate (g)	Energy (kcal)
Isocal per 100 ml	3.2	4.2	12.6	101
Clinifeed Iso per 100 ml	2.8	4.1	13.0	100
Fortison per 100 ml	4.0	4.0	12.0	100
Ensure per 100 ml	3.7	3.7	14.5	105
per 100 g powder	17.5	17.5	69.0	500
Enteral 400 per 100 ml	2.8	3.9	14.3	100
per 100 g powder	13.2	18.1	66.7	465
Vita Nova				
per 100 ml	2.1	5.1	6.6	81
per 100 g powder	14.0	34.0	44.0	540
Compleat per 100 ml	4.3	4.3	14.1	107
Fortisip per 100 ml	4.0	4.0	12.0	100
Build up per 100 ml	7.0	9.2	13.5	120

Energy supplements				
Fortical per 100 ml (Cow & Gate)	—	—	61.5	246
Hycal per 100 ml (Beechams)	—	—	49.5	242

III.3 High energy and high protein milk drinks

1. 20 g milk powder ⎫ puree together
   180 ml full cream milk ⎭
   provides 13 g protein and 190−215 kcal[a]
2. 100 ml canned evaporated milk ⎫
   100 ml full cream milk ⎬
   5 g sugar or glucose polymer ⎭
   provides 12 g protein and 245 kcal
3. 30 g ice cream ⎫
   10 g milk powder ⎬
   160 ml full cream milk ⎭
   provides 10 g protein and 200 kcal
4. 100 g natural yoghourt ⎫ OR 100 g sweetened yoghourt
   10 g sugar or glucose polymer ⎬ without sugar
   100 ml full cream milk ⎭
   provides 9 g protein 160 kcal
5. 30 g thick (double) cream ⎫ stir together
   170 ml full cream milk ⎭
   provides 6 g protein and 245 kcal
6. 50 g (1 medium) egg[b] ⎫
   5 g sugar or glucose polymer ⎬ puree together
   140 ml full cream milk ⎭
   provides 12 g protein and 180 kcal
7. 100 g soft canned fruit (e.g. peaches) ⎫
   20 g milk powder ⎬ puree together
   80 ml full cream milk ⎭
   provides 10 g protein and 190−220 kcal[a]

All of the above recipes (except no. 7) may be flavoured with milk shake syrup or milk shake powder to taste.

[a] Higher energy value using dried whole milk powder; lower value assumes skimmed milk powder.

[b] Not more than one raw egg per day.

III.4 High energy and high protein soups

1. 30 g soft cooked meat ⎫ puree together
   100−120 ml meat or vegetable soup ⎭
   provides approx. 8−10 g protein and 150−170 kcal
2. 20 g dried milk powder ⎫ puree together
   100−120 ml vegetable soup ⎭
   provides approx. 8−10 g protein and 150−170 kcal
3. 80 g canned baked beans ⎫ puree together
   100−120 ml tomato soup ⎭
   provides approx. 6.5 g protein and 120 kcal
4. 40 g thick (double) cream ⎫ puree together
   100−120 ml vegetable type soup ⎭ (do not boil after adding cream)
   provides approx. 2−4 g protein and 240−260 kcal

III.5 High energy fruit drinks

These drinks all provide approximately 120 kcal per 200 ml serving.
A negligible amount of protein is provided by nos. 1–3.
See also section on commercially produced enteral feeds on p. 242.

1. 190 ml natural unsweetened fruit juice
   10 g sugar or glucose polymer

2. 100 g soft canned fruit (e.g. peaches)
   10 g sugar or glucose polymer } puree together
   90 ml water

3. 20 ml fruit flavoured squash or cordial
   25 g sugar or glucose polymer
   160 ml water

4. 50 g (1 medium) egg[a]
   150 ml sweetened or unsweetened orange juice } puree together
   provides 7 g protein

5. 40 g ice cream
   150 ml Cola or fizzy drink } stir together just before drinking
   provides 1.5 g protein

[a] Not more than one raw egg per day.

III.6 Fluid diet

Example suitable for 5-year-old child, weight 19 kg.
RDA: fluid 1600 ml; protein 40 g; energy 1600 kcal (from Appendices I.1–I.6).

	Protein (g)	Energy (kcal)
On waking: orange juice } 1 raw egg } total 200 ml	7.7	115
Breakfast: 20 g smooth breakfast cereal } 150 ml full cream milk } puree 20 g sugar/glucose polymer }	7.4	250
Mid-morning: lemon squash } 40 g sugar/glucose polymer } total 200 ml	—	160
Mid-day: 30 g soft meat } 150 ml chicken soup } puree	8.6	150
Early afternoon: 40 g stewed apple } 10 g sugar/glucose polymer } puree 150 g ice cream }	5.7	275
Mid-afternoon: 20 ml blackcurrant cordial } 180 ml water }	—	45
Evening: 150 ml tomato soup } 50 g thick (double) cream } puree	2.0	305
Bedtime: 10 g drinking chocolate } 10 g sugar/glucose polymer } 180 ml full cream milk }	6.6	200
Total:	38.0	1500

NB If vitamin C enriched drinks are not consumed, a supplement of ascorbic acid will be required.
If meat is not consumed a supplement of iron and B vitamins is necessary.
A folic acid supplement is advisable with this regimen.

III.7 One litre of maintenance feed for children with severe protein–energy malnutrition

Dried skimmed milk (g)	Sugar (g)	Oil (g)
15	100	40

Mix with water to make up to 1 litre (1000 ml)
Provides 80 kcal (335 MJ), 0.5 g protein/100 ml

III.8 High-energy feed based on cows' milk (for other children)

Milk	Amount (g)	Added carbohydrate[a] (g)	Added fat[b] (g)	Water (ml)
Liquid cows' milk	900	60	50	—
Evaporated milk	400	60	50	500
Dried skimmed milk	90	60	80	800
Formula milk, e.g. Pelargon (Nestlé)	190	—	50	800

Adapted from Ashworth A (1980). Practical aspects of dietary management during rehabilitation from severe protein−energy malnutrition. *J. Human Nutr.*, **34**, 360−369.

1 litre provides 30 g protein, 100 g carbohydrate, 80 g fat, 1275 kcal.

[a] Carbohydrate: sugar or glucose polymer.

[b] Fat: vegetable oil. Use double this quantity if modular fat emulsion is used. If vegetable oil is used delivery must be by bolus and the feed vigorously shaken to disperse the fat.

In addition, a supplement for the RDA of vitamins A and C, thiamine (B_1) and pyridoxine (B_6) should be given, plus supplemental iron if this feed is the sole source of nutrition.

III.9 High-energy feed based on whey-type formula

Recipe for 1000 ml	Protein (g)	Fat (g)	Carbohydrate (g)	Energy (kcal)
130 g powder, dialysed whey babymilk	15.0	38.0	70.0	650
30 g sugar/glucose[a]	—	—	30.0	120
40 ml fat emulsion or 20 ml oil[b]	—	20.0	—	180
Water to make up to a final volume of 1000 ml				
	15.0	58.0	100.0	950

[a] Glucose polymer or milk shake powder/syrup can be used. Added carbohydrate can be gradually increased to a total of 80 g if tolerated.

[b] Can be gradually increased to 80 ml emulsion, 40 ml oil.

III.10 High-protein, minimal-fat formula for infants

	Protein (g)	Fat (LCTs) (g)	CHO (g)	Energy (kcal)	Na^+ (mg)
30 g dried powder dialysed whey infant milk (SMA)	3.6	8.4	16.8	153	36
130 g dried skimmed milk powder	44.8	0.4	63.9	424	780
20 g glucose polymer	—	—	20.0	80	—
Water to make up to 1000 ml					
Totals	48.2	8.8	100.7	657	816 (35.5 mmol)
Per kg body weight fed at 120 ml/kg	5.8			79	4.3 mmol
Per kg body weight fed at 150 ml/kg	7.2			99	5.3 mmol

III.11 Low fat milk drink with MCTs

Moderate protein

	Protein (g)	Fat (g)	Energy (kcal)	Sodium (mmol)
300 ml cows' milk	10.2	11.1	198	6.5
or 140 ml evaporated milk				
or 40 g dried whole milk powder				
60 g skimmed milk powder	20.7	0.2	196	15.6
80 ml Liquigen (p. 270)	—	40.0[a]	332[b]	Trace
80 g glucose polymer *or* sugar	—	—	320	Trace
Milkshake flavouring				
Water to make up to 100 ml				
	31.0	51.3	1—46	22.1

[a] Fat is MCT.
[b] MCT energy value = 8.3 kcal/g.

High protein

  62 g protein
  51 g fat (40 g MCTs)
  1179 kcal
  45.6 mmol sodium
300 ml cows' milk
  or 140 ml evaporated milk
  or 40 g dried powder
150 g skimmed milk powder
80 ml Liquigen
40 g glucose polymer *or* sugar
Milkshake flavouring and water to make up to 1000 ml

Low sodium

To reduce the sodium content of either of these recipes substitute a modular protein with a low electrolyte content, such as Maxipro HBV (p. 268).

III.12 High-protein, moderate sodium milk for salt-restricted diets

The following products are high in protein and low in sodium and are suitable for inclusion in a high protein, high energy, restricted salt diet: Casec, Casilan, Maxipro, Propac. Details of the composition of these powders will be found in the section on protein modules (p. 268.)

Recipe for 1000 ml	Protein (g)	Fat (g)	Carbohydrate (g)	Energy (kcal)	Sodium (mmol)
130 g powder, dialysed whey babymilk	15.0	38.0	70.0	650	7.8
30 g Casilan powder	27.0	Trace	Trace	113	Trace
30 g sugar/glucose	—	—	30.0	120	Trace
40 ml fat emulsion or 20 ml oil	—	20.0	—	180	—
Water to make up to 1000 ml					
	42.0	58.0	100.0	1063	7.8

The protein in the milk can be increased to a total of 60 g protein per litre, provided that enough extra non-protein energy is provided in the form of, for example, high energy drinks.

Appendix IV: Diets used in the treatment of gastrointestinal and allergic conditions and disorders of fat metabolism

IV.1 Formulae with a reduced lactose content

Almiron A.B. Powder   *Nutricia*

Free of sucrose and gluten. Contains milk protein (casein and whey), a reduced amount of lactose, and long chain vegetable fats. Complete feed, no supplements recommended by manufacturer. Iron content (0.585 mg/100 ml feed) is below the FAO recommendations for a supplemented milk; cholecalciferol content (2.25 mg/100 ml feed) is above the maximum recommendation.
Preparation 15% solution. 1 scoop (4.5 g) powder added to 30 ml water.
This product is not recommended for the treatment of galactosaemia.

Almiron A.B. Ready to Use. As for Almiron A.B. powder, except that it requires no dilution with water.

Farilon   *Nutricia*

Acidified formula, free of sucrose and gluten. Contains milk protein (casein and whey), a reduced amount of lactose, long chain milk and vegetable fats. Complete feed, no supplements recommended. Iron content (0.54 mg/100 ml feed) is below FAO recommendations for a supplemented milk; cholecalciferol (2.1 mg/100 ml feed) is above the maximum recommended by FAO.
Preparation 15% solution. 1 scoop (4.5 g) powder added to 30 ml water.
This product is not recommended for the treatment of galactosaemia.

Galactomin 17   *Cow & Gate*

Free of sucrose, starch and gluten. Contains milk protein (casein) a minimal amount of lactose and long chain vegetable fats. Galactomin 17 is not a complete feed. The manufacturers recommend that a complete vitamin supplement is given, including retinol, cholecalciferol, thiamine, riboflavin, pyridoxine, cyanocobalamin, ascorbic acid, tocopherol, biotin, folic acid, nicotinamide and pantothenate (*see* Vitamin supplements, p. 226). In addition a trace metal supplement, including iron, copper, zinc, manganese, aluminium, cobalt, molybdenum and iodine is also recommended (*see* Mineral supplements, p. 226). The sodium content is below the FAO guidelines:
Preparation 12.5% solution. Four scoops (each containing 3.5 g powder) made up to a total volume of 100 ml with water.

AL 100   *Nestlé*

Free of sucrose, starch and gluten. Contains milk protein (casein), a small amount of lactose and long chain milk and vegetable fats. Complete formula, no supplements recommended.
Preparation 13.3% solution. 1 scoop (4.4 g) powder added to 30 ml water.

Lactalac V   ***Friesland Products***

Lactase-treated full cream milk powder. Nutrient content as for whole milk. Contains small amounts of lactose. Not adapted as an infant formula.
Preparation 11.7% solution. Four scoops (26 g) powder added to 200 ml warm boiled water.

Lactalac M

As for Lactalac V, except that skimmed milk is used.

IV.2 Composition of low lactose milks

Milk	Protein (g)	Fat (g)	Total CHO (g)	Lactose	Energy (kcal)	Sodium (mmol)	Osmolality (mosmol/kg)
Almiron AB 100 g powder	11.5	26.8	57.1	9.2 g	519	6.52	
100 ml feed	1.5	3.5	7.4	1.3 g	67	0.98	160
Farilon 100 g powder	14.0	19.9	60.8	8.5 g	482	6.52	
100 ml feed	2.0	2.8	8.5	1.2 g	67	0.98	260
Galactomin 17							
100 g powder	22.3	22.8	50.2	100 mg	478	4.5	
100 ml feed	2.8	2.8	6.3	12.5 mg	60	0.56	198
AL 110 110 g powder	14	25	55.5	<75 mg	502	7.4	
100 ml feed	1.9	3.3	7.4	<10 mg	80	1.00	150
Lactalac V 100 g powder	26.0	28.0	37.0		2108		
100 ml feed	3.1	3.3	4.4	ns	252	ns	ns

See also — milks containing MCTs, formula free of milk protein and modular feeding.
ns = not stated.

IV.3 Formulae based on soy

Infants who have shown a severe reaction to one or more food proteins should not be given a full strength feed initially. A half-strength formula is suggested for the first 12 hours. If the infant is receiving parenteral glucose and electrolytes, then the diluted feed can safely be made up with water. To improve the energy and electrolyte content of the diluted feed half of the fluid volume used to make up the feed can be in the form of an oral glucose—electrolyte mixture, p. 225.

Feeds based on soy protein isolate

Prosobee Powder   ***Mead Johnson***

Free of milk protein, lactose, sucrose and gluten. Contains long chain vegetable fats. Complete feed, no supplements recommended. Meets FAO criteria.

Preparation — 13% solution. 1 scoop (8.6 g) powder added to 60 ml water.

Prosobee Liquid — as for powder.

Preparation — one part Prosobee concentrated liquid added to one part water.

I-Soyalac Concentrate   *Loma Linda*

Free of milk protein, lactose and gluten. Contains sucrose and long chain vegetable fats. Complete feed, no supplements recommended. Meets FAO criteria.
Preparation — one part I-Soyalac concentrated liquid added to one part liquid.

I-Soyalac Ready to Serve. As for concentrate, but requires no dilution with water.

Formula 'S' (Export)   *Cow & Gate*

Free of milk protein, lactose, sucrose and gluten. Contains long and medium chain fats. Complete feed, no supplements recommended. Meets FAO criteria.
Preparation — 13% solution. One scoop (4.5 g) powder added to 30 ml water.

Formula 'S' (UK)   *Cow & Gate*

As for Export product.

Nutri-Soja   *Nutricia*

Free of milk protein, lactose, sucrose and gluten. Contains long chain vegetable fats. Complete feed, no supplements recommended. Meets FAO criteria.
Preparation — 13.7% solution. One scoop (4.5 g) powder added to 30 ml water.

Isomil Powder   *Abbott Laboratories*

Free of milk protein, lactose and gluten. Contains sucrose and long chain vegetable fats. Complete feed, no supplements recommended. Meets FAO criteria.
Preparation — 13.2% solution. One scoop (9 g) powder added to 60 ml water.

Isomil Ready to Feed — as for powder, but needs no dilution with water.

Isomil Concentrated Liquid

Free of milk protein, lactose and gluten. Contains starch, sucrose and long chain vegetable fats. Complete feed, no supplements recommended. Meets FAO criteria.

Preparation — one part concentrated liquid added to one part water.

Isomil SF Concentrated Liquid

Free of milk protein, lactose, sucrose and gluten. Contains long chain vegetable fats.
Preparation — one part concentrated liquid added to one part water.

Feeds based on soy flour or soybean

Bebe-Nago   *Galactina*

Free of milk protein, lactose and gluten. Contains sucrose, starch and long chain vegetable fats. Complete formula, no supplements recommended by manufacturers. Fat content lower and carbohydrate content higher than FAO guidelines. Calcium : phosphorus ratio (1.0) lower than FAO guidelines (not less than 1.2); vitamin C (4.3 µg/100 ml) lower than, and vitamin A (217 µg/100 ml) and vitamin D (1.45 µg/100 ml) higher than FAO guidelines.
Preparation — 14.5% solution. One scoop (8 g) added to 50 ml water.

Soyalac Powder   *Loma Linda*

Free of milk protein, lactose and gluten. Contains sucrose and long chain vegetable fats. Complete formula, no supplements recommended. Meets FAO criteria.
Preparation — 13% solution. One scoop (8.5 g) added to 60 ml water.

Soyalac Concentrate — as for Soyalac powder.
Preparation — one part Soyalac concentrate added to one part water.

Soyalac Ready To Serve — as for concentrated liquid except needs no dilution with water.

IV.4 Composition of soy milks

Soy milk		Protein (g)	Fat (g)	Carbohydrate (g)	Energy (kcal)	Sodium (mmol)	Osmolality (mosmol/kg)
Prosobee	100 g powder	15.6	28.0	51.6	522	8.5	
	100 ml feed	2.0	3.6	6.7	67	1.1	160
I-Soyalac	100 ml feed	2.1	3.7	6.6	67	1.47	280
Formula 'S' Export							
	100 g powder	16.0	21.2	58.3	492	6.5	
	100 ml feed	2.2	2.9	8.0	67	0.87	200
Formula 'S' UK							
	100 g powder	16.0	24.0	54.0	483	10.4	
	100 ml feed	2.2	3.2	7.3	65	1.4	230
Nutri-Soja	100 g powder	16.0	21.2	58.3	492	6.5	
	100 ml feed	2.2	2.9	8.0	67	0.87	200
Isomil + Isomil SF							
	100 g powder	15.2	27.3	51.6	513	9.9	
	100 ml feed	2.0	3.6	6.8	68	1.3	250
Wysoy, Nursoy and Infasoy							
	100 g powder	16.0	27.0	52	505	6.52	
	100 ml feed	2.1	3.6	6.9	67	0.87	242
Infasoy 18% solution							
	100 ml feed	2.5	4.3	8.3	80	1.0	290
Alsoy	100 g powder	14.0	25.0	55.0	500	7.4	
	100 ml feed	1.9	3.3	7.4	67	1.0	189
Bebe-Nago	100 g powder	19.0	12.0	63.0	450	7.0	
	100 ml feed	2.7	1.7	9.1	65	1.01	244
Soyalac	100 g powder	16.0	28.0	49.0	509	10.8	
	100 ml feed	2.1	3.7	6.6	67	1.47	210

IV.5 Formulae containing hydrolysed protein

The complete formulae containing hydrolysed proteins that are currently being marketed are based on milk protein. This has been enzymatically hydrolysed into short chain peptides and amino acids thus reducing the allergenic properties of intact milk protein. Allergic reactions have been thought to occur in a small proportion of milk-sensitive infants fed on hydrolysed milk protein. The osmolar load of hydrolysates is of necessity higher than formulae containing intact protein, due to the high osmotic effect of the small peptide and amino acid molecules. For these reasons it is prudent to commence feeding on a half-strength or a quarter-strength formula. If the infant is receiving glucose and electrolytes parentally then the diluted feeds can be made up with water. If fluids are administered solely by the oral route the low carbohydrate, sodium and potassium content of the feed can be improved by using an oral electrolyte formula (p. 225) to replace half or three-quarters of the water in the feed. Reports of acidosis occurring in infants with low birth weight or prolonged malabsorption have been published, and careful monitoring of blood gases is important, particularly in the first few days. Sodium bicarbonate (2—3 mmol daily) may be administered if necessary.

Nutramigen   *Mead Johnson*

Casein hydrolysate. Free of whole milk protein, lactose sucrose and gluten. Contains sucrose, starch and long chain vegetable fats. Complete formula, no supplements recommended. Meets FAO criteria for all nutrients.
Preparation — 14% solution. One scoop (4.9 g) Nutramigen powder plus 30 ml water.

Pregestimil Powder   *Mead Johnson*

Casein hydrolysate. Free of whole milk protein, lactose, sucrose and gluten. Contains starch, medium and long chain vegetable fats. Complete feed, no supplements recommended. Meets FAO criteria for all nutrients.

This formula contains 42% of the total fat in the form of medium chain triglycerides (MCTs). If MCTs are introduced too rapidly abdominal cramp and diarrhoea can result. See section on MCT milks, p. 257.
Preparation — 14% solution. One scoop (4.9 g) Pregestimil powder plus 30 ml water.

IV.6 Composition hydrolysate milks

Milk		Protein (g)	Long-chain fat (g)	Medium-chain fat (g)	Carbohydrate (g)	Energy (kcal)	Sodium (mmol)	Osmolality (mosmol/kg)
Nutramigen	100 g powder	13.3	18.3	—	64.1	458	9.6	
	100 ml feed	1.9	2.6	—	9.1	65	1.37	320
Pregestimil	100 g powder	16.0	10.5	7.7	61.6	464	9.3	
	100 ml feed	2.4	1.5	1.1	9.1	69	1.38	338

IV.7 Formulae containing medium chain triglycerides

Because of the smaller particle size, medium chain triglycerides (MCTs) exert a higher osmotic effect than long chain fats. Rapid administration of MCTs can cause symptoms such as abdominal cramp, nausea and diarrhoea. This may lead paediatricians to believe that a particular feed is not being tolerated. In infants the feeds for the first 24 hours should not contain more than 1% MCTs (i.e. 1 g MCTs/100 ml prepared feed). In effect this usually means a quarter-strength formula. If this appears not to have caused problems then the concentration can be increased to half and then three-quarter strength. This can be achieved in several ways. If the infant is receiving parenteral nutrition, then the diluted feeds can be made up using water in the usual way. If, however, the infant is being fed entirely by the oral route then the quarter-strength feed should be prepared by using a quarter of the required volume as MCT milk, with a glucose electrolyte mixture (p. 225) providing three-quarters of the feed volume. This can be succeeded by a half-strength formula which consists of half MCT milk and half glucose–electrolyte mixture.

MCT (1) Milk Powder   *Cow & Gate*

Free of sucrose, gluten and long chain fats. Contains a small amount (7.6 mg/100 ml, 0.95 mg/100 ml) lactose, milk protein (casein) and medium chain vegetable fats.

MCT (1) is not a complete feed. The manufacturers recommend that a vitamin supplement which includes retinol, cholealciferol, thiamine, riaboflavin, pyridoxine, cyanocobalamin, ascorbic acid, tocopherol, biotin, folic acid, nicotinamide and pantothenate be given (*see* Vitamin supplements, p. 226). In addition, a trace metal supplement of iron, copper, zinc, manganese, aluminium, cobalt, molybdenum and iodine is also recommended (*see* Mineral supplements, p. 226). The sodium content is below the FAO guidelines; the protein content is higher than the FAO guidelines; the carbohydrate is lower than the ESPGAN recommendations of 8 g/100 ml feed. The linoleic acid content appears to fall below the FAO guidelines of 200 mg/100 ml feed.
Preparation — 12.5% solution. Four scoops (each containing 3.1 g powder) made up to a total volume of 100 ml by the addition of water.

Caprilon   *Nutricia*

Free of sucrose, starch and gluten. Contains milk protein (whey and casein), a reduced amount of lactose (9.2 g/100 g powder, 1.2 g/100 ml feed), medium and long chain vegetable fats.

Complete feed, no supplements recommended by manufacturers. Linoleic acid content (64 mg/100 ml) lower than FAO guidelines of 200 mg/100 ml feed. Iron content (0.585 mg/100 ml feed) is below the FAO recommendations for a supplemented milk; cholecalciferol content (2.25 µg/100 ml) is above the maximum recommended, tocopherol content (0.18 mg/100 ml feed), is below FAO guidelines.

Preparation — 15% solution. One scoop (4.5 g) powder added to 30 ml water.

This product is not recommended for the treatment of galacto-saemia.

Portagen Powder   *Mead Johnson*

Free of lactose, starch and gluten. Contains milk protein (casein), sucrose, medium chain vegetable fats and a small amount of long chain vegetable fats. Complete feed, no supplements recommended. Meets FAO criteria for all nutrients.
Preparation — 14% solution. 50 g powder added to 315 ml water.

IV.8 Composition of MCT milks

Milk		Protein (g)	LCTs (g)	MCTs (g)	Carbohydrate (g)	Energy (kcal)	Sodium (mmol)	Osmolality (mosmol/kg)
MCT (1)	100 g powder	25.6	—	28.0	40.6	507	4.3	
	100 ml feed	3.2	—	3.5	5.1	63	0.54	162
Caprilon	100 g powder	11.5	0.7	26.1	57.1	498	6.52	
	100 ml feed	1.5	0.1	3.4	7.4	65	0.85	160
Portagen	100 g powder	16.5	2.9	19.0	54.3	488	9.61	
	100 ml feed	2.5	0.4	2.8	8.2	74	1.46	236

See also Pregestimil, Alfare and Modular Feeding Regimes.

IV.9 Elemental or chemically defined formulae

This type of formula usually is designed to bypass the normal digestive processes, as it is said to be 'pre-digested'. The use of elemental feeds should be considered as a safer alternative to intra-venous nutrition wherever bowel sounds are present but gut function is likely to be poor. Because there is no intact protein these formulae are hypoallergenic and can also be used if there is intolerance to milk and other protein or as the basis for an elimination diet for food allergy (*see* Chapter 10 and Appendix IV.33).

The protein consists of short chain peptides or free amino acids which require little or no hydrolysis by intestinal peptidases. Preparations containing peptides are considered to have advantages over amino acid preparations because they have a lower osmolality and are thought to be more rapidly absorbed, although clinical trials have failed to demonstrate any convincing benefits of one type of feed over the other.

Carbohydrate is generally in the form of hydrolysed corn starch or short chain glucose polymers. Such products are almost all free of lactose and other disaccharides.

Elemental formulae are usually low in fat, though there should be a small proportion of linoleic acid present to prevent the development of a deficiency of essential fatty acids. Where extra triglyceride is present, a proportion of it is in the form of medium chain triglycerides (MCTs).

There are several products available in powder or ready to feed form. Alternatively a modular preparation can be designed using a protein source that consists of peptides or amino acids (*see* Appendix IV.12).

Most complete formulae are designed for use in adults and, although the preparations contain vitamins, minerals and trace elements, an adequate intake of these will only be achieved if a large volume of feed is taken. Where such products are used for infants and small children, extra supplements will be required.

There have been few reports on the long-term use of elemental or chemically defined diets in children in situations where no 'natural' foods are taken. If such use is contemplated for periods of longer than 3–4 weeks careful monitoring of growth and other nutritional parameters should be undertaken on a regular basis.

Although this type of product has been found to be useful in conditions such as short gut, inflammatory bowel disease and pre- and postsurgery to the gut they have several disadvantages and consideration should be given to the use of a non-elemental formula that has been adapted to overcome a specific digestive problem, such as low lactose or low fat formulae before an elemental feed is started.

The major disadvantage of elemental products is the high osmolality caused by the large number of small particles in the formula. Introduction of elemental feeds should be very slow, an the initial feed must be a small volume of a dilute formula. Even quarter-strength feeds may have the same osmolality as a full-strength normal milk feed.

In sick or young children the suggested starting formula is one-eighth strength for at least 12 hours, increasing to quarter strength only if there are no symptoms such as vomiting, abdominal discomfort or diarrhoea. Half-strength feeds should be continued for at least 24 hours and progression from half- to full-strength feeds should be carried out particularly slowly because the feed will be hyperosmolar at this concentration. A three-quarter strength feed will be necessary for at least 24 hours, and an intermediate dilution between three-quarter and full strength may be required.

A further disadvantage of elemental formulae is the unpalatable taste of most products. This is unlikely to cause major problems in infants feeding from a bottle, but older children will need considerable persuasion to take this type of feed from a cup. Toddlers may accept the feed more readily from a feeding bottle or beaker and older children through a straw. If the feed is chilled prior to offering it to the child, the taste is less obvious. Flavourings are available for some products or milk shake flavouring can be added. Both types of flavourings will increase both the osmolality and the allergenicity of the feed.

Neocate   *Scientific Hospital Supplies*

Powder. Free of lactose, sucrose, gluten, milk and all intact protein. Protein: synthetic L-amino acids; pattern based on human breast milk. Contains fat, including a small amount of MCTs. Carbohydrate: maltodextrin. Unflavoured; flavouring available but not recommended for infants of less than 6 months of age.

Designed for use in neonates and infancy. Normal vitamin, mineral and trace element requirements met in 25 g Neocate powder/kg body weight per day.

Preparation — 15% solution. One scoop (5 g) Neocate powder plus 30 ml water.

Pepdite 0−2   *Scientific Hospital Supplies*

Powder. Free of lactose, sucrose, gluten, milk and intact protein. Protein: low-molecular-weight peptides (hydrolysed non-milk protein) and L-amino acids. Contains long chain fat. Carbohydrate: maltodextrin. Unflavoured; flavourings available.

Designed for use in the 0−2 year age range. Normal vitamin, mineral and trace element requirements met in 25 g/kg body weight per day.

Preparation — 15% solution. One scoop (5 g) Pepdite 0−2 plus 30 ml water.

MCT Pepdite 0−2

As for Pepdite 0−2, except fat component consists mainly of MCTs.

Pepdite 2+   *Scientific Hospital Supplies*

Composition as for Peptide 0−2.
Designed for use in children over the age of 2 years.
Preparation — 20% solution. One sachet (100 g) plus 400 ml water gives 500 ml.

MCT Pepdite 2+

As for Pepdite 2+, except 50% fat component consists of MCTs.

Elemental 028   *Scientific Hospital Supplies*

Powder. Free of lactose, sucrose, gluten, milk and all intact protein. Protein: synthetic L-amino acids; pattern based on human breast milk. Contains long chain fat. Carbohydrate: maltodextrin. Orange flavour and unflavoured versions available.

Designed for use in adults; not recommended for use in infants aged less than one year. Normal adult vitamin, mineral and trace element requirements contained in 500 g powder.

Preparation. One sachet (100 g) Elemental 028 powder plus 650 ml water to give a final volume of 750 ml.

Alfare   *Nestlé*

Powder. Free of lactose, sucrose, gluten and intact milk protein.

Protein: whey hydrolysate; 80% peptides, 20% free amino acids. Contains 50% long chain fat and 50% MCTs. Carbohydrate: glucose polymer and potato starch. Unflavoured.

Designed for use in infants. Contains full range of vitamins, minerals and trace elements.

Preparation — 15% solution. Three scoops (15 g) Alfare powder plus 90 ml water.

Flexical   *Mead Johnson*

Powder. Free of lactose, sucrose, gluten and intact milk protein. Protein: casein hydrolysate, 70% free amino acids, 30% small peptides. Contains long chain fat and MCTs. Carbohydrate: corn syrup solids and tapioca starch. Unflavoured.

Designed for use in adults. Normal adult vitamin, mineral and trace element requirements contained in 454 g powder.

Preparation. One can (454 g) Flexical powder plus water to make up to final volume of 2000 ml.

Criticare Liquid   *Mead Johnson*

Free of lactose, sucrose, gluten and intact milk protein. Protein: casein hydrolysate and L-amino acids. Contains long chain fats. Carbohydrate: maltodextrin and corn starch. Unflavoured.

Designed for use in adults. Normal adult mineral, vitamin and trace element requirements contains in 1900 ml volume.

Preparation. Ready to feed.

Vivonex Powder   *Eaton Laboratories*

Free of lactose, sucrose, gluten, milk and all intact protein. Protein: synthetic L-amino acids. Contains minimal fat as linoleic acid. Carbohydrate: glucose solids. Unflavoured; flavourings available.

Designed for use in adults. Normal adult requirements of vitamins, minerals and trace elements contained in 480 g powder.

Preparation. One sachet (80 g) Vivonex powder plus 250 ml water gives final volume of 300 ml.

Vivonex HN

Composition as for Vivonex; contains approximately twice the quantity of amino acids.

Pregomin   *Milupa*

Semi-elemental formula. Free of lactose, sucrose, gluten and milk protein. Protein: hydrolysed bovine collagen and hydrolysed soy protein. Contains long-chain vegetable fats. Carbohydrate: maltodextrin and precooked starch.

Designed for use in infants and children. Conforms to FAO/WHO recommendations for infant formulae.

Preparation — 15% solution. Four scoops (4.5 g per scoop) Pregomin powder plus 100 ml water.

IV.10 Composition of elemental or chemically defined formulae

Product	Protein (g)	Fat LCT (g)	MCTs (g)	Carbohydrate (g)	Energy (kcal)	Osmolality (mosmol)
Neocate						
per 100 g powder	13.5	22.9	0.6	56.0	475	
per 100 ml feed	2.0	2.8	0.1	8.4	71	320/kg
Pepdite 0–2						
per 100 g powder	13.8	22.9	0.6	56.0	475	
per 100 ml feed	2.1	3.4	0.1	8.4	70	195/kg
MCT Pepdite 0–2						
per 100 g powder	13.8	3.2	15.6	62.6	450	
per 100 ml feed	2.1	0.5	2.3	9.4	67	337/kg
Pepdite 2+						
per 100 g powder	13.9	11.8	6.3	63.0	450	
per 100 ml feed	2.8	2.4	1.3	12.6	90	288/kg
MCT Pepdite 2+						
per 100 g powder	13.9	3.2	15.6	62.4	460	
per 100 ml feed	2.8	0.6	3.2	12.5	92	360/kg
Elemental 028						
per 100 g powder	12.0	6.6	0	77.8	400	
per 100 ml feed	1.6	0.9	0	10.4	53	520/l
Alfare						
per 100 g powder	16.5	14.3	11.5	51.7	480	
per 100 ml feed	2.5	2.1	1.7	7.8	72	220/kg
Flexical						
per 100 g powder	9.7	12.0	3.0	67.0	440	
per 100 ml feed	2.2	2.7	0.7	15.2	100	550/kg
Criticare						
per 100 ml feed	3.8	0.3	0	22.2	100	650/kg
Vivonex						
per 100 g powder	7.5	0.6	0	86.5	376	
per 100 ml feed	2.0	0.1	0	23.0	100	550/l
Vivonex HN						
per 100 g powder	16.5	0.3	0	79.3	376	
per 100 ml feed	4.4	Trace	0	21.1	100	800/l
Pregomin						
per 100 g powder	13.3	24.2	0	57.0	499	
per 100 ml feed	2.0	3.6	0	8.6	75	210/l

IV.11 Modular feeding preparations

Despite the large numbers of specialized formulae that have become available, a situation arises on many occasions when no preparation appears to be exactly suitable, or the preparation is not available.

In these cases it is possible to formulate a recipe using modules which supply one or more of the major nutrients: a feed can be 'tailored' to match an individual's requirements and idiosyncracies. The formulation and preparation of modular feeds requires a great deal of time and expertise, so it is wise to try a number of the large range of complete feeds available in the first instance.

Most of the complete specialized formulae available on the market adhere to the WHO recommendations for a complete baby milk (p. 218) for all nutrients. An adequate volume of the full-strength recipe of any of these products will contain sufficient vitamins, minerals and trace elements. There is no such safeguard when individual modules are used. Some formulations will contain no added micronutrients; others, designed primarily for use with adults, will contain a balance of vitamins and minerals that is unsuitable for the young child. Care must be taken to ensure that minimum recommendations for all nutrients (Appendix I) are met.

Protein

Protein modules currently available contain intact or hydrolysed milk protein, amino acids, chicken meat or soy protein isolate.

The method or preparation given for these preparations will give a protein content of 2.4–2.7 g/100 ml prepared feed, in accordance with WHO recommendations; 100 ml fluid/kg body weight will thus provide a young infant with his protein requirement.

The FAO recommendation of 2.2–2.4 g protein/kg per day from birth to 3 months and 1.85–2.2 g protein/kg daily from 3 to 5 months can be exceeded provided that there is no renal or hepatic impairment. If protein is well tolerated then it is possible to improve the energy intake by using protein to provide energy in the diet. It is most important to monitor both blood urea nitrogen and renal and liver function if this course is chosen, as an inappropriately high protein intake will result in vomiting and failure to thrive, as well as more serious consequences. The protein intake should be calculated on an actual weight basis, not on expected weight for a given age, because, except where the weight deficit is due to dehydration, weight is a reflection of the actively metabolizing kidney and liver tissue. It is possible for protein intakes of up to 10 g/kg daily to be tolerated in this way, providing that deamination and urea synthesis can keep pace with the protein load. If a protein intake of greater than 15% of total energy or 3 g/kg daily is continued for some time, the extra pyridoxine (vitamin B_6) is advisable.

The choice of protein will depend upon the suspected food intolerance, but the choice will also affect the osmolality of the final feed. Due to the direct relationship between the osmolar load and the number of particles in the solution, intact protein modules will have a lower osmolality than hydrolysates and amino acid mixtures.

Fats

Fat modules provide energy in the form of long chain or medium chain vegetable fats. Unless fat intolerance is proven, it is generally preferable to use a long chain fat, due to the problems of introduction of MCTs rapidly into a feed (p. 257). If MCTs are used as the sole source of fat, a linoleic acid supplement should be given. Fat

modules are available in two forms: oils or water miscible emulsions. If an oil is used, a measured quantity should be added to
individual feeds, and these should be shaken at intervals during
administration to aid dispersion of the oil. The use of 50% w/v
emulsion of oil and water will overcome the problems of separ-
ating out.

These preparations do not contain any intrinsic or added micronutrients; they are designed as a feed supplement.

A fat concentration similar to that found in normal milk formulae (i.e. 2.0–4.0 g/100 ml feed) is likely to be tolerated by most
infants. Above 4 g fat/100 ml, extra fat should be introduced
cautiously, increasingly by no more than 1 g fat/100 ml daily. A
concentration above 6 g fat/100 ml is usually not tolerated by
young infants, who will develop steatorrhoea. If a particularly high
fat intake is achieved (more than 40% of the total energy intake),
then an extra tocopherol supplement is recommended. It is most
important that the energy intake from fat (both parenteral and
oral) does not equal or exceed the combined energy intake from
protein and carbohydrate. Under these circumstances ketosis and
hypoglycaemia are likely to occur, particularly if MCTs are used.

Carbohydrate

Sucrose, glucose or fructose can be used to supplement protein and
fat modules, if no intolerance is suspected. The disadvantages of
these is their relatively high osmolality. Most of the carbohydrate
modules available are based on hydrolysed corn starch and consist
of maltodextrins and higher polymers.

A solution containing 5 g carbohydrate/100 ml is usually well
tolerated. Concentrations in excess of 8 g/100 ml can be achieved
by gradually increasing the carbohydrate concentration by no more
than 1 g/100 ml per 24 hours. If monosaccharides are used then an
initial concentration of 5 g/100 ml is suggested, increasing gradually as described up to 7 or 8 g/100 ml. Care should be taken if the
carbohydrate source is fructose alone as acidosis may result. If di-
or polysaccharides are used an initial concentration of 7 g/100 ml
can be used, gradually increasing up to 10 g/100 ml. If a high
carbohydrate intake (greater than 50% of the total energy intake)
is achieved then extra supplements of thiamine may be necessary
and the infant should be monitored for hyperglycaemia and
glycosuria.

It is vital that sufficient carbohydrate is given to maintain a
normal blood glucose level. Small and malnourished infants lack
the enzymic pathways for efficient gluconeogenesis and are particularly prone to hypoglycaemia. Under no circumstances should
an infant receive a carbohydrate-free regimen without frequent
blood glucose monitoring. If a complete gastrointestinal intolerance to all carbohydrate is suspected then fat and protein oral
modules can be introduced while the infant receives intravenous
dextrose.

Minerals and vitamins

The inclusion of sodium and potassium in adequate amounts, either orally or intravenously, is vital at all times. The recommendations on p. 200 give a generalized guideline. If the modules chosen do not contain other minerals such as calcium, phosphorus and magnesium then these must be added according to requirements no longer than 48 hours after commencing the regimen. The protein modules derived from milk protein generally contain calcium in fairly large quantities. Hypercalcaemia can result if a calcium containing supplement is also given. Trace elements should be added after 48 hours if the regimen does not contain them. Suitable preparations are listed on p. 225.

Small and malnourished infants and children have few reserves of vitamins, particularly the water-soluble ones, and these should be added after 48 hours if the regimen does not contain them. Suitable multivitamin preparations are listed on p. 225, but the individual vitamin requirements should be assessed if anything other than a normal balance of nutrients is used.

Protein modules

Derived from whole milk protein

Casec Powder   *Mead Johnson Nutritionals*

Calcium caseinate. Contains traces of lactose and a small quantity of butterfat. No added vitamins or minerals; high calcium and low sodium content.
Preparation. 30 g Casec powder plus carbohydrate and fat, made up to a final volume of 1000 ml with water.

Casilan Powder   *Glaxo-Farley*

Calcium caseinate. Contains traces of lactose and butterfat. No added vitamins or minerals; high calcium and minimal sodium content.
Preparation. 30 g Casilan powder plus carbohydrate and fat, made up to a final volume of 1000 ml with water.

Maxipro   *Scientific Hospital Supplies*

Whey protein supplemented with amino acids. Contains butterfat and a trace of lactose. No added vitamins or minerals; low calcium and sodium content.
Preparation. 30 g Maxipro powder plus carbohydrate and fat, made up to a final volume of 1000 ml with water.

Propac   *Biosearch Medical Products*

Whey protein with some butterfat and lactose. No added vitamins or minerals; moderate calcium and sodium content.
Preparation. 39 g (2 sachets) Propac powder plus carbohydrate and fat made up to a final volume of 1000 ml with water.

Protifar   *Nutricia*

Skimmed milk concentrate. Very low lactose. Low fat. Requires full vitamin and mineral supplement, except calcium.

Preparation. 30 g (12 scoops) Protifar powder plus carbohydrate and fat if made up to a final volume of 1000 ml with water.

Hydrolysed protein

Albumaid Complete Powder   *Scientific Hospital Supplies*

Beef serum hydrolysate, free of fat and carbohydrate. Product is supplemented with a full range of vitamins, minerals and trace elements, but the supplementation is not appropriate for young infants — levels of most added nutrients are in excess of the WHO recommendations. In particular the low calcium (25 mg/100 ml), high phosphorus (37 mg/100 ml) and a calcium : phosphorus ratio of 0.68 indicate that blood levels of these nutrients should be checked regularly. In very small infants who may be prone to hypocalcaemia this produce is best avoided.
Preparation. 30 g Albumaid complete powder plus a fat and carbohydrate source, made up to a final volume of 1000 ml with water.

Amirge Powder   *Nutricia*

Lactalbumin hydrolysate. Contains a small amount of lactose and a trace of butterfat. Vitamins and minerals not added; moderate calcium and adequate sodium content.
Preparation. 30 g Amirge Powder plus fat and carbohydrate made up to a final volume of 1000 ml with water.

Meat-based products

Comminuted Chicken   *Cow & Gate, Nutricia*

Liquidized ground chicken meat in water. Contains some fat and no carbohydrate. Vitamins and minerals not added.
Preparation. 330 g (3 jars) plus fat and carbohydrate source made up to a final volume of 1000 ml.

Amino acids

Aminutrin   *Geistlich Sons Ltd*

Synthetic amino acids, free of fat and carbohydrate. Vitamins and minerals not added.
Preparation. 30 g (2 sachets) Aminutrin powder plus fat and carbohydrate, made up to a final volume of 1000 ml.

Modules containing more than one nutrient

Protein and fat

Product 3232 A powder   *Mead Johnson*

Protein—casein hydrolysate; contains medium and long chain vegetable fats and some starch. Complete feed apart from carbohydrate — meets with WHO recommendations for vitamins, minerals and trace elements.
Preparation. 88 g 3232 A powder plus carbohydrate made up to a final volume of 1000 ml.

Ross Carbohydrate Free (RCF) concentrated Liquid   Abbott Laboratories

Protein—soy protein isolate; contains long chain vegetable fats and a trace of carbohydrate. Free of lactose. Complete feed apart from carbohydrate — meets with WHO recommendations for vitamins, minerals and trace elements. Manufacturers advise the addition of an iron supplement.
Preparation. One tin (384 ml) RCF concentrated Liquid plus carbohydrate made up to a final volume of 770 ml with water, or 500 ml (1.33 tins) plus carbohydrate made up to a final volume of 1000 ml with water.

Protein and carbohydrate

Prosol Extra Powder, Protifar Powder   *Cow & Gate, Nutricia*

Modified skimmed milk powder, containing lactose. Some vitamins and minerals not added; high calcium and low-normal sodium content. Requires supplementation with most vitamins and trace elements.
Preparation. 45 g Prosol or Protifar plus carbohydrate and a fat source made up to a final volume of 1000 ml.

Maxamine Complete   *Scientific Hospital Supplies*

Synthetic amino acids and maltodextrins. Vitamins and minerals added. WHO recommendations generally exceeded. Sodium content (2.5 mmol per 100 ml) is higher than recommended; a calcium: phosphorus ratio of 1.1 is lower than suggested and the retinol content of 35 µg/100 ml is below the recommendation of 50–100 µg/100 ml.
Preparation. Maxamine complete powder (90 g) plus a fat source made up to 1000 ml with water.

Fat and carbohydrate

Product 80056 powder   *Mead Johnson*

Free of protein. Contains glucose polymers and some starch; fat is in the form of long chain vegetable fats. Vitamins and minerals added; conforms to WHO recommendations, apart from sodium, which the manufacturers advise should be added.
Preparation. 117.5 g 80056 powder plus protein made up to a final volume of 1000 ml with water.

Duocal Powder   *Scientific Hospital Supplies*

Free of protein. Contains hydrolysed starch, long chain fats and medium chain fats in the form of an emulsion; 34% of the total lipid content is in the form of MCTs. Vitamins, minerals and trace elements have not been included.
Also available — Duocal liquid.

Duocal MCT Powder   *Scientific Hospital Supplies*

Free of protein. Contains hydrolysed starch, a small amount of LCTs, linoleic acid and medium chain fats in the form of an emulsion. Vitamins, minerals and trace elements have not been included.

IV.12 Composition of protein modules

Product (per 100 g powder)	Protein (g)	Fat (g)	Carbohydrate (g)	Energy (kcal)	Sodium (mmol)	Calcium (mg)	Supplementation
Intact milk protein							
Casec	88	2	—	372	6.5	1600	Full supplement required except Ca
Casilan	90	2	Trace	383	0.3	1200	As for Casec
Maxipro	88	4	Trace	390	10.0	300	Full supplement required
Propac	77	8	5	402	10.0	600	As for Casec
Protifar	88.5	1.0	0.5	377	1.3	1350	As for Casec
Hydrolysed protein							
Albumaid Complete	74	—	—	300	34.8	850	Vitamins + minerals added (*see* text)
Amirge	83	Trace	3	354	30.4	800	As for Casec
Meat based (per 100 g liquid)							
Comminuted Chicken	7.5	3	—	60	0.4	9	Full supplement required
Amino acids (per 100 g powder)							
Aminutrin	77	—	—	257	—	—	Full supplement required

IV.13 Composition of two nutrient modules

Product per 100 g powder or per 100 ml liquid concentrate	Protein (g)	Fat LCTs (g)	MCTs (g)[a]	Carbohydrate (g)	Energy (kcal)	Sodium (mmol)	Calcium (mg)	Vitamin and mineral supplementation required
Product 3232A	22	15.0	18.0	33.0	500	15.6	719	Not required
Ross CHO free (per 100 ml) concentrate	4.0	7.2	—	0.1	81	2.6	140	Requires iron
Product 80056	0	22.5	—	71.8	490	3.1	540	Requires sodium
Duocal	0	14.8	7.5	72.7	421	1.2	30/100 ml (0.8 mmol)	Requires full supplement
Duocal MCT	0	4.0	19.2	74.0	474	7.6	30/100 ml (0.8 mmol)	Requires full supplement
Prosol Extra	60.0	1.0	—	29.1	365	13.0	1300	*See* text

na = not available.

IV.14 Composition of non-protein modules

Product and manufacturer	Form	Fat (g)	Carbohydrate (g)	Energy (kcal)	Sodium (mmol)
Carbohydrate — per 100 g powder sugar, glucose, fructose		—	100	400	Trace
Calonutrin (Geistlich)	Polysaccharides, disaccharides, monosaccharides	—	100	410	4.0
Fantomalt (Nutricia)	Maltodextrin	—	97	385	2.2
Maxijul (SHS) Maxijul (LE)	Hydrolysed food starch — 5 glucose polymers	—	96	375	0.1 0.01
Moducal (Mead Johnson)	Hydrolysed corn starch	—	100	376	3.0
Polycose (Abbott)	Hydrolysed corn starch	—	100	376	5.4
Sumnacal (Biosearch)	Hydrolysed corn starch	—	95	382	4.3
Fats — per 100 ml liquid Vegetable oil	LCT oil	99	—	830	Trace
Calogen (SHS)	LCT arachis oil emulsion	50	—	450	0.9
Microlipid (Biosearch)	LCT safflower oil emulsion	50	—	450	—
Liquigen (SHS)	MCT emulsion	52	—	407	1.7
MCT oil (Mead John, Cow & Gate, Nutricia)	MCT oil	98	—	818	—

IV.15 Full-strength modular feed using meat protein
Example of feed for 6-kg infant

Feed		Protein (g)	Fat (g)	Carbohydrate (g)	Energy (kcal)	Sodium (mmol)	Potassium (mmol)	Calcium (mg)	Iron (mg)
Comminuted Chicken	300 g	22.5	9.0	0	181	1.3	3.8	27	1.2
Calogen	45 ml	0	22.5	0	203	0.4		0	0
Moducal	70 g	0	0	70	281	2.1		0	0
Mineral Mixture	6 g	0	0	0	0	10.3	12.7	492	3.8
Water to make up to a total volume of 860 ml									
Feed totals:		22.5	31.5	70	665	14.1	16.5	519	5.0
per 100 ml feed		2.6	3.7	8.1	77	1.6	1.9	60	0.58
per kg body weight		3.7			110	2.3	2.7		

Because none of the modules used contains vitamins or minerals, a complete supplement, Metabolic Mineral Mixture (Scientific Hospital Supplies) 1 g/kg body weight was used. Additional iron may also be required.
In addition a full vitamin supplement such as Ketovite tablets and liquid (Paines & Byrne) is required.

IV.16 High-energy modular feed

Many small infants will not thrive unless they receive an energy intake approaching 140 kcal/kg actual weight. Because feeds which supply more than 1.0 kcal/ml are not well tolerated, a generous fluid intake of 150–200 ml/kg body weight may be required.
Example of high energy density feed for 6-kg infant

Feed		Protein (g)	Fat (g)	Carbohydrate (g)	Energy (kcal)	Sodium (mmol)	Potassium (mmol)
Comminuted Chicken	440 g	33	13	0	260	1.9	5.6
Calogen	50 ml	0	25	0	226	0.4	Trace
Moducal	95 g	0	0	95	382	3.0	Trace
Mineral Mixture	8 g	0	0	0	0	13.8	17.0
Water to make up to 950 ml							
Feed totals		33	38	95	868	19.1	22.6
per 100 ml feed		3.5	4	10	79	2.0	2.4
per kg body weight		5.5			145	3.2	3.7

Extra sodium and potassium are recommended in this feed; in addition a high intake of B vitamins is also required. If a mutivitamin preparation such as Ketovite is used this can be achieved by increasing the dose from three tablets to four tablets daily.
Transition from the normal full strength feed, providing 77 kcal/ml to the high energy feed should be a gradual planned one, taking place over a period of 5–7 days.

IV.17 Full-strength modular feed using hydrolysate

Example of feed for a 3-kg infant

Ingredient	Protein (g)	Fat (g)	Carbohydrate (g)	Energy (kcal)	Na$^+$ (mmol)	K$^+$ (mmol)
15 g Albumaid Complete	11.7	—	—	45	5.2	0.6
60 g Maxijul	—	—	60.0	240	—	—
30 ml Calogen	—	15.0 (LCTs)	—	135	—	—
30 ml Liquigen	—	15.0 (MCTs)	—	124	—	—
3.0 g Metabolic Mixture[a]	—	—	—	—	5.2	6.3
Totals:	11.7	30.0	60.0	544	10.4	6.9
Per kg:	3.9	(5%)	(10%)	181	3.5	2.3

[a] Mineral supplement is Metabolic Mineral Mixture.

IV.18 Transfer from parenteral to oral modular feed

A 3-kg infant initially fed on 200 ml/kg parenteral fluids. The volume of intravenous fluids is decreased as oral fluids increased

Day	Oral fluids (ml)	Carbohydrate (g)	Protein (g)	Fat (g)	Mineral supplement[a] (g)	Energy (kcal)
1 (am)	30	0.5 (1.6%)	—	—	—	
(pm)	30	1.0 (1.6%)	—	—	—	6
2 (am)	50	1.5 (3.3%)	—	—	—	
(pm)	50	2.5 (5%)	—	—	—	16
3 (am)	100	5.0 (5%)	—	—	—	
(pm)	100	5.0 (5%)	—	2 ml Calogen (1.0 g LCT)		49
4 (am)	150	7.5 (5%)	—	1.5 (LCTs)	0.25	
(pm)	150	7.5 (5%)	—	1.5 (LCTs) 1.5 (MCTs)	0.25	99
5 (am)	200	10.0 (5%)	—	2.0 (LCTs) 2.0 (MCTs)	0.5	
(pm)	200	10.0 (5%)	3.0 g Albumaid	2.0 (LCTs) 2.0 (MCTs)	0.5	159
6 (am)	250	12.5 (5%)	4.0 g Albumaid	2.5 (LCTs) 2.5 (MCTs)	0.75	
(pm)	250	15.0 (6%)	5.0 g Albumaid	3.5 (LCTs) 3.5 (MCTs)	0.75	241
7 (am)	300	18.0 (6%)	5.5 g Albumaid	4.0 (LCTs) 4.0 (MCTs)	1.0	
(pm)	300	22.0 (7%)	5.5 g Albumaid	5.5 (LCTs) 5.5 (MCTs)	1.0	357[b]

[a] Mineral supplement is Metabolic Mineral Mixture.

[b] This feed is approximately three-quarter strength full volume, and parenteral fluids can be discontinued if the infant tolerates this feed.

IV.19 Lactose content of foods

Foods with a high lactose content (>1 g/100 g)	Foods with a low lactose content (<1 g/100 g)	Foods free of lactose
Milks of all species; milk-based desserts; single cream; yoghurt; ice cream Some processed infant savoury dishes Cream soups	Hard cheese; double cream; butter; margarines Some processed meat and fish dishes — e.g. burgers, sausage, fish fingers	Most coffee whiteners/creamers; soy milks; margarines prepared from vegetable products; ghee; oils; cooking fats Meat; poultry; fish; egg; offal
Some artificial sweetners Milk chocolate	Toffee; filled chocolate products; some fizzy drinks and 'pop'	Saccharin; cyclamate; glucose; fructose; sucrose; jam; jelly; jello; clear fruit-type sweets and gums Gelatin; most fruit drinks
Processed milk/cheese based fruit, vegetable and pasta dishes; white sauce (sweet and savoury) Most infant breakfast cereals and rusks	Some adult breakfast cereals Some breads; biscuits and baked goods Some flavoured crisps and savoury snacks	Vegetables; potato; peas; beans; lentils; nuts Fruit Rice; wheat; barley; oats; maize; sago; semolina; tapioca; cornflour Most breads; most adult-type breakfast cereals; pasta

IV.20 Foods which may contain milk

Protein foods: sausages, burgers, frozen and canned meat and fish in sauce, meat and fish coated with batter or breadcrumbs.
Cereal products: infant cereals and rusks, biscuits and cookies, milk bread, buns, cakes, pastries, canned spaghetti with cheese.
Dairy products: margarines, canned, dehydrated and frozen desserts and ice creams, canned and dehydrated baby desserts, powdered coffee whiteners and cream substitutes, malted milks.
Fruit and vegetables: canned and dehydrated vegetables in sauce.
Confectionary: milk chocolate, filled chocolates and chocolate bars, toffees and soft sweets or candies, lemon curd, chocolate-type spreads.
Miscellaneous: canned and dehydrated soups, mustard, pickles in sauce, flavoured crisps and similar snack items, salad dressings.

IV.21 Glucose and galactose content of foods

Foods with a high glucose or galactose content (>1 g/100 g)	Foods with a low glucose or galactose content (<1 g/100 g)	Foods free of glucose and galactose
Milk-based foods	Hard cheese; double cream; butter; margarine Liver; shellfish	Oils; cooking fats; ghee Meat; poultry; fish; egg
Lactose-based artificial sweeteners Sucrose and foods containing sucrose Starch and foods containing starch		Saccharin; cyclamate; fructose (laevulose) powder; Aspartame
Root vegetables; starchy vegetables; peas; beans; lentils; nuts Most fruits and fruit drinks	Green leafy vegetables; asparagus; bamboo shoots; brussel sprouts; celery; herbs; marrow; mushrooms; squash Cantaloupe melon; lemon	Salt; pepper; vinegar; spices Gelatin
Rice; wheat; oats; maize; barley; soya; sago; semolina; tapioca Pasta; breakfast cereal; bread; baked goods		

IV.22 Fructose content of foods

Foods with a high fructose content (>1 g/100 g)	Foods with a low fructose content (<1 g/100 g)	Foods free of fructose
Some infant formulae; some soy milks Flavoured yoghurts; milk-based desserts; ice cream		Milk; cream; cheese; butter; plain (unflavoured) yoghurt Margarine; ghee; fats; oils Meat; poultry; fish; egg
Sucrose and foods containing sucrose, i.e. preserves and confectionary		Glucose; glucose polymer; cornstarch; dextrins Saccharin; cyclamate
Root vegetables; sweetcorn; tomato Peas; beans; lentils Most fruits and fruit drinks Corn (maize); soya; soy flour Some infant and adult breakfast cereals; biscuits and baked goods; rusks	Potato (old) Nuts; olives; avocado pear Green leafy vegetables; asparagus; bamboo shoots; broccoli; brussel sprouts; cauliflower; celery; mushrooms; squash; herbs Cranberries; lemon; loganberries; rhubarb	Rice; wheat; oats; barley; cornflour Pasta; most breads and flours Cornflour; sago; semolina; tapioca Salt; pepper; herbs; spices Gelatin

IV.23 Sucrose and starch content of foods

Foods containing added sucrose	Foods containing starch	Foods containing natural sucrose	Foods free or low in sucrose and starch
Processed milk-based desserts and puddings; ice cream Processed meat products — e.g. sausages[a], burgers[a] Processed fish products — e.g. fish fingers[a]			Milk; cream; cheese; butter; ghee; margarines; fats; oils Meat; poultry; offal; fish; egg
Some artificial sweeteners Sweets; candies; jam; jelly; jello; preserves; some honey		Some brands of pure honey	Glucose; lactose; fructose; saccharin; cyclamate; Aspartame
Canned vegetable and bean dishes[a] Some flavoured crisps and savoury snacks[a]	Potato; plain crisps; savoury snacks Soy beans; soy flour Peas; beans; lentils; nuts	Root vegetables[a], e.g. carrot, turnip Tomato; onion Banana[a] Fruits; unsweetened fruit juice	Green leafy vegetables; asparagus; celery; cauliflower; green beans; marrow; mushrooms Lemon; blackberries; cherries; cranberries; currants; gooseberries; grapes; raspberries; strawberries
Baked goods[a] — e.g. biscuits; cookies; cakes Canned pasta[a] and milk puddings Some adult[a] and infant breakfast cereals Wine; beer; cider; fruit drinks Sauces and ketchups Fizzy drinks; 'pop'	Rice; wheat; oats; barley; maize; tapioca; sago; semolina Pasta; bread; pastry Cornflour/cornstarch		Salt; pepper; herbs; spices; vinegar Spirits — e.g. gin, whisky Gelatin

[a] These foods also contain starch.

IV.24 Foods free of lactose and sucrose

Glucose (dextrose); fructose (laevulose) powders
Margarines prepared entirely from vegetable products; ghee;
cooking fats; cooking oils
Gelatin
Meat; poultry; fish; offal; egg
Salt; pepper; herbs; spices (not monosodium glutamate)
Potato[a]
Grapes; cherries; rhubarb[b]
Green leafy vegetables; green beans; celery[b]
Mushrooms; cauliflower; broccoli[b]
Rice; (wheat; oats; barley;) cornflour/cornstarch[a]
Sago; semolina; tapioca[a]
Some adult and infant type breakfast cereals (check ingredients)[a]
Most varieties of bread (check ingredients)[a]

[a] Contain starch.
[b] Contain traces of sucrose.
NB Wheat, oats, barley, semolina and breads contain gluten.

IV.25 Fat content of foods

Foods with a high fat content (6 g per adult sized portion)	Foods with a moderate fat content (2–6 g per adult sized portion)	Foods with a low fat content (2 g per adult sized portion)
Doughnuts	Biscuits, pastry, cakes, cookies	Breakfast cereals, flour, bread, rice, pasta
Whole milk, cream	Semi-skimmed milk, ice cream	Skimmed milk, low fat yoghurt
Beef, pork, lamb, sausages, hamburgers, meat pies	Chicken, oily fish, shellfish, packet soups	White fish, consommé, meat extracts
Egg, cheese, nuts, butter margarine	Low fat spreads	Egg white, cottage cheese, quark
Cooking fats and oils	Salad dressings	
Fried foods	Avocado pear, olives	Vegetables, fruits
Chocolate	Toffee	Clear fruit sweets and candies
	Malted milk powders	Fruit juice and squash, sugar, jam, preserves, jelly

IV.26 Cholesterol content of foods (mg/100 g food)

High cholesterol (>100 mg per adult size portion)		Moderate cholesterol (20–100 mg per adult size portion)		Low cholesterol (up to 20 mg per adult size portion)		Cholesterol free
Cream, double	140	Cream, single	66			
		Ice cream, dairy	21	Ice cream, non-dairy	11	
		Milk, whole	14	Milk, skim	2	Vegetable oil
		Butter and ghee	230			Vegetable margarine
		Cheese, cheddar	70	Cottage cheese	13	
		Cheese, stilton	120	Low fat yoghurt	7	
Egg, whole	450					Egg white
Kidney	400	Beef, raw	65			
Liver	370	Lamb and mutton	78			
		Pork	72			
		Chicken	69			
		Frankfurters	46			
		Sausage, raw	40			
		Salami	79			
		Beefburgers	59			
Cod roe	500–700	Cod	50			Fruit
Whiting	110	Plaice	70			Vegetables
Sardines	100					Cereals
Crab	100					Sugar
Prawns	200					
Shrimps	200					

IV.27 Uses of medium chain triglycerides

Medium chain triglycerides (MCTs) are oils containing fatty acids with a chain length of C_8–C_{12}.

The energy value of MCTs is 8.3 kcal/g (9 kcal/g other triglycerides). Fatty acids with these chain lengths normally constitute approximately 1% of naturally occurring fats. Commercially MCT is derived from coconut oil.

Because of their particle size they are more easily hydrolysed than other triglycerides and, once absorbed, enter directly into the bloodstream via the hepatic portal vein, thus providing a rapidly utilizable source of energy even in conditions where there is impairment of fat digestion and absorption.

MCT preparations are available as oils and water miscible emulsions (Appendix IV.13), and with the MCTs incorporated into milk formulae (Appendix IV.7 and IV.8).

MCTs exert a higher osmotic pressure than other triglycerides, and care must be taken not to introduce MCTs too rapidly into the diet, resulting in abdominal cramps, nausea and diarrhoea. The introduction of MCT milk formulae in infants is dealt with in Appendix IV.7. For older children foods containing a small amount of MCTs should be given initially, and portion size or MCT quantity built up over a period of days. Tolerance to the high osmolality develops with time.

For older children and adults, MCT oil can be used for cooking in a similar way to other edible oils.

It can be used for frying to add variety and energy to the diet, although the technique of cooking with MCTs is slightly different to that of using other oils. It has a low smoke point compared to other oils used for cooking and care must be taken that it does not burn. The optimum cooking temperature for MCTs is 160°C, compared to 210°C for corn oil.

Foods need to be cooked for a few minutes longer than normal because of the lower temperatures used.

If MCTs are heated above 20°C, they develop a bitter taste and an unpleasant odour and should be discarded if this happens.

As a consequence of the lower cooking temperature, the colour of items such as fried potato or chips is paler than that of foods cooked in other oils. Users should be warned not to cook for too long in the hope of achieving a more intense colour, as foods will become dry and hard in texture. Fat-containing foods such as bacon or meat can be fried using MCTs, but because these foods will leak long chain triglycerides into the MCTs the oil should be discarded after use. It can be re-used once or twice if it has been used for fat-free items such as potato or bread.

MCTs can also be used to make cakes, biscuits and pastry by following recipes which use oils such as corn in place of solid fats.

IV.28 Gluten content of foods

Gluten-free foods	Gluten-containing foods
Pure wheat starch (*see* special products)	Wheat, wheat based breakfast cereals, bread, flour, pastry, semolina, pasta and canned spaghetti
Corn (maize), sweetcorn, cornstarch, cornflour, cornflakes	
Rice, rice-based breakfast cereals, tapioca and sago	Oats, oat-based breakfast cereals, oatmeal and porridge
Buckwheat, cassava and arrowroot	Triticale, millet and sorghum
Soy beans and soy protein isolate, nuts, beans, pulses and lentils	Rye, rye breads and crispbreads
Fresh meat, poultry, offal, fresh fish and shellfish	Barley, beer, malted drinks and cereals
Potatoes, unflavoured potato crisps, fresh fruit and vegetables	
Milk, fresh cream, coffee whitener, cheese and eggs	
Butter, margarine, fats and oils	
Sugar, jams, jello, jelly and honey	
Clear fruit sweets or candies, ice lollies or popsicles	
Tea, coffee, fruit drinks, 'pop', wines and spirits	
Salt, ground pepper, powdered mustard, yeast extract, monosodium glutamate, herbs, powdered spices and bicarbonate of soda	

IV.29 Processed foods which may contain gluten

(Check the label)

Dessert mixes, custard and blancmange mixes, sweet and savoury sauce mixes, dessert toppings, artificial creams and aerosol packed creams

Canned, frozen or prepared fruit and vegetable products in sauce or pastry. Malted 'bedtime' drinks and chocolate-type drinks

All sweets and candies, filled chocolate, chocolate bars and ice cream

Textured vegetable protein and hydrolysed vegetable protein, soy-based meat extenders. Packaged suet, gravy powders and granules. Thickeners and improvers

Canned, frozen or prepared meat products in sauce, gravy or pastry. Smoked or processed meats, cold cuts, sausage, salami and products in breadcrumbs

Canned, frozen or prepared fish and shellfish products in sauce, mayonnaise, butter or breadcrumbs

Savoury spreads — meat pastes, fish paste, cheese based spreads. Packaged and canned soups. Savoury snacks and flavoured crisps

Ketchup, bottled and canned savoury sauces, mustards (unless powder), baking powder, mayonnaise and salad creams

---

IV.30 Special products available for wheat-free diets (low protein and gluten free)

Products manufactured from wheatstarch may be suitable for use in a gluten-free or a low protein diet. However, while low protein products are generally suitable for a gluten-free diet, the reverse is not true. Gluten free products may have milk and/or egg included in the ingredients, thus significantly increasing the protein content.

Product	Supplier	Gluten-free	Low protein
Rite-Diet/Wel-Plan	Welfare Foods (UK)		
	Anglo-Dietetics (USA)		
Gluten-free flour mix		Y	N
Gluten-free white bread mix		Y	N
Gluten-free brown bread mix		Y	N
Gluten-free white bread[a]		Y	N
Gluten-free brown bread[a]		Y	N
Gluten-free high fibre bread[a]		Y	N
Soy bran		Y	N
Gluten-free sweet and savoury biscuits		Y	N
Low protein flour mix		Y	Y
Low protein white bread[a]		Y	Y
Low protein bread with bran[a]		Y	Y
Low protein sweet biscuits		Y	Y
Paygel-P	General Mills		
Wheatstarch		Y	Y
Baking Mix		Y	Y
Aproten	General Mills (USA)		
	Carlo Erber (Ultrapharm, UK)		
Pasta		Y	Y
Rusks		Y	Y
Semolina		Y	Y

[a] Bread available in cans and/or sealed plastic packs.

IV.31 Soy content of foods

Foods which may include soya as an ingredient include:
1. Protein foods: sausages, burger, canned and frozen meat dishes in a sauce, shaped and minced (ground) meat products.
2. Cereal products: bread (information should be sought from individual bakeries), biscuits, cakes, pastries.
3. Dairy products: malted milk type beverages.
4. Miscellaneous: meat and vegetable extracts, savoury canned and bottled sauces, canned and dehydrated soups, soy sauce.

IV.32 Fibre content of foods

Good fibre sources (g fibre/100 g food)		Lesser sources (g fibre/100 g food)	
Cereals			
Bran (wheat)	44.0		
Bread		Bread — white	2.7
wholemeal	8.5		
brown	5.1		
Chapatti — wholemeal	8.0	Chapatti — chapatti flour	3.7
Rice, boiled — wholegrain	1.5	Rice, boiled — white	0.8
Biscuits/'cookies' —		Biscuits/'cookies' —	
wholemeal, e.g. 'Digestive'	5.5	white flour	2.3
Crispbread — rye	11.7	Crackers	3.0
Breakfast cereals		Breakfast cereals —	
bran based	26.7	rice based	4.0
wholewheat	12.7–15.4		
corn based	11.0		
muesli type	7.5		
Fruits			
Berry fruits	4.2–8.2	Strawberries	2.2
Banana	3.4	Apple — raw	2.0
Dates — fresh	8.5	Grapes	0.9
Damsons — raw	4.1	Orange	2.0
Prunes — stewed	8.1	Mango	1.5
Raisins, sultanas	7.0	Melon	1.0
Nuts			
Peanuts	8.1		
Peanut butter	7.6		
Coconut — fresh	13.6		
Other nuts	5.2–14.3		
Vegetables			
Potatoes, boiled		Cucumber	0.4
old	1.0	Lettuce	1.5
new	2.0	Tomato	1.5
Potato crisps	11.9		
(1 packed=approx 20 g)			
Root vegetables	2.8–3.1		
Leafy vegetables	2.5–3.0		
Spinach	6.3		
Beans			
green	3.4		
dried, boiled	5.1–7.4		
baked beans	7.3		
Peas — boiled	5.2		
Lentils, boiled — dhal	2.4		

IV.33 Minimal and low residue foods

Foods free of fibre	Low fibre foods (g fibre/100 g food)	
Egg	Cornstarch or cornflour	0.3
Fish and shellfish	White polished rice (boiled)	0.8
Meat[a]	Tapioca	Trace
Milk[a]	Spaghetti (white)	0.2
Cheese[a]		
Butter and margarine[a]		
Cooking fats and oils[a]		
Ice cream[a]		
Plain yoghourts[a]		
Meringues	Sponge cake (plain)	1.0
Jelly/Jello		
Sugar	Asparagus	0.8
Honey	Cucumber	0.4
Jam (no pips)		
Clear sweets/candies	Pumpkin	0.5
	Tomato flesh (no skin and pip)	0.9
Clear soups and broths	Grapes (no skin and pips)	0.9
	Melon	0.9
Fruit flavoured squash	Fresh/canned fruit juice	Trace
Fizzy drinks		
Tea and coffee		

[a] Although animal foods such as meat, milk and milk products contain no dietary fibre, they are incompletely digested in the small intestine. Food residue passes into the large intestine providing a substrate for bacterial action, and increasing the bulk of intestinal contents. These foods cannot be regarded as being residue free therefore. Milk and milk products result in appreciable quantities of stool bulk and may need to be restricted if a very low residue diet is required.

In malabsorption syndromes all foods are likely to result in food residue passing into the large bowel and thus increasing stool bulk.

IV.34 Elimination regimen

Stage I

Until symptoms have been absent for one week use foods of low reported allergenicity:

1. Lamb — cooked without the addition of meat or yeast extracts or manufactured 'gravy mixes'.
2. Green vegetables — such as cabbage or green beans, boiled in water.
3. Potatoes — boiled in water.
4. Rice — boiled in water, or ground rice cooked with water and sweetened with glucose as a cereal substitute.
5. Table salt may be added to taste.
6. Fluids should consist only of water sweetened with glucose.
7. Fresh pears — may be poached in water and sweetened with glucose.

No other foods or drinks should be taken. An elemental diet may be used to supplement this regimen and to supply minerals, vitamins and trace elements.

The ten stages of the elimination diet need not be introduced in the order given. Only one item of food should be introduced in any one day and a record should be kept of any symptoms that arise.

Stage II
Other foods of low allergenicity.
Sugar, root vegetables (e.g. carrot, turnip, swede), olive oil (for frying), other green vegetables (e.g. lettuce, brussel sprouts, cauliflower, broccoli).

Stage III
Citrus fruits and foods containing salicylate.
Apple, apricots, banana, cucumber, grapes, oranges, peaches, rhubarb, tomato.

Stage IV
Yeast.
Yeast extract, e.g. Marmite, used as gravy.

Stage V
Cereals.
Home-made yeast bread, flour, cornflour, corn oil, oats, wholemeal pasta.

Stage VI
Protein foods.
Chicken, egg, pork, ham, bacon (not sausages).

Stage VII
Dairy products.
Butter (not margarine), cheese, evaporated milk, whole milk, beef, veal.

Stage VIII
Pulses.
Peas (if Stage III tolerated), broad beans, soy milk, peanuts, vegetable oil, lentils.

Stage IX
Chocolate (if VII and VIII tol 5.1 ed), fish.

Stage X
Food additives.
Bread, biscuits, colourings (red, yellow and green), soft drinks, sausages (if beef, yeast and wheat tolerated), fish fingers (if fish and wheat tolerated).

Other items which appear on the initial diet record can then be introduced at the rate of one per day. In this way the true allergens in foods containing many ingredients can be pinpointed, rather than whole classes of foods being arbitrarily removed from the diet.

IV.35 Salicylates and additives in foods

Foods which contain natural salicylate

1. Vegetables: cucumber, peas, tomato
2. Fruit and nuts: almonds, apples, apricots, bananas, blackcurrants, berry fruits including raspberries, strawberries, cherries, grapes including sultanas, raisins, currants, oranges and similar fruits, peaches, prunes, rhubarb.

Foods which may contain additives (check the label)

1. Protein foods: canned, dehydrated and frozen meat or fish products, fresh products coated with breadcrumbs such as ham and fried fish, sausages, luncheon meats, burgers.
2. Cereal products: breakfast cereals, bought cakes, biscuits, bread, cookies and pastry, cake mixes, popcorn, non-wholemeal pastas, noodles, tinned spaghetti in sauce.
3. Daily products: ice cream, milk shakes, processed cheese, dessert mixes and puddings, flavoured yoghurts, margarines.
4. Confectionery: hard and soft sweets or candies, chocolate containing fruit or almonds, mints, cough sweets, fruit squash drinks, carbonated or 'fizzy' drinks, chewing gum, jams, lemon curd.
5. Miscellaneous: canned and dehydrated soups, sauces, vinegar, pickles, salad dressings, crisps and similar products, vegetables in sauce (e.g. baked beans), beer, wine, cider.
6. Non-food items: aspirins and similar drugs, toothpaste, mouthwashes, throat lozenges, perfumes, any pills or tablets with coloured surround, coloured medicines or cough mixtures.

IV.36 Quantification of tyramine in cheeses

Type	Quantity (µg/g)
Cottage cheese	
Quark (skimmed milk soft cheese)	
Cream cheese	Not detectable
Curd cheese	
Edam	216
Brie	240
Wensleydale	312
Leicester	312
Lancashire	360
Melbury	456
Processed cheddar	552
Goat's cheese	576
Vegetarian cheddar	601
Derby	648
Mild cheddar	768
Lymeswold	787
Swiss emmental	864
Low calorie cheddar	912
Mature cheddar	1036
Italian gorgonzola	1248
Fully matured cheddar	1440
Danish blue	3840
Blue stilton	4200

By kind permission of S Gray and CS Evans, London.

Appendix V: Diets used for modification of nitrogen and mineral intake

V.1 Protein content of foods and protein exchanges
V.2 Sodium content of foods
V.3 Potassium content of foods
V.4 Phosphorus content of foods
V.5 Low phenylalanine protein substitutes
V.6 Composition of low phenylalanine protein substitutes
V.7 Phenylalaine content of foods
V.8 Phenylalanine exchanges
V.9 Protein substitutes for inborn errors of metabolism
V.10 Minimal protein regimen for infants to give 1.5 g protein/kg body weight
V.11 Emergency protein-free regimen for inborn errors of protein metabolism (pre-diagnosis or during infection)

V.1 Protein content of foods and protein exchanges

High protein foods (weight of food which contains 6 g protein)	Moderate protein foods (weight of food which contains 2 g protein)	Low protein foods (allowed freely, except on minimum protein diets)
Cows' milk 180 ml	Single cream 80 g	Fruit
Dialysed Whey Infant Formula reconstituted milk 400 ml dry powder 50 g	Ice cream 50 g	Vegetables — green leafy, salad and root varieties
	Uncooked potato 100 g	
	Uncooked fresh peas 30 g	Cornstarch, cornflour, low protein flour, wheatstarch, sago, tapioca
Canned evaporated milk 80 ml	Wheat flour 25 g	
Uncooked fresh/frozen/canned meat 25 g	Bread 25 g	
	Uncooked pasta 20 g	Double cream, butter, lard, margarines, oils, fat emulsions
Uncooked fresh/frozen/canned fish 30 g	Uncooked rice 30 g	
	Sweet biscuits (cookies) 40 g	Sugar, jam, syrup, glucose polymers, clear fruit sweets or candies
Egg — (1 small) 50 g		
Cheese 25 g		Alcoholic beverages, fruit juice, fruit cordials, fizzy drinks
Uncooked lentils 25 g		
Uncooked dried beans 30 g		Herbs, spices

V.2 Sodium content of foods

High sodium foods (excluded on 'no added salt' regimen)	Moderate sodium foods (excluded on 'low salt' regimen)	Low sodium foods (generally allowed freely)
Salt can be used in cooking, but should not be added at the table	Salt should not be used at any stage of preparation or serving	
Canned savoury pasta and rice dishes, savoury 'nibbles', canned and packet soups	Ordinary breads[a], breakfast cereals[a], biscuits, cakes, pastries, crispbreads	Plain flours, dietectic low salt bread, rice, pasta
Canned, smoked, dried and fermented meat and fish, sausages, 'cold cuts', savoury spreads, meat extracts	Eggs[a] Shellfish Cows' milk and milk products[a] Fermented milks and yoghurts (depends on local customs)	Fresh meat, poultry, offal and fish Dialysed whey infant formulae
Cheeses		
Canned dried and fermented vegetables and pulses, olives, pickles, tomato juice, crisps, salted nuts		Fresh and frozen vegetables, nuts pulses, fresh, frozen and canned fruit, fruit juice
	Salted butter and margarines	Unsalted butter, double cream, lard, cooking and salad oils
Sauces, ketchup, relish, salad dressing, food additives, flavour enhancers, stock and gravy makers	Golden syrup, treacle, chocolate filled sweets and candies, fruit cordials, instant tea and coffee, malted milk, mineral water, fizzy drinks	Sugar, jam, jelly etc., clear sweets or candies, ice lollies or popsicles Yeast, herbs, spices, pepper, vinegar
Baking aids, baking powder, bicarbonate of soda	Drinking water (depends on area)	Cocoa powder, tea, coffee
Monosodium glutamate, yeast extracts		Distilled water Salt substitutes (contain potassium or ammonium salts)

[a] These moderate sodium foods are generally allowed in limited quantities on a low salt diet. One or more foods (depending on the degree of restriction required), in a quantity that is appropriate to the age of the child, can be taken each day, e.g. one egg daily, 1 cup, 200 ml, cows' milk daily etc.

V.3 Potassium content of foods

High potassium foods (more than 100 mg per average adult sized portion)	Moderate potassium foods (50–100 mg per average adult sized portion)	Low potassium foods (less than 50 mg per average adult sized portion)
Wholemeal cereals and bread, bran, soy flour and soy products	Refined (white) cereals, breads and pasta	Cornflour, wheatstarch, tapioca, sago, low protein breads and flours Boiled rice
Potatoes, tomatoes, leafy green vegetables, vegetable juices, pulses, nuts, fresh fruit and fruit juices, dried fruits	Runner and French beans, celery, cauliflower, root vegetables (e.g. carrot), apple, pear, canned fruits	Butter, margarine, fats, oils, double cream Sugar, glucose and glucose polymers, jams, honey etc., clear sweets and candies
Milk and milk products Meat and fish, meat extracts Salt substitutes, stock and gravy makers, low salt canned dietetic products, yeast extract	Egg Dialysed whey infant formulae	Herbs, spices, salt, pepper, vinegar
Blackcurrant cordials, malted milks, chocolate	Ground and instant coffee, instant tea, drinking water[a]	Tea, fruit cordials and fizzy drinks, distilled water

[a] Drinking water may contain high quantities of potassium in some areas.
NB The potassium content of cooked foods can be significantly reduced by prior soaking of the food in a large volume of water. This water is discarded and the food is cooked in a further large volume of water. Sauces and gravies should not be prepared from the cooking water. This process also reduces the vitamin C content of foods.

V.4 Phosphorus content of foods

High phosphorus foods (more than 150 mg per average adult sized portion)	Moderate phosphorus foods (50–150 mg per average adult sized portion)	Low phosphorus foods (less than 50 mg per average adult sized portion)
Wholemeal bread, flours and cereals, bran, soy flour and products	Refined (white) bread, flours, cereals and pasta	Cornflour, wheatstarch, tapioca, sago, rice
Offal, game, meat extracts, sardines, fatty fish, fish roe and offal Cows' milk and products, cheese, milk chocolate	Meat, fish, egg Dialysed whey infant milk formulae, single cream, cream cheese	Butter, margarine, fats, oils, double cream Sugar glucose and glucose polymer, jam, honey, clear sweets and candies
Peas, beans, spinach, mushrooms, dried fruit, nuts	Potato, fresh, frozen and canned green and root vegetables, lentils, dates, figs	Fresh, frozen and canned fruit
Malted milks, cocoa powder	Instant coffee, mineral water, drinking water (dependent on area)	Tea, coffee, fruit cordials and fizzy drinks, distilled water
Yeast extract, baking powder, baking aids	Stock and gravy makers	Herbs, spices, salt, pepper, vinegar

V.5 Low phenylalanine protein substitutes

Hydrolysates

These products are enzymatic hydrolysates of whole protein in which most of the phenylalanine has been removed. Additional amino acids, especially tyrosine, are added. None of these preparations contain adequate phenylalanine and a natural protein must be given in addition. Some preparations are complete feeds while others require the addition of fat or carbohydrate modules. It is important to follow the manufacturers' instructions regarding minerals and vitamins because some products are deficient. Hydrolysates have an unpleasant taste and odour and are likely to be rejected by older children although they are accepted by bottle-fed infants.

Albumaid XP   *Scientific Hospital Supplies*

Recommended age 0–2 years. Requires the addition of energy modules. Additional iron and a source of vitamins A, D, E and C, also essential fatty acids and vitamin K.
Preparation. 50 g Albumaid XP made up to a total of 1000 ml with water.

Albumaid XP concentrate   *Scientific Hospital Supplies*

Recommended age — over 2 years. Vitamin and mineral supplements required as for Albumaid XP.
Preparation. 40 g Albumaid concentrate powder made up to a total of 1000 ml with water.

Lofenalac   *Mead Johnson*

Recommended from birth onwards. Complete feed, no additions recommended.
Preparation. Infants — 147 g Lofenalac powder made up to a total of 1000 ml with water; children — 200 g Lofenalac made up to 1000 ml with water.

Minafen   *Cow & Gate*

Recommended age 0–2 years. Requires supplementation with vitamins A, D, C and B_{12}.
Preparation. 125 g Minafen powder made up to 1000 ml with water.

Phenyldon A.M.   *Nutricia*

Recommended from birth onwards. Complete feed, no supplements recommended.
Preparation. 13% solution. One scoop (4.5 g) Phenyldon AM powder plus 30 ml water.

Synthetic amino acid mixtures

Although hydrolysates are widely used they do have a number of disadvantages for older children. Apart from their unpleasant taste often large quantities need to be taken in order to achieve an adequate protein intake. Their energy density is frequently high, leading to obesity. These disadvantages are largely overcome by the use of a synthetic phenylalanine-free amino acid mixture; the amino acid pattern is generally based on that of cows' milk. Extra fat and carbohydrate modules need to be added if these products are used for infants but, for older children, additional energy should be provided in the form of low-protein foods, thus allowing a diet which appears more normal. Manufacturers' instructions regarding vitamin and mineral supplementation must be followed.

Aminogran Food Supplement *Allen & Hanbury*

Recommended from birth onwards. Requires energy modules when used as an infant food as well as complete mineral, vitamin and trace element supplement. Manufacturers recommend Aminogran Mineral Supplement (p. 233) and Ketovite tablets and liquid (p. 226).

Preparation. Infants 20 g Aminogran Food Supplement powder plus recommended supplements made up to a total of 1000 ml with water; children — estimated protein requirements made up to a paste or drink with flavourings, given three times daily.

Maxamaid XP *Scientific Hospital Supplies*

Recommended from age 2years. Requires additional vitamin K if no dietary source.

Preparation. One part Maxamaid powder by weight to 5 parts water by volume (i.e. 10 g powder plus 50 ml water).

Phenylfree *Mead Johnson*

Recommended for older infants and children. No supplements required provided that some natural foods are taken.

Preparation. 217 g Phenylfree powder made up to a total of 1000 ml with water.

PK Aid 1 *Scientific Hospital Supplies*

Recommended age 0–2 years. Requires additional energy modules if used as an infant feed and complete mineral, vitamin and trace element supplement. Manufacturers recommend Metabolic Mineral Mixture (p. 233) and Ketovite tablets and liquid (p. 226).

PKU Mix *Milupa*

Recommended from birth onwards. Requires supplements of vitamin D (and vitamin K if no natural foods taken) and the addition of a fat module if used as an infant feed.

Preparation. 150 g PKU Mix powder made up to 1000 ml with water.

PKU 1 *Milupa*

Recommended for older infants. Requires the addition of energy modules, vitamin D (and vitamin K if no natural foods taken).

Preparation. 50–100 g PKU 1 powder made up to 1000 ml with water.

PKU 2 *Milupa*

Recommended for children. Requires supplementation with vitamin D.

Preparation. Daily requirement made into a paste or drink with flavourings and given three times daily.

PKU 3   *Milupa*

Recommended for adolescents and pregnancy. Does not require supplements.
Preparation — as PKU 2.

V.6 Low phenylalanine protein substitutes

	per 100 g powder						
	Protein equiv. (g)	Phenylalanine (mg)	Tyrosine (mg)	Fat (g)	Carbohydrate (g)	Energy (kcal)	Vitamin, mineral or trace element supplementation
Hydrolysates							
Albumaid XP	33.0	<10	3200	0	50.0	323	*See* text
Albumaid XP Conc	70.0	<25	6690	0	0	287	*See* text
Lofenalac	15.0	74	805	18.0	59.6	460	None recommended
Minafen	12.5	<20	810	31.0	47.9	510	*See* text
Amino acids							
Aminogran	83.0	0	6420	0	0	335	Complete supplement recommended
Maxamid XP	25.0	0	2700	0	62.0	360	None recommended
Phenylfree	20.3	0	934	6.8	66.0	403	None recommended
PKAid I	83.0	0	6000	0	0	335	Complete supplement recommended
PKU Mix	12.0	<5	800	0	80.9	378	Vit. D required (and vit. K)
PK1	50.3	0	3400	0	17.6	276	Vit. D required (and vit. K)
PK2	66.8	0	4500	0	7.1	300	Vit. D required
PK3	68.0	0	6000	0	2.3	285	None recommended

V.7 Phenylalanine content of foods

Low protein foods	Fruits and vegetables
Usually allowed freely in diet:	*These may be allowed freely:* 1 average sized portion contains 15–20 mg phenylalanine.
Sugar, glucose, glucose polymer, jam, jello, honey	
Clear fruit sweets and candies, vegetarian jelly[a]	Asparagus, beansprouts, broccoli, beans — green beans only
Ice lollies, popsicles, saccharin[a]	
Fruit juice, fruit flavoured squash, 'pop'	Brussel sprouts, cabbage, carrots, cauliflower, celery, cucumber, aubergine, kale, leeks, lettuce, okra, onion, parsley, parsnips, peppers, pumpkin, radishes, squash, tomato, turnip, spring greens, swede
Tea, coffee	
Vegetarian margarine, pure white shortening, cooking and salad oils, protein-free fat emulsion (e.g. Calogen)	
Salt, pepper, mustard, vinegar, herbs, spices	Apple, apricot, avocado, banana, berries, dates, figs, grapes, guava, mango, melon, oranges, peaches, pears, pineapples, plum
Flavourings and colourings, baking powder[a]	
Special low protein products prepared from wheatstarch[b], e.g. low protein flour, low protein bread and bread mix, low protein biscuits or cookies, low protein pasta	

[a] The artificial sweetener Aspartame or Nutrisweet is a dipeptide and is hydrolysed in the small intestine to phenylalanine and so cannot be used for this diet. The level of Aspartame in soft drinks may be up to 700 mg/l (400 mg phenylalanine per litre) and in sweetening tablets 18 mg (10 mg phenylalanine).
[b] Gluten-free products may contain protein.

V.8 Phenylalanine exchanges

Food	Phenylalanine (mg per 100 g food)	Weight (g) of food containing 1 × 50 mg Phe exchange (UK)	Weight (g) of food containing 1 × 30 mg Phe exchange (USA)
Cows' milk	180	30	15
Double cream	82	60	35
Breakfast cereal			
Cornflakes	430	15	10
Rice Krispies	300	15	10
Puffed Wheat	680	10	5
Wheatflour			
white	630	10	5
wholemeal	520	10	5
Potato			
raw	92	55	30
boiled	62	80	50
chipped	170	30	20
crisps	270	20	10
Rice			
raw	330	15	10
boiled	110	45	25
Peas			
raw	270	20	10
boiled	230	20	15
Lentils			
dried, raw	1250	5	2.5
boiled, split	400	10	10
dhal	260	20	10
Beans, dried — most varieties, gram	1130−1170 (av. 1150)		
Sweetcorn/maize kernels, boiled	150	35	20

V.9 Protein substitutes for inborn errors of metabolism

Only the major products used are listed. Usually the manufacturers can supply a specific formula for other inborn errors.

Condition	Product	Manufacturer
Maple syrup urine disease	MSUD Diet Powder	Mead Johnson
	MSUD 1 and 2	Milupa
	Leucidon	Nutricia
	MSUD Aid	Scientific Hospital Supplies
Urea cycle defects	UCD 1 and 2	Milupa
	Keto/Amino Mix	Scientific Hospital Supplies
Histidinaemia	HIST 1 and 2	Milupa
	Histidon	Nutricia
	Histidine free AA mix	Scientific Hospital Supplies
Hereditary tyrosinaemia	Product 3200AB	Mead Johnson
	TYR 1 and 2	Milupa
	Tyrosidon	Nutricia
	Met/Tyr/Phen-free AA mix	Scientific Hospital Supplies
Homocystinuria	Product 3200K	Mead Johnson
	HOM 1 and 2	Milupa
	Methionine free AA mix	Scientific Hospital Supplies

V.10 Minimal protein regimen for infants to give 1.5 g protein/kg body weight

12.0 dialysed whey babymilk powder per kg body weight (p. 221)
15.0 g glucose polymer per kg (p. 270)
120 ml fluid per kg
For example for a 3-kg infant

	Protein (g)	Energy	
		(kcal)	(kJ)
36.0 g dialysed whey powder	4.5	213	890
45.0 g glucose polymer powder	—	180	752
Water to make up to total volume of 360 ml			
Total	4.5	393	1643
per kg	1.5	131	548

NB In addition a full vitamin supplement, e.g. Ketovite tablets and Liquid (p. 226), and a mineral/trace element supplement containing electrolytes, iron and calcium (p. 233) should be given.

V.11 Emergency protein-free regimen for inborn errors of protein metabolism (pre-diagnosis or during infection)

Day 1 10% dextrose saline
100 ml/kg actual body weight = 40 kcal/kg = 167 kJ/kg

Day 2 15% carbohydrate with electrolytes

	Carbohydrate (g)
1 sachet Infalyte (p. 225) or similar	23
130 g glucose polymer (p. 270)	130
Water to make total volume of 1000 ml	
Total	153

100 ml/kg = 60 kcal/kg
170 ml/kg = 102 kcal/kg

Day 3 20% carbohydrate with electrolytes

	Carbohydrate (g)
1 sachet Infalyte etc.	23
180 g glucose polymer	180
Water to make total volume of 1000 ml	
Total	203

plus 3 Ketovite tablets and 5 Ketovite Liquid (p. 226)
100 ml/kg = 80 kcal/kg
130 ml/kg = 104 kcal/kg

Appendix VI: Diets used for modification of energy or cabohydrate intake

VI.1 Advice for reducing diets
VI.2 Low carbohydrate low energy foods
VI.3 Low carbohydrate foods containing energy
VI.4 Carbohydrate exchanges of cereals and vegetables
VI.5 Carbohydrate exchanges of milk and fruits
VI.6 Carbohydrate distribution in diabetes

VI.1 Advice for reducing diets

Choose meals from these foods:

Lean meat	Vegetables: all varieties of green and root vegetables, salads	Fruit: all varieties of fresh fruit or fruit canned in natural juice
Poultry		
Fish		
Eggs		
Cheese		

Drinks:
  Low calorie squash and cola
  Unsweetened fruit juice
  Tea, coffee without sugar
  Unthickened soups

Cereals: include *one* portion from exchange list at each meal.

Seasonings, herbs, spices and artificial sweeteners if desired.

Allowances:
  0.5−1 pint milk daily
  0.5 lb (240 g) butter or margarine weekly
Useful isocaloric exchanges (70 kcal or 293 kJ):
  1 slice bread (preferably wholemeal)
  or 1 tablespoon boiled rice
  or 3 tablespoons unsweetened breakfast cereal
  or 1 potato (not fried)
  or 2 crispbreads
  or 4 tablespoons cooked porridge

Foods to avoid:

Sugar	Fruit squash	Cream
Sweets	Cordials	Fried foods
Chocolate	Fizzy drinks, e.g. Cola	Crisps
Glucose		
Honey	Cakes	Proprietary
Syrup	Pastries	slimming and
Treacle	Pies	diabetic foods except
Jam	Sweet biscuits	fruit squash
Marmalade		
Sorbitol		

VI.2 Low carbohydrate, low energy foods

Vegetables

Group A — negligible energy or carbohydrate, 1–3 g fibre per small portion. Allowed freely:

Asparagus	Green leafy vegetables and salads
Brussel sprouts	Mushrooms
Cauliflower	Peppers
Celery	Radish
Cucumber	Tomato
French, runner or snap beans	

Group B — contain approximately 5 g carbohydrate, 45 kcal (188 kJ), 3–5 g fibre per small portion. May be allowed freely:

Beetroot	Peas
Carrots	Squash
Onions	Turnip

Fruits

Contain approximately 5 g carbohydrate, 45 kcal (188 kJ), 2–6 g fibre per small portion. May be allowed freely:

Berry fruits	Lemon
Blackcurrants	Rhubarb
Cranberries	Watermelon
Grapefruit	

Other foods

Negligible content, allowed freely:

Artificial sweeteners	Sugar-free, low energy drinks
saccharin	Stock or bouillon cubes
Aspartame (Nutri-sweet)	Tea
Coffee	Vinegar
Gelatin	
Herbs, spices, seasonings	

VI.3 Low carbohydrate foods containing energy

Animal foods

Allowed in moderation by the British Diabetic Association, not measured as exchanges.

Measured as meat exchanges by the American Diabetic Association.
One meat exchange contains 75 kcal (314 kJ), 7 g protein, 5 g fat.

	Quantity = 1 exchange (g)
Bacon, lean, grilled	25
Cheese (cheddar)	30
Cottage cheese[a]	50
Egg (1 medium)	50
Fish — white, e.g. cod (cooked)[a]	80
Fish — oily, e.g. tuna	30
Frankfurter	60
Meat — beef, lamb, pork (raw)	30
Offal — liver, kidney	30
Poultry — chicken, turkey[a]	50
Sausage (raw)[b]	25

[a] Low fat foods — contain less than 5 g fat per exchange
[b] 1 sausage contains 5 g carbohydrate and also counts as a cereal exchange

Fatty foods

Allowed in small quantities by the British Diabetic Association, not measured as exchanges.

Measured as fat exchanges by the American Diabetic Association.
One fat exchange contains 45 kcal (188 kJ), 5 g fat, no protein.

	Quantity = 1 exchange (g)	*Measurement*
Butter, margarine or ghee	6 g	1 teaspoon
Low fat margarine substitute	10 g	2 teaspoons
Cooking or vegetable oil	5 g	1 teaspoon
Cream		
single (light)	20 g	2 tablespoons
double (heavy)	10 g	1 tablespoon
Nuts	10 g	6 small

VI.4 Carbohydrate exchanges of cereals and vegetables

British system : 1 CHO exch. = 50 kcal (210 kJ), 10 g CHO, 1.5 g protein				American system : 1 CHO exch. = 70 kcal (293 kJ), 15 g CHO, 2 g protein			
Bread and cereals		Weight (g)	Fibre (g)			Weight (g)	Fibre (g)
Bread			0.5	Bread			
white	⅔ medium slice	20		white	1 medium slice	30	0.8
wholemeal			1.7	wholemeal			2.5
Chapatti		20	0.7	Chapatti		30	1.1
Biscuit, semisweet	2 small biscuits	12	0.3	Biscuit/cookie, semisweet	3 small	20	0.5
Biscuit, digestive	1 large	12	0.6	Biscuit/cookie		20	1.0
Rye crispbread	2 crispbreads	12	1.4	Rye crispbread	3 crispbreads	20	2.3
Breakfast cereals		12		Breakfast cereals		20	
wheat			1.5	wheat			2.5
rice	2 tablespoons		0.5	rice	3 tablespoons		0.9
corn			1.3	corn			2.2
Flour				Flour	1 heaped		
white	1 tablespoon	15	0.4	white	tablespoon	20	0.6
wholemeal			1.4	wholemeal			1.9
Pasta — cooked		40		Pasta — cooked		60	
Rice, polished, cooked	2 tablespoons	30	0.3	Rice, polished, cooked	3 tablespoons	60	0.5
Beans — baked/cooked	2 tablespoons	60	4.4	Beans — baked/cooked	3 tablespoons	90	6.6
Lentils — dhal	2 tablespoons	60	1.4	Lentils — dhal	3 tablespoons	90	2.2
Parsnip — cooked		70	1.7	Parsnip — cooked		110	2.7
Potato				Potato			
cooked	1 small potato	50	1.0	cooked	1 medium potato	75	1.6
chips	6 medium chips	30	1.0	chips	10 medium chips	45	1.5
crisps	small packet	20	2.3	crisps		30	3.6
Sweetcorn kernels	2 tablespoons	60	3.4	Sweetcorn kernels	3 tablespoons	90	5.1

VI.5 Carbohydrate exchanges of milk and fruits

Milk-based foods

One exchange = 170 kcal (710 kJ), 10 g carbohydrate.
One milk exchange (American Diabetic Association) also contains 8 g protein, 12 g fat.

	1 exchange (g)	Measurement
Milk, liquid, whole	200	1 cup (USA), 7 fl. oz (Imp)
Dried whole milk powder	25	1 heaped tablespoon
Dried skimmed milk powder[a]	20	1 rounded tablespoon
Evaporated milk	80	4 tablespoons
Ice cream	90	2 tablespoons or scoops
Plain yoghurt, unsweetened	150	1 (5 oz) tub
Fruit-flavoured yoghurt, sweetened	60	½ (5 oz) tub

[a] Low in fat: less than 1 g fat/10 g carbohydrate exchange.

Fruits

One exchange = 40 kcal (167 kJ), 10 g carbohydrate.

	1 exchange (g)	Measurement	Fibre (g)
Apple	120	1 small	2.4
Apricot			
fresh	150	2 medium	3.1
dried	25	4 halves	3.1
Banana (no skin)	50	½ medium	3.9
Dates, fresh	20	2 large	1.7
Figs, fresh	100	3 large	2.5
Grapes	60	12	0.2
Mango	100	½ medium	1.4
Melon (except watermelon)	150	1 slice	1.0
Orange and tangerine (no skin)	120	1 large	2.4
Papaya	70	⅓ medium	0.3
Peach	100	1 small	1.4
Pear	100	1 medium	2.3
Pineapple	100	⅛ medium fruit	1.2
Raisins, sultanas etc.	20	2 tablespoons	1.3
Unsweetened fruit juice	100	½ cup (USA)	0

VI.6 Carbohydrate distribution in diabetes

Age of child: 8 years.
Sex: male.
Weight: 25 kg (50th percentile).
Energy intake: 2000 kcal (8.36 MJ) (assessed by diet history).

Insulin: soluble and isophane 50:50.   07.30—14 units
                                                     17.00—10 units

Peak insulin action time: 09.00—14.00
                           18.30—22.00

Dietary prescription: 2000 kcal (8.36 MJ)

50% energy should derive from carbohydrate = 250 g carbohydrate (1000 kcal; 4.18 MJ)

Using a 10 g carbohydrate exchange system = 25 × 10 g exchanges.

These should be divided into three main meals and three snacks, the quantity to coincide with times of peak insulin action.

Morning: Breakfast 08.00   6 × 10 g exchanges
         Snack 10.30   3 × 10 g

Mid-day: Lunch 12.30   6 × 10 g
          Snack 15.30   1 × 10 g

Evening: Dinner 17.30   6 × 10 g
          Snack 20.00   3 × 10 g

Appendix VII: Names, addresses of manufacturers and availability of their products

Not every product manufactured by a company is available in all areas indicated below. There are likely to be formulation differences between products of the same name marketed in different countries; in addition, the size of scoops produced with some milk substitutes may differ from country to country. It is important to read the manufacturer's instructions for each product prior to use.

Addresses of manufacturer	Availability
Abbott International Ltd, Abbott Park, North Chicago, Illinois 60064, USA	Africa, Asia, Australia, Canada, Caribbean, Europe, Far East, Middle East, New Zealand, S. Africa, S. America, USA
Abbot Laboratories Ltd Distributors (Ross Laboratories USA), Queenborough, Kent ME11 5EL, UK	UK
Allen & Hanbury Ltd, Horsenden House, Oldfield Lane North, Greenford, Middx UB6 0HB, UK	UK
Anglo-Dietetics, PO Box 333, Wilton, Connecticut 06897, USA (*see also* Welfare Foods Ltd)	Canada, USA
Armour Pharmaceutical Co. Ltd, Hampden Park, Eastbourne, Sussex BN21 3YG, UK	Africa, Middle East, UK
Astra, Astra Pharmaceuticals Ltd, Home Park Estate, Kings Langley, Herts WD4 8DH, UK	Australia, Cananda, Europe
Beecham Products, Stoke Poges Lane, Slough, Berks SL1 3NW, UK	Asia, Europe, Middle East, S. Africa, UK
Bencard, Great West Road, Brentford, Middx TW8 9BD, UK	Africa, Australia, Europe, Middle East, UK
Biosearch Inc., 35 Industrial Parkway, PO Box 1700, Somerville, New Jersey 08876, USA	Canada, USA

Addresses of manufacturer	Availability
Boots Hospital Products, Thane Road West, Nottingham NG2 3AA, UK	UK
Bristol-Myers Co., 345 Park Avenue, New York 10154, USA (*see also* Mead Johnson Nutritionals)	Asia, Australia, Canada, Caribbean, Europe, Middle East, Far East, New Zealand, S. Africa, S. America, USA
Carlo Erber *see* Ultrapharm Ltd	
Carnation, 36 Park Street, Croyden, Surrey CR9 1 TT, UK	UK
Cow & Gate Babyfoods Ltd, Cow & Gate House, Trowbridge, Wilts BA14 8YX, UK (*see also* Nutricia)	Australia, Europe, Middle East, UK
Ciba, CIBA Laboratories, Wimblehurst Road, Horsham, West Sussex RH12 4AB, UK	Africa, Asia, Australia, Europe, Middle East, New Zealand, S. America, UK
The Doyle Pharmaceutical Co., Minneapolis, Minnesota 55416, USA	USA
Eaton Laboratories, Norwich Eaton, Regent House, The Broadway, Woking, Surrey GU21 5AP, UK	Africa, Asia, Australia, Europe, Middle East, New Zealand, S. America, UK, USA
Farley Health Products Ltd, Torr Lane, Plymouth, Devon PL3 5UA, UK	UK
Fisons Ltd, Pharmaceutical Division, 12 Derby Road, Loughborough, Leics LE11 0BB, UK	Australia, Canada, Europe, S. Africa, UK, USA
Friesland Products, PO Box 226, 8901 MA Leeuwarden, The Netherlands	The Netherlands
Geistlich Sons Ltd, PO Box 37, Newton Bank, Long Lane, Chester CH2 3QZ, UK	UK
Gerber Products Co., 445 State Street, Freemont, Michigan 49412, USA	Europe, USA

Addresses of manufacturer	*Availability*
KabiVitrum Ltd, Kabivitrum House, Riverside Way, Uxbridge, Middx UB8 2YF	Australia, Europe, Middle East, S. Africa, UK
Lederle Laboratories, Cyanmid Plaza, Wayne, New Jersey 07470, USA	USA
Loma Linda Foods, 11503 Pierce Street, Riverside, California 92515, USA	Canada, USA
Mead Johnson Nutritionals, Division of Bristol-Myers Co. Ltd, Station Road, Slough, Middx SL3 6EB, UK (*see also* Bristol-Myers)	UK
E. Merck Ltd, Winchester Road, Four Marks, Alton, Hants GU34 5HG, UK (*see also* Pfrimmer & Co.)	Asia, Europe, Far East, UK
Milupa AG, 6382 Friedrichsdorf, West Germany	Australia, Canada, Europe, Middle East, USA
Milupa Ltd, Milupa House, Hercies Road, Hillingdon, Middx UB10 9NA, UK	UK
MyPlan Ltd, 96 Worchester Road, Malvern, Worcs WR14 1NY, UK	UK
Napp, Napp Laboratories Ltd Cambridge Science Park, Milton Road, Cambridge CB4 4BH, UK	Australia, UK
The Nestlé Co. Ltd, St George's House, Croyden, Surrey CR9 1NR, UK	Australia, Europe, UK
Nutricia Laboratories, PO Box 1, 2700 MA Zoetermeer, The Netherlands (*see also* Cow & Gate)	Asia, Europe, Far East, UK
Paines & Byrne Ltd, Pabryn Laboratories, Bilton Road, Perivale, Greenford, Middx UB6 7HG, UK	Africa, Asia, Australia, Caribbean, Europe, Middle East, Far East, New Zealand, S. America, UK, USA

Addresses of manufacturer	*Availability*
Parke Davies Research Laboratories Mitchell House, Southampton Road, Eastleigh, Hants SO5 5RY, UK	Asia, Middle East, S. America, UK
Pfrimmer & Co., Erlangen, West Germany (*see* Merck)	West Germany
Penwalt Corporation, PO Box 1710, Rochester, New York 14623, USA	USA
Reckitt & Coleman Pharmaceutical Division, Dansom Lane, Hull, York HU8 7DS, UK	UK
Ross Laboratories *see* Abbot Laboratories Ltd	
Roussel Laboratories Ltd, Broadwater Park, North Orbital Road, Denham, Uxbridge, Middx UB9 5HP, UK	Africa, Middle East, UK
Sandoz Products Ltd, Pharmaceuticals Division, Sandoz House, 98 The Centre, Feltham, Middx TW13 4EP, UK	Australia, Canada, Europe, UK
Scientific Hospital Supplies Ltd 38 Queensland Street, Liverpool L7 3JG, UK	Australia, Europe, New Zealand, UK
SHS Inc., 110 Deer Park Way, Gaitherburg, Maryland 20877, USA	USA
Searle Laboratories, Division of G.D. Searle Co. Ltd, PO Box 53, Lane End Road, High Wycombe, Bucks HP12 4HL, UK	Africa, Asia, Caribbean, Middle East, S. Africa, S. America, UK
United Dairymen, PO Box 222, 3340 AE Woerden, The Netherlands	Europe
Wallace Mfg, Wallace Manufacturing Chemists Ltd, 1a Frognal, London NW3 6AN, UK	Africa, Caribbean, Middle, East, Far East, UK
Wander AG, Postfach 2747, 3001 Berne, Switzerland	Europe

Addresses of manufacturer	*Availability*
Welfare Foods Ltd, 63 London Road South, Poynton, Stockport, Cheshire SK12 1YD, UK (*see also* Anglo-Dietetics)	Europe, Middle East
Wyeth International Ltd, Philadelphia PA 19101, USA	Australia, Canada, Middle East, Far East, S. Africa, S. America, USA
Wyeth Laboratories, Huntercombe Lane South, Taplow, Maidenhead, Berks SL6 0PH, UK	UK, USA
Ultrapharm Ltd, 5 Beaconfield Road, Royal Leamington Spa, Warwickshie CV31 1DH, UK (Also Carlo Erber)	UK

References

Chapter 1

Aggett, PJ (1985) Physiology and metabolism of essential trace elements; an outline. In: *Clinics in Endocrinology and Metabolism*, Vol. 14/3, *Trace Elements in Human Disease*, A Taylor (ed.), pp. 513–543. WB Saunders, Philadelphia.

American Academy of Pediatrics, Committee on Nutrition (1976) Commentary on breast feeding and infant formulas, including proposed standards for formulas. *Pediatrics* 57: 278–285.

Anon (1987a) Advice about milk for infants and young children. *Lancet* i: 843–844.

Anon (1987b) Vitamin D: new perspectives. *Lancet* i: 1122–1123.

Arneil GC and Crosbie JC (1963) Infantile rickets returns to Glasgow. *Lancet* ii: 423–425.

Benton D and Roberts G (1988) Effect of vitamin and mineral supplementation of intelligence of a sample of schoolchildren. *Lancet* i: 140–143.

Cordano A (1978) Copper deficiency in clinical medicine. *Proceedings of the Seventeenth Annual Meeting of the American College of Nutrition*, KM Hambidge and BL Nichols Jr (eds) SP Medical and Scientific Books, Montreal.

Danks DM, Cartwright E, Stevens BJ and Townley RRW (1973) Menkes' kinky hair disease. *Science* 179: 1140–1142.

DHSS (1979) Recommended daily amounts of food energy and nutrients for groups of people in the United Kingdom. *Report on Health and Social Subjects, No. 15*. HMSO, London.

DHSS (1980) Artificial feeds for the young infant. *Report on Health and Social Subjects, No. 18*. HMSO, London.

DHSS (1987) *Milk for Infants and Young Children*. Committee on the Medical Aspects of Food Policy, Panel on Child Nutrition. HMSO, London.

FAO (1985) Energy and protein requirements. Report of Joint FAO/WHO/UNU Expert Committee. *Technical Report Series 724*, WHO, Geneva.

Fell, HB (1970) The direct action of vitamin A on skeletal tissue *in vitro*. In: *The Fat-Soluble Vitamins*, HF De Luca and JW Suttie (eds), pp. 187–202. University of Winconsin Press, Madison.

Fomon, SJ (1974) *Infant Nutrition*. WB Saunders, Philadelphia.

Ford JE and Scott KJ (1968) The folic acid activity of some milk foods for babies. *J. Dairy Res.* 35: 85–90.

Gillis J, Murphy FR, Boxall LBH and Pencharz PB (1982) Biotin deficiency in a child on long-term TPN. *J. Parent. Ent. Nutr.* 6: 308–310.

Goel KM, Sweet EM, Campbell S, Attenburrow A,

Logan RW and Arneil GC (1981) Reduced prevalence of rickets in Asian children in Glasgow. *Lancet* ii: 405–407.

Gräsbeck R, Gordin R, Kantero I and Kuhlbäck B (1960) Selective vitamin B_{12} malabsorption and proteinuria in young people. A Syndrome. *Acta Med. Scand.* 167: 289–296.

Greer FR, Mummah-Schendel LL, Marshall S and Suttie JW (1988), Vitamin K_1 (phylloquinone) and vitamin K_2 (menaquinone) status in newborns during the first week of life. *Pediatrics* 81: 137–140.

Hambidge KM (1976) The importance of trace elements in infant nutrition. In: *Current Medical Research and Opinion*. Symposium Issue: New concepts of infant nutrition. Volume 4, Supplement 1, pp. 44–53.

Imerslund O (1960) Idiopathic chronic megaloblastic anaemia in children. *Acta Paediatr.* 49 (Suppl.): 119.

Johnston PK (1984) Getting enough to grow on. *Am. J. Nursing* 3: 336–339.

Keenan WJ, Jewett T and Glueck HI (1971) Role of feeding and vitamin K in hypoprothrombinemia of the newborn. *Am J. Dis. Child.* 121, 271–277.

Lanzkowsky P (1978) Megaloblastic anemias and other nutritional anemias. In *Smith's Blood Diseases of Infancy and Childhood*, DR Miller, HA Pearson, RL Baehner and CW McMillan. (eds) pp. 173–211. CV Mosby, St Louis.

Lawson DEM (1981) Dietary vitamin D: is it necessary? *J. Human Nutr.* 35: 61–63.

Lewis JS (1969) An E/PUFA ratio of 0.4 maintains normal plasma tocopherol levels in growing children. *Fed. Proc.* 28: 758.

Lifshitz F (1980) (Ed.) *Pediatric Nutrition*. Dekker Inc, New York.

McLaren DS and Burman D (Eds) (1982) *Textbook of Paediatric Nutrition*. Churchill Livingstone, Edinburgh.

Mock, DM, deLorimer AA, Liebman WM, Sweetman L and Baker H (1981) Biotin deficiency: An unusual complication of parenteral alimentation. *N. Engl. J. Med.* 304: 820–823.

National Academy of Sciences (1980) Food and Nutrition Board. Recommended dietary allowances. National Academy of Sciences, Washington.

Raghuramulu N and Reddy V (1980) Serum 25-hydroxyvitamin D levels in malnourished children with rickets. *Arch. Dis. Child.* 55: 285–287.

Russell JGB and Hill LF (1974). True fetal rickets. *Br. J. Radiol.* 47: 723–734.

Shaw JCL (1973) Parenteral nutrition in the management of sick low birthweight infants. *Pediatr. Clins N. Am.* 20: 333–358.

Suskind RM (1981) *Textbook of Pediatric Nutrition*. Raven Press, New York.

Vanier TM and Tyas JF (1966) Folic acid status in normal infants during the first year of life. *Arch. Dis. Child.* 41: 658–665.

Walker WA and Wakkins JB (eds) (1985) *Nutrition in Pediatrics*. Little, Brown & Co., Boston.

WHO (1974) *Handbook on Human Nutritional Requirements.* Monograph Series 61, WHO, Geneva.

WHO (1976) Joint WHO/FAO Food Standards Programme, Codex Alimentarius Commission. Recommended International Standards for Foods for Infants and Children. FAO, Rome.

Ziegler EE, Biga RL and Fomon SJ (1981) Nutritional requirements of the premature infant. In *Textbook of Pediatric Nutrition.* RM Suskind (ed.) pp. 29–39. Raven Press, New York.

Zlotkin SH, Stallings VA and Pencharz PB (1985) Total parenteral nutrition in children. In *Nutrition*, PB Pencharz, ed., *Pediatric Clinics of North America*, Vol. 32, No. 2, pp. 381–400. WB Saunders, Philadelphia.

Chapter 2

Bellanti J (1983) *Acute Diarrhea: Its Nutritional Consequences in Children. Nestlé Nutrition Workshop Series Volume 2.* Raven Press, New York.

Bentley D, Lynn J and Laws JW (1985) Campylobacter colitis with intestinal aphthous ulceration mimicking obstruction. *Br. Med. J.* 291: 634.

Bishop RF, Davidson GP, Holmes IH and Ruck BJ (1973) Virus particles in epithelial cells of duodenal mucosa from children with acute non-bacterial gastroenteritis. *Lancet* ii: 1281–1283.

Booth IW and Harries JT (1984) Regulatory mechanisms of secretory diarrhea and electrolyte imbalance. In: *Acute and Chronic Diarrhea in Infancy*, E Lebenthal (ed.), pp. 307–317. Raven Press, New York.

Ebrahim, GJ (1987) Looking beyond oral rehydration therapy. *Br. Med. J.* 297: 1222–1223.

Egemen A and Bertan M (1980) A study of oral rehydration therapy by midwives in a rural area near Ankara. *Bull. W. H. O.* 58 (2): 333–338.

Elliot EJ, Walker-Smith JA and Farthing MJ (1987) The role of bicarbonate and base precurors in the treatment of acute gastroenteritis. *Arch. Dis. Child.* 62: 91–95.

Farthing MJG (1987) Traveller's diarrhoea. *Gastroenterol Pract.* 3: 24–30.

Finberg L (1986) Too little water has become too much. *Am. J. Dis. Child.* 140: 524.

Francis D (1986) *Nutrition for Children.* Blackwells, Oxford.

Francis D (1987) *Diets for Sick Children.* Blackwells, Oxford.

Gryboski J. and Walker WA (1983) *Gastrointestinal Problems in the Infant.* WB Saunders, Philadelphia.

Kovacs A, Chan L, Hotrakitya C, Overturf G and Portnoy B (1987) Rotavirus gastroenteritis. Clinical and laboratory features and use of the Rotazyme test. *Am. J. Dis. Child.* 141: 161–166.

Lancet (1983) Oral hydration in context. *Lancet* ii: 118.

Lebenthal E (1984) *Chronic Diarrhea in Children. Nestlé Nutrition Workshop Series Volume 6.* Raven Press, New York.

McLaren DS and Cutting WAM (1986) The global magnitude of diarrhoeal disease in young children. In: *Diarrhoea and Malnutrition in Childhood*, JA Walker-Smith and AS McNeish (eds), pp. 203–205. Butterworths, London.

Mehta MN and Subramaniam S (1986) Comparison of rice water, rice electrolyte solution, and glucose electrolyte solution in the management of infantile diarrhoea. *Lancet* i: 843–845.

Mir NA and Elzouki AY (1984) Oral rehydration solutions and electrolyte content of water. *Arch. Dis. Child.* 59: 903.

Morley D (1985) The state of the world's children. *Arch. Dis. Child.* 60: 693–694.

Oral Rehydration Therapy (1980) An annotated bibliography. A collaborative project by Pan American Health Organisation US Agency for International Development, Office of Nutrition, US Center for Disease Control, Bureau of Epidemiology, US Office of International Health.

Paneth N (1980) Hypernatremic dehydration of infancy. *Am. J. Dis. Child.* 134: 785–792.

Pizarro D, Castillo GP et al. (1987) Efficacy comparison of oral rehydration solutions containing either 90 or 70 ml sodium per litre. *Pediatrics* 79: 190–194.

Sandhu BK, Horn J, Farmer G, Habel A, Bentley D and Brueton M (1987a) In search of optimal oral rehydration therapy for acute infantile diarrhoea in developed countries: results of a multicentre trial using three solutions with differing sodium content and a fourth containing glycine and glucose. *Gastroenterology*, 92, 1613.

Sandhu BK, Horn J, Cristobel FL, Burston D, Bentley D and Brueton M (1987b) Glycine based and other oral rehydration solution—experimental and clinical studies. *Z. Gastroenterol.* 25, 644–645.

Silverman A and Roy CC (1983) *Pediatric Clinical Gastroenterology.* CV Mosby, St Louis.

Stites DP, Stobo JD, Fudenberg HH and Wells JV (1984) *Basic and Clinical Immunology.* Lange, California.

Stryer L (1975) *Biochemistry.* WH Freeman and Co., San Francisco.

Tamer AM, Friedman LB, Maxwell SR, Cynamon HA, Perez HN and Cleveland WW (1985) Oral rehydration of infants in a large urban US Medical Center. *J Pediatr.*, 107, 14–22.

Thomas HC and Jewell DP (1979) *Clinical Gastrointestinal Immunology.* Blackwell Scientific, Oxford.

Tripp JH and Candy DCA (1984) Oral rehydration fluids. *Archs Dis. Child.* 59: 99–101.

Turner AM, Lawrence LB et al. (1983) Oral rehydration of infants in a large urban US medical centre. *J. Pediatr.* 107: 14–26.

Vesikari T and Isolauri E (1986) Glycine supplemented

oral rehydration solutions for diarrhoea. *Arch. Dis. Child.* **61**: 372–376.

Walker-Smith JA and McNeish AS (1986) *Diarrhoea and Malnutrition in Childhood.* Butterworths, London.

Wharton BA, Pugh RE Taitz LS, Walker-Smith JA and Booth IW (1988) Dietary management of gastroenteritis in Britain. *Br. Med. J.* **296**: 450–452.

Williams CD and Jelliffe DB (1972) *Mother and Child Health: Delivering the Services.* pp. 62–65. Oxford University Press, Oxford.

Wood DJ (1988). Adenovirus gastroenteritis. *Br. Med. J.* **296**: 229–230.

Yates DW (1987) Volume replacement: The choice of fluid. *Hosp. Update* **13**: 297–306.

Chapter 3

American Academy of Pediatrics Committee on Nutrition, 1982–1983 (1983) Commentary on parenteral nutrition. *Pediatrics*, **71**: 547–552.

Andersson G, Brohult J and Sterner G (1969) Increasing metabolic acidosis following fructose infusion in two children. *Acta Paediatr. Scand.* **58**: 301–304.

Anon (1987) Chronic diarrhoea in children — a nutritional disease. *Lancet* **i**: 143–144.

Auty B (1988) Enteral feeding pumps. *Intens. Ther. Clin. Monitor.* **9**: 6.

Aynsley-Green A (1983) Plasma hormone concentrations during enteral and parenteral nutrition in the human newborn. *J. Pediatr. Gastroenterol. Nutr.* **2** (Suppl. 1): S108–S112.

Bivins, BA (1982) Reducing the risks of I. V. Therapy. Summary of the Proceedings of a Seminar, Millipore (UK) Ltd, pp. 1–15.

Brown MR, Thunberg BJ, Golub L, Maniscalco WM and Shapiro DL (1987) Decreased cholestasis with oral instead of intravenous protein in the very low birth weight (VLBW) infant. *J. Parent. Ent. Nutr.* **II** (no 1/suppl.): 1.

Candy DC (1980) Parenteral nutrition in paediatric practice: a review. *J. Human Nutr.* **34**: 287–296.

Clark ML (1977) Elemental and parenteral nutrition. *Proc. R. Soc. Med.* **70**: 475–477.

Courtney Moore M and Greene HL (1985) Tube feeding of infants and children. *Pedian. Clins N. Am.* **32**(2): 401–417.

Downie G, McRae N and Will I (1985) Leaching of plasticisers by fat emulsion from polyvinyl chloride. *Br. J. Parent. Ther.* **6**: 142–144.

Dudrick SJ, Wilmore DW, Vars HM and Rhoads JE (1968) Long-term parenteral nutrition with growth, development and positive nitrogen balance. *Surgery* **64**: 134–142.

Easton LB, Halata MS and Dweck HS (1982) Parenteral nutrition in the newborn: a practical guide. In *Symposium on the Newborn.* W. Oh (ed.) *Pediatric Clinics of North America*, vol. 29, pp. 1171–1190. WB Saunders, Philadelphia.

Filer RM (1981) Parenteral support of the surgically ill child. In *Textbook of Pediatric Nutrition*, RM Suskind (ed.) pp. 341–355. Raven Press, New York.

Harries JT (1971a) Intravenous feeding in infants. *Arch. Dis. Child.* **46**: 855–863.

Harries JT (1971b) Metabolic acidosis during intravenous feeding of infants. In: *International Congress on Parenteral Nutrition*, London. April 29–May 1, 1971.

Heird WC, Hay W, Helms RA, Storm MC, Kashyap S and Dell RB (1988) Pediatric parenteral amino acid mixture in low birth weight infants. *Pediatrics* **81**: 41–50.

Helfrick FW and Abelson NM (1944). Intravenous feeding of a complete diet in a child: report of a case. *J. Pediatr.* **25**: 400–403.

Jones B and Silk D (1980) Enteral nutrition. *Hospital Doctor*, January 17, 8–9.

Kanarek KS, Williams PR and Curran JS (1982) Total parenteral nutrition in infants and children. In: *Advances in Pediatrics*, LA Barness (ed.) pp. 151–181. Year Book Medical Publishers Inc., London.

Koo WWK, Kaplan L, Horn J, Tsang RC and Steichen JJ (1986) Aluminum in parenteral nutrition solution: sources and possible alternatives. *J. Parent. Ent. Nutr.* **10** (1, suppl.): 94.

McGraw M, Bishop N, Jameson R, Robinson MJ, O'Hara M, Hewitt CD and Day JP (1986) Aluminium content of milk formulae and intravenous fluids used in infants. *Lancet* **i**: 157.

Meek JH and Pettit BR (1985) Avoidable accumulation of potentially toxic levels of benzothiazoles in babies receiving intravenous therapy. *Lancet* **ii**: 1090–1092.

Metz G, Dilawari J and Kellock TD (1978) Simple technique for naso-gastric feeding. *Lancet* **ii**: 454.

Panter-Brick M (1983) Principles of parenteral nutrition in infancy. In: *A Manual of Central Venous Catheterization and Parenteral Nutrition*, JL Peters (ed.), pp. 231–240. John Wright and Sons Ltd, Bristol.

Puntis JWL (1987) Percutaneous insertion of silastic central venous feedings catheters. *Intens. Ther. Clin. Monitor.* **8**: 7–10.

Rosbotham S (1986) Total parenteral nutrition. *Pharmaceut. J.* **237**: 99.

Sahebjami H and Scalettar R (1971). Effects of fructose infusion on lactate and uric acid metabolism. *Lancet* **i**: 366–369.

Silk DBA and Keohane PP (1982) Formulation of enteral diets. In: *Clinical Nutrition 81*. RIC Wesdorp and PB Soeters (eds), pp. 125–132. Churchill Livingstone, Edinburgh.

Zlotkin SH, Stallings VA and Pencharz PB (1985) Total parenteral nutrition in children *Pediatr. Clins. N. Am.* **32**(2): 381–400.

Chapter 4

Alvear J, Artaza C, Vial M, Guerrero S and Muzzo S (1986) Physical growth and bone age of survivors of protein energy malnutrition. *Arch. Dis. Child.* **61**: 257–262.

Ashworth A (1979) Progress in the treatment of protein–energy malnutrition. *Proc. Nutr. Soc.* **38**: 89–97.

Ashworth A (1980) Practical aspects of dietary management during rehabilitation from severe protein–energy malnutrition. *J. Human Nutr.* **34**: 360–369.

Briend A, Wojtyniak B and Rasland MGM (1987) Arm circumference and other factors in children at high risk of death in rural Bangladesh. *Lancet* ii: 725–728.

Cameron M and Hofvander Y (1983) *Manual on Feeding Infants and Young Children*, 3rd edn. Oxford University Press, Oxford.

Editorial (1970) Classification of infantile malnutrition. *Lancet* ii: 302–303.

Editorial (1979) The campaign against malnutrition. *Lancet* ii: 833.

Editorial (1982) The malnourished child: cure better than prevention? *Lancet* i: 1106–1107.

Harland PSEG (1983) The treatment of kwashiorkor. In: *Topics in Paediatric Nutrition*, JA Dodge (ed.). Pitman Books Ltd, London.

Hendrickse RG, Coulter JBS and Lamplugh, SM (1982) Aflatoxins and kwashiorkor: a study in Sudanese children. *Br. Med. J.* **285**: 843–846.

Herbst JJ, Sunshine P and Kretchmer N (1969) Intestinal malabsorption in infancy and childhood. In: *Advances in Pediatrics*, I Schulman (ed.), pp. 11–31. Year Book Medical Publishers Inc., Chicago.

Lindqvist BG, Mellander O and Svanberg U (1981) Dietary bulk as a limiting factor for nutrient intake in pre-school children. *J. Trop. Pediatr.* **27**(2): 68–73.

Walia BN, Rugmini PS and Khurana S (1982). Refeeding the malnourished child *Ind. J. Pediatr.* **49**: 219–225.

Waterlow JC (1972) Classification and definition of protein-calorie malnutrition. *Br. Med. J.* **3**: 566–569.

WHO (1981) International code of marketing of breast-milk substitutes. p. 36. World Health Organisation, Geneva.

Chapter 5

Aggett PJ, Atherton DJ, More J, Davey J, Delves HT and Harries JT (1980) Symptomatic zinc deficiency in a breast-fed, preterm infant. *Arch. Dis. Child.* **55**: 547–550.

American Academy of Pediatrics, Committee on Nutrition (1977) Nutritional needs of low-birthweight infants. *Pediatrics* **60**: 519–530.

American Academy of Pediatrics, Committee on Nutrition (1983) Soy-protein formulas: recommendations for use in infant feeding. *Pediatrics* **72**: 359–363.

American Academy of Pediatrics, Committee on Nutrition (1985) Nutritional needs of low-birthweight infants. *Pediatrics* **75**: 976–986.

Andrews BF and Lorch V (1974) Improved fat and Ca absorption in LBW infants fed a medium chain triglyceride containing formula. *Pediatr. Res.* 8:378/104

Bell SJ, Molnar JA, Krasker WS and Burke JF (1984) Dietary compliance for pediatric burned patients. *J. Am. Diet. Assoc.* **84**: 1329–1333.

Brooke OG (1982) Low birth weight babies: Nutrition and feeding. *Br. J. Hosp. Med.* **28**: 462–465.

Brooke OG, Onubogu O, Heath R and Carter ND (1987) Human milk and preterm formula compared for effects on growth and metabolism. *Arch. Dis. Child.* **62**: 917–923.

Carter AC, Lefkon BW, Farlin M amd Feldman EB (1975) Metabolic parameters in women with metastatic breast cancer. *J. Clin. Endocrinol. Metab.* **40**: 260–264.

Cleghorn G, Durie P, Benjamin L and Dati F (1988). The ontogeny of serum immunoreactive pancreatic lipase and cationic trypsinogen in the premature human infant. *Biol. Neonates* **53**: 10–16.

Curreri PW, Richmond D, Marvin J and Baxter CR (1974) Dietary requirements of patients with major burns. *J. Am. Diet. Assoc.* **65**: 415–417.

Davies MRQ, Rode H, Cywes S and van der Riet RLeS (1981) Burn wound management. *Progr. Pediatr. Surg.* **14**: 33–61.

de Curtis M and Brooke OG (1987) Energy and nitrogen balances in very low birthweight infants. *Arch. Dis. Child.* **62**: 830–832.

Department of Health and Social Security (1977) *Report on Health and Social Subjects, No. 12. The Composition of Mature Milk.* HMSO, London.

Dobbing J and Sands J (1973) Quantitative growth and development of human brain. *Arch. Dis. Child.* **48**: 757–767.

Donaldson SS, Wesley MN, DeWys WD, Suskind RM, Jaffe N and Van Eys J (1981) A study of the nutritional status of pediatric cancer patients. *Am. J. Dis. Child.* **135**: 1107–1112.

Drew JH, Johnston R, Finocchiaro C, Taylor PS and Goldberg HJ (1979) A comparison of nasojejunal with nasogastric feedings in low-birth-weight infants. *Austr. Paediatr. J.* **15**: 98–100.

Editorial (1987) Copper and the infant. *Lancet* i: 900–901.

Engelke SC, Shah BL, Vasan U and Raye JR (1978) Sodium balance in very low-birth-weight infants. *J. Pediatr.* **93**: 837–841.

Friel JK, Gibson RS, Peliowski A and Watts J (1984) Serum zinc, copper, and selenium concentrations in preterm infants receiving enteral nutrition or parenteral nutrition supplemented with zinc and copper. *J. Pediatr.* **104**: 763–768.

Gonzales C and Villasanta U (1982) Life threatening hypocalcaemia and hypomagnesaemia associated with cis-platin therapy. *Obstet. Gynecol.* **59**: 732–734.

Herndon DN, Thompson PB, Desai MH and Van Osten

TJ (1985) Treatment of burns in children in Symposium on Pediatric Surgery. *Pediatr. Clins. N. Am.* **32**: 1311–1332.

Hildreth M and Carvajal HF (1982) A simple formula to estimate daily caloric requirements in burned children. *J. Burn Care Rehabil.* **3**: 78–80.

Hyams JS, Batrus CL, Grand RJ and Sallan SE (1982) Cancer chemotherapy-induced lactose malabsorption in children. *Cancer* **49**: 646–650.

Jensen TG, Long JM, Dudrick SJ and Johnston DA (1985) Nutritional assessment indications of post-burn complications. *J. Diet. Assoc.* **85**: 68–72.

Kibirige MS, Morris Jones PH and Stevens RF (1987) Indicators of malnutrition in leukemic children. *Arch. Dis. Child.* **62**: 845–846.

Laing IA, Lang MA, Callaghan O and Hume R (1986) Nasagastric compared with nasoduodenal feeding in low birth weight infants. *Arch. Dis. Child.* **61**: 138–141.

Lindblad BS, Hagelberg S and Lundsjö A (1982) Blood levels of critical aminoacids in very low birth weight infants on a high human milk protein intake. *Acta Paediatr. Scand. Suppl.* **296**: 24–27.

Lucas A (1982) Human milk banks. *Lancet* **i**: 103.

Lucas A and Roberts CD (1979) Bacteriological quality control in human milk-banking. *Br. Med. J.* **1**: 80–82.

Lucas A, Gibbs JAH, Lyster RL and Baum JD (1978) Creamatocrit: simple clinical technique for estimating fat concentration and energy value of human milk. *Br. Med. J.* **1**: 1018–1020.

Lundholm M, Bennegard K, Eden E, Edstrom S and Schersten T (1982) Glucose metabolism in cancer disease. In: *Clinical Nutrition '81*, RIC Wesdorph and PB Soeters (eds), pp. 153–167. Churchill Livingstone, Edinburgh.

McLaurin NK, Goodwin CW, Zitzkca CA and Hander EW (1983) Computer generated graphic evaluation of nutritional status in critically injured patients. *J. Am. Diet. Assoc.* **82**: 49–52.

Melegh B, Kerner J, Sandor A, Vincellér M and Kispál G (1987) Effects of oral L-carnitine supplementation in low birthweight premature infants maintained on human milk. *Biol. Neonate* **51**: 185–193.

Novak I, Broz L, Konigova R and Spatenka J (1983) More experience with burn shock treatment in children. *Acta Chirur. Plast.* **25**: 179–187.

Okamoto E, Muttart CR, Zucker CL and Heird WC (1982) Use of medium-chain triglycerides in feeding the low-birth-weight infant. *Am. J. Dis. Child.* **136**: 428–431.

Pittard III WB and Bill K (1981) Human milk banking. *Clin. Pediatr.* **20**: 30–33.

Raffles A, Schiller G, Erhardt P and Silverman M. (1983) glucose polymer supplementation of feeds for very low birth weight infants. *Br. Med. J.* **286**: 935–936.

Räihiä NCR, Heinonen K, Rassin DK and Gaull GE (1976) Milk protein quantity and quality in low-birthweight infants: 1. Metabolic reponses and effects on growth. *Pediatrics* **57**: 659–674.

Rickard KA, Coates TD, Grosfeld JL, Weetman RM, Provisor AJ and Baehner RL (1983) Role of nutrition support in the management of children with cancer. In: *13th International Cancer Congress, Part D. Research and Treatment*, pp. 179–192. Alan R. Liss Inc., New York.

Schanler RJ, Garza C and Nicholls BL (1985a) Fortified mother's milk for low birthweight infants: results of growth and nutrient balance studies. *J. Pediatr.* **107**: 437–444.

Schanler RJ, Gaza C and Smith EO (1985b) Nasogastric compared with nasoduodenal feeding in low birth weight infants. *Arch. Dis. Child.* **61**: 138–141.

Sivan Y, Dinari G, Wielunski E, Marcus H, Rosenbach Y, Zahavi I and Nitzan M (1985) Protein conservation by the immature intestine. *Biol. Neonate* **47**: 32–35.

Solomon JR (1981) Nutrition in the severely burned child. *Progr. Pediatr. Surg.* **14**: 63–79.

Stern LM and Davey RB (1985) A team approach with severely burned children in a multi-disciplinary rehabilitation setting. *Burns* **11**: 281–284.

Strauss RG (1978) Iron deficiency, infections and immune function: a reassessment. *Am. J. Clin. Nutr.* **31**: 660–666.

Sutherland AB (1955) The nutritional care of the burned patient. *Br. J. Plast. Surg.* **8**: 68–74.

Toce SS, Keenan WJ and Homan SM (1987) Enteral feeding in very low birth weight infants. *Am. J. Dis. Child.* **141**: 439–444.

Weaver LT, Laker MF and Nelson R (1986) Neonatal intestinal lactase activity. *Arch. Dis. Child.* **61**: 896–899.

Wharton BA (ed.) (1987) *Nutrition and Feeding of Preterm Infants*. Blackwell Scientific, Oxford.

Whitelaw A (1986) Feeding the very low birthweight infant. *Hum. Nutr. Appl.* **40A** (Suppl.): 19–26.

Whyte RK, Campbell D, Stanhope R, Bayley HS and Sinclair JC (1986) Energy balance in low birthweight infant fed formula of high or low medium chain triglyceride content. *J. Pediatr.* **108**: 964–971.

Yuen P, Lin HJ and Hutchison JH (1979) Copper deficiency in a low birthweight infant. *Arch. Dis. Child.* **54**: 553–555.

Zipursky A, Brown EJ, Watts J, Milner R, Rand C, Blanchette VS, Bell EF, Paes B and Ling E (1987). Oral vitamin E supplementation for the prevention of anemia in premature infants: A controlled trial. *Pediatrics* **79**: 61–68.

Zoeren-Grobben DV, Schijver J, Van den Berg H and Berger HM (1987) Human milk vitamin content after pasteurisation, storage or tube feeding. *Arch. Dis. Child.* **62**: 161–165.

Chapter 6

Ariagno RL, Guilleminault C, Baldwin R and Owen-Boeddiker M (1982) Movement and gastroesophageal reflux in awake term infants with 'near miss' SIDS, unrelated to apnea. *J. Pediatr.* **100**: 894–897.

Balistreri WF and Farrell MK (1983) Gastroesophageal reflux in infants. *N. Engl. J. Med.* **309**: 790–792.

Boix-Ochoa J, Lafuente JM and Gil-Vernet JM (1980) Twenty-four hour esophageal pH monitoring in gastroesophageal reflux. *J. Pediatr. Surg.* **15**: 74–78.

Carré I (1979) Gastroesophageal reflux. In: *Report of the Seventy-Sixth Ross Conference on Pediatric Research.* SS Gellis (ed.), pp. 1–22. Ross Laboratories, Columbus, Ohio.

Carré I (1985) Management of gastro-oesophageal reflux. *Arch. Dis. Child.* **60**: 71–75.

Christie DL (1978) Methylene blue test for gastroesophageal reflux. *Lancet* **ii**: 474.

Euler AR and Ament M. (1977) Value of esophageal manometric studies in the gastroesophageal reflux of infancy. *Pediatrics* **59**: 58.

Gellis SS (ed.) (1979) *Report of the 76th Ross Conference on Pediatric Research.* Ross Laboratories, Columbus, Ohio.

Gordon I (1986) Gastrointestinal scintigraphy in paediatrics. In: *Nuclear Gasteroenterology*, PJA Robinson (ed.), pp. 170–176. Churchill Livingstone, Edinburgh.

Herbst JJ (1981) Medical progress. Gastroesophageal reflux. *J. Pediatr.* **98**: 859–870.

Herbst JJ, Book LS and Bray PF (1978) Gastroesophageal reflux in the 'near miss' sudden infant death syndrome. *J. Pediatr.* **92**: 73–75.

Keipert JA (1979) The mode of action and complications of infant gaviscon. *Austr. Paediatr. J.* **15**: 263–265.

Leape LL, Holder TM, Franklin JD, Amoury RA and Ashcraft KW (1977) Respiratory arrest in infants secondary to gastroesophageal reflux. *Pediatrics* **60**: 924–928.

Meyers WF and Herbst JJ (1982) Effectiveness of positioning therapy for gastroesophageal reflux. *Pediatrics* **69**: 768–772.

Moroz SP, Espinoza J, Cumming WA and Diamant NE (1976) Lower esophageal sphincter function in children with and without gastroesophageal reflux. *Gastroenterology* **71**: 236–241.

Orenstein SR, Whitington PF and Orenstein DM (1983) The infant seat as treatment for gastroesophageal reflux. *N. Engl. J. Med.* **309**: 760–763.

Vandenplas Y and Sacré L (1986) Continuous 24 hour eosophageal pH monitoring in 200 asymptomatics. *Pediatr. Res.* **20**: 692.

Vandesplas Y and Sacré L (1987) *Clin. Pediatr.* **26**: 66–71.

Chapter 7

Anand BS and Truelove SC (1977) Skin test for coeliac disease using a subfraction of gluten. *Lancet* **i**: 118–120.

Ashkenazi A, Idar D, Handzel ZT, Ofarim M and Levin S (1978) An in-vitro immunological assay for diagnosis of coeliac disease. *Lancet* **i**: 627–629.

Baker PG (1975) Facts about gluten. *Lancet* **i**: 1307.

Benson CD (1955) Resection and primary anastomosis of the jejunum and ileum in the newborn. *Ann. Surg.* **142**: 478–485.

Besterman HS, Bloom SR, Sarson DL, Blackburn AM, Johnston DI, Patel HR, Stewart JS, Modigliani R, Guerin S and Mallinson CN (1978) Gut-hormone-profile in coeliac disease. *Lancet* **i**: 785–788.

Branski D and Lebenthal E (1981) Celiac disease. In: *Textbook of Gastroenterology and Nutrition in Infancy*, E Lebenthal (ed.), pp. 1013–1025. Raven Press, New York.

Cacciari E, Volta U, Lazzari R, Feliciani M, Partesotti S, Tassoni P, Bianchi FB, Salardi S, Biasco G, Corazza GR, Cicognani A, Azzaroni D, Pirazzoli P and Pisi E (1985) Can antigliadin antibody detect symptomless coeliac disease in children with short stature. *Lancet* **i**: 1469–1471.

Cashel KM, Thomas MP and Properjohn J (1978) Hyperosmolar infant formulae: potential problems in clinical use. *J. Human Nutr.* **32**: 264–269.

Christie DL and Ament ME (1975) Dilute elemental diet and continuous infusion technique for management of short bowel syndrome. *J. Pediatr.* **87**: 705–708.

Colaco J, Egan-Mitchell B, Stevens FM, Fottrell PF and McCarthy CF (1987) *Arch. Dis. Child.* **62**: 706–708.

Cooper A, Floyd TF, Ross AJ, Bishop HC, Templeton JM Jr and Ziegler MM (1984) Morbidity and mortality of short bowel syndrome acquired in infancy: An update. *J. Pediatr. Surg.* **19**: 711–718.

Dicke WK (1950) Coeliakie. *MD thesis*, Utrecht or Zurich, International Congress of Pediatrics.

Dorney SF, Ament ME, Brequist WE, Vargas JH and Hassall E (1985) Improved survival in very short small bowel of infancy with use of long term parenteral nutrition. *J. Pediatr.* **107**: 521–525.

Dowling RH (1982). Small bowel adaptation and its regulation. *Scand. J. Gastroenterol.* **17** (Suppl. 74): 53–74.

Drummey GD, Benson JA and Jones CM (1961) Microscopical examination of the stool for steatorrhea. *N. Engl. J. Med.* **264**: 85–87.

Flint JM (1912) The effect of extensive resections of the small intestine. *Bull. Johns Hopkins Hosp.* **23**: 127–144.

Gee S (1888) On the coeliac affection. *St Bartholomew's Hospital Reports* **24**: 17–20.

Holt D, Easa D, Shim W and Suzuki M (1982) Survival after massive small intestinal resection in a neonate. *Am. J. Dis. Child.* **136**: 79–80.

Katz AJ and Falchuk ZM (1978) Definitive diagnosis of gluten-sensitive enteropathy. *Gastroenterology* **75**: 695–700.

Kendall MJ, Cox PS, Schneider R and Hawkins CF (1972) Gluten subfractions in coeliac disease. *Lancet* **ii**: 1065–1067.

Kurz R and Sauer H (1983) Treatment and metabolic findings in extreme short-bowel syndrome with 11 cm jejunal remnant. *J. Pediatr. Surg.* **18**: 257–263.

Lin C-N, Rossi TM, Heitlinger LA, Lerner A, Riddlesberger MM and Lebenthal E (1987) Nutritional assessment of children with short-bowel syndrome receiving home parenteral nutrition *Am. J. Dis. Child.* **141**: 1093–1098.

McCarthy DM and Kim YS (1973) Changes in sucrase enterokinase, and peptide hydrolase after intestinal resection. *J. Clin. Invest.* **52**: 942–951.

Mäki M, Hällström O, Vesikari T and Visakorpi JK (1984) Evaluation of a serum IgA-class reticulin antibody test for the detection of childhood celiac disease. *J. Pediatr.* **105**: 901–905.

Mann DL, Katz SI, Nelson DL, Abelson LD and Strober W (1976) Specific B-cell antigens associated with gluten-sensitive enteropathy and dermatitis herpetiformis. *Lancet* **i**: 110–111.

Meeuwisse GW (1970) European Society for Paediatric Gastroenterology Meeting in Interlaken September 18, 1969. Diagnostic criteria in coeliac disease. *Acta Paediatr. Scand,* **59**: 461–464.

Milla PJ (1986) The management of massive intestinal resection. *Mat. Child. Hlth* **11**: 43–48.

Postuma R, Moroz S and Friesen F (1983) Extreme short bowel syndrome in an infant. *J. Pediatr. Surg.* **18**: 264–268.

Richards AJ, Condon JR and Mallinson CN (1971) Lactose intolerance following extensive small intestinal resection. *Br. J. Surg.* **58**: 493–494.

Rickham PP (1967) Massive small intestinal resection in newborn infants. *Ann. R. Coll. Surg. Engl.* **41**: 480–492.

Rolles CJ, Anderson CM and McNeish AS (1975) Confirming persistence of gluten intolerance in children diagnosed as having coeliac disease in infancy. *Arch. Dis. Child.* **50**: 259–263.

Sagor GR, Al-Mukhta MYT, Ghatel MA, Wright NA and Bloom SR (1982) The effect of altered luminal nutrition on cellular proliferation and plasma concentration of enteroglucagon and gastrin after small bowel resection in the rat. *Br. J. Surg.* **69**: 14–18.

Seah PP, Fry L, Holborow EJ, Rossiter MA, Doe WF, Magalhaes AF and Hoffbrand AV (1973) Antireticulin antibody: incidence and diagnostic significance. *Gut* **14**: 311–315.

Stevens FM, Egar-Mitchell B, Cryan E, McCarthy CF and McNicholl B (1987) Decreasing incidence of coeliac disease. *Arch. Dis. Child.* **62**: 465–468.

Touloukian RJ and Gertner JM (1981) Vitamin D deficiency rickets as a late complication of the short gut syndrome during infancy. *J. Pediatr. Surg.* **16**: 230–235.

Unsworth DJ, Manuel PD, Walker-Smith JA, Campbell CA, Johnson GD and Holborow EJ (1981) New immunoflourescent blood test for gluten sesitivity. *Arch. Dis. Child.* **56**: 864–868.

Visakorpi JK and Immonen P (1967) Intolerance to cow's milk and wheat gluten in the primary malabsorption syndrome in infancy. *Acta Paediatr. Scand.* **56**: 49–56.

Walker-Smith JA (1970) Transient gluten intolerance. *Arch Dis. Child.* **45**: 523–526.

Walker-Smith JA (1986). Food sensitive Enteropathies. In: *Clinics,* **15**, no. 1. *Gastroenterology,* JA Walker-Smith (ed.), pp. 55–69 WB Saunders Co., London.

West R and Shaw A (1981) Lipoprotein disorders in childhood. *Hosp. Update* **7**: 379–389.

Wilmore DW (1972) Factors correlating with a successful outcome following extensive intestinal resection in newborn infants. *J. Pediatr.* **80**: 88–95.

Wilmore DW, Dudrick SJ, Daly JM and Vars HM (1971) The role of nutrition in the adaptation of the small intestine after massive resection. *Surg. Gynecol. Obstet.* **132**: 673–680.

Young WF and Pringle EM (1971) 110 children with coeliac disease, 1950–1969. *Arch. Dis. Child.* **46**: 421–436.

Chapter 8

Crossley JR and Elliott RB (1977) Simple method for diagnosing protein-losing enteropathies. *Br. Med. J.* **1**: 428–429.

Hill RE, Hercz A, Corey ML, Gilday DL and Hamilton JR (1981) Fecal clearance of α_1-antitrypsin: a reliable measure of enteric protein loss in children. *J. Pediatr.* **99**: 416–418.

Keaney NP and Kelleher J (1980) Faecal excretion of α_1-antitrypsin in protein-losing enteropathy. *Lancet* **i**: 711.

Waldman TA (1966) Protein-losing enteropathy. *Gastroenterology* **50**: 422–443.

Tift WL and Lloyd JK (1975) Intestinal lymphangiectasia: long-term results with MCT diet. *Arch. Dis. Child.* **50**: 269–276.

Vardy PA, Lebenthal E and Shwachman H (1975) Intestinal lymphangiectasia: a reappraisal. *Pediatrics* **55**: 842–850.

Chapter 9

Anon (1987) What has happened to carbohydrate intolerance following gastroenteritis? *Lancet* **i**: 23–24.

Auricchio S, Rubino A and Mürset G (1965) Intestinal glycosidase activities in the human embryo, fetus and newborn. *Pediatrics* **35**: 944–954.

Biller JA, King S, Rosenthal A and Grand RJ (1987) Efficacy of lactase-treated milk for lactose in tolerant pediatric patients. *J. Pediatr.* **111**: 91–94.

Chambers RA and Pratt RTC (1956) Idiosyncracy to fructose. *Lancet* **ii**: 340.

Froesch ER (1972) Essential fructosuria and hereditary fructose intolerance. In: *The Metabolic Basis of Inherited*

Disease, 3rd edn, JB Stanbury, JB Wyngaarden and DS Fredrickson (eds), p. 124. McGraw-Hill, New York.

Gray GM, Conklin KA and Townley RRW (1976) Sucrase–isomaltase deficiency. *N. Engl. J. Med.* **294**: 750–753.

Holzel A, Schwarz V and Sutcliffe KW (1959) Defective lactose absorption causing malnutrition in infancy. *Lancet* **i**: 1126–1128.

Johnson JD, Kretchemer N and Simoons FJ (1974) Lactose malabsorption: its biology and history. In: *Advances in Pediatrics*, I Schulman (ed.), pp. 197–237. Year Book Medical Publishers Inc., Chicago.

Kerry KR and Anderson CM (1964) A ward test for sugar in faeces. *Lancet* **i**: 981–982.

Lebenthal E and Rossi TM (1981) Lactose malabsorption and intolerance. In *Textbook of Gastroenterology and Nutrition in Infancy*, E Lebenthal (ed.) pp. 675–683. Raven Press, New York.

Lindquist B, Meeuwisse GW and Melin K (1962) Glucose–galactose malabsorption. *Lancet* **ii**: 666.

McNair A, Gudmand-Hyer E, Jarnum S and Orrild L (1972) Sucrose malabsorption in Greenland. *Br. Med. J.* **2**: 19–21.

Metz G, Gassull MA, Leeds AR, Blendis LM and Jenkins DJA (1976) A simple method of measuring breath hydrogen in carbohydrate malabsorption by end-expiratory sampling. *Clin. Sci. Mol. Med.* **50**: 237–240.

Plimmer RHA (1906–7) On the presence of lactase in the intestine of animals and on the adaptation of the intestine to lactose. *J. Physiol.* **35**: 20–31.

Walker-Smith J (1979) *Diseases of the Small Intestine in Childhood*, pp. 412. Pitman Medical Publishing Co. Ltd, London.

Chapter 10

Adams RF, Murray KE and Earl JW (1985) High levels of faecal *p*-cresol in a group of hyperactive children. *Lancet* **i**: 1313.

Ament ME and Rubin CE (1972) Soy protein—another cause of the flat intestinal lesion. *Gastroenterology* **62**: 227–234.

Ashkenazi A, Levin S, Idar D, Or A, Rosenberg I and Handzel ZT (1980) *In vitro* cell-mediated immunology assay for cows' milk allergy. *Pediatrics* **66**: 399–402.

Axelsson I and Jakobsson I (1986) Macromolecular absorption in the pre-term infant. *Pediatr. Res.* **20**: 689.

Bahna SL and Heiner DC (1980) *Allergies to Milk*. Grune and Stratton Inc., New York.

Bentley D, Katchburian A and Brostoff J (1984) Abdominal migraine and food sensitivity in children. *Clin. Allergy* **14**: 499–500.

Bjarnason I, Peters TJ and Veall N (1983) A persistent defect in intestinal permeability. *Lancet* **i**: 323–325.

Bleumink E and Young E (1968) Identification of the atopic allergen in cows' milk. *Int. Arch. Allergy Appl. Immunol.* **34**: 521–534.

Bock S (1985) Natural history of severe reactions to food in young children. *J. Pediatr.* **107**: 676–680.

Brostoff J, Carini C and Wraith DG (1983) The presence of immune complexes containing IgE following food challenge and the effect of sodium cromoglycate. In: *Proceedings of the Second Fisons Food Allergy Workshop*, pp. 30–34. Medicine Publishing Foundation, Oxford.

Cant A (1986) The diagnosis and management of food allergy. *Arch. Dis. Child.* **61**: 730–731.

Coca AF (1943) *Familial Nonreaginic Food-Allergy*, pp. 300. Charles C. Thomas, Springfield, Illinois.

Conners CK, Goyette CH, Southwick DA, Lees JM and Andrulonis PA (1976) Food additives and hyperkinesis: a controlled double blind experiment. *Pediatrics* **58**: 154–166.

David TJ (1987a) Unorthodox allergy procedures. *Arch. Dis. Child.* **62**: 1060–1062.

David TJ (1987b) Dietary reactions to tartrazine. *Arch. Dis. Child.* **62**: 119–122.

Dwyer JT (1978) *Year Book of Pediatrics*, pp. 326–327. Year Book Medical Publishers, London.

Eastham EJ, Lichauco T, Pang K and Walker WA (1982) Antigencity of infant formulas and the induction of systemic immunological tolerance by oral feeding: cows' milk and soya milk. *J. Pediatr. Gastroenterol. Nutr.* **1**: 23–28.

Editorial (1979) Is there a hyperkinetic syndrome? *Br. Med. J.* **1**: 506–507.

Editorial (1986) Does hyperactivity matter? *Lancet* **i**: 73–74.

Egger J, Carter CM, Wilson J, Turner MW and Soothill JF (1983) Is migraine food allergy? *Lancet* **ii**: 865–869.

Egger J, Carter CM, Graham PJ, Gumley D and Soothill JF (1985) Controlled trial of oligoantigenic treatment in the hyperkinetic syndrome. *Lancet* **i**: 540–545.

Endre L and Osvath P (1975) Antigen-induced lymphoblast transformation in the diagnosis of cows' milk allergic disease in infancy and early childhood. *Acta Allergol.* **30**: 34–42.

Fälth-Magnusson K, Kjellman N-IM, Magnusson K-E and Sundqvist T (1984) Intestinal permeability in healthy and allergic children before and after sodium cromoglycate treatment assessed with different sized polyethyleneglycols (PEG 400 and PEG 1000). *Clin. Allergy* **14**: 277–286.

Feingold BF (1975) Hyperkinesis and learning disabilities linked to artificial food flavors and colors. *Am. J. Nursing* **75**: 797–803.

Firer MA, Hosking CS and Hill DJ (1988) Possible role for rotavirus in the development of cows' milk enteropathy in infants. *Clin. Allergy* **18**: 53–61.

Forsythe WI and Redmond A (1974) Two controlled trials of tyramine in children with migraine. *Develop. Med. Child Neurol.* **16**: 794–799.

Freier S and Berger H (1973) Disodium cromoglycate in gastrointestinal protein intolerance. *Lancet* **i**: 913–915.

Gell PGH and Coombs RRA (1963) *Clinical Aspects of Immunology*, 1st edn. Blackwell Scientific, Oxford.

Gibb C, Glover V and Sandler M (1986) Inhibition of phenolsulphotransferase P by certain food constituents. *Lancet* i: 794.

Glaser J and Johnstone DE (1953) Prophylaxis of allergic disease in the newborn. *J. Am. Med, Assoc.* **153**: 620−622.

Goldman AS, Anderson DW Jr, Sellers WA, Saperstein S, Kniker WT and Halpern SR (1963) Milk allergy. I. Oral challenge with milk and isolated milk proteins in allergic children. *Pediatrics* **32**: 425−443.

Gryboski JD (1967) Gastrointestinal milk allergy in infants. *Pediatrics* **40**: 354−362.

Halpern SR, Sellars WA, Johnson RB, Anderson DW, Saperstein S and Reisch JS (1973) Development of childhood allergy in infants fed breast, soy, or cow milk. *J. Allergy Clin. Immunol.* **51**: 139−151.

Halpin TC, Byrne WJ and Ament ME (1977) Colitis, persistent diarrhea and soy protein intolerance. *J. Pediatr.* **91**: 404−407.

Harrison M, Kilby A, Walker-Smith JA, France NE and Wood CBS (1976) Cows' milk protein intolerance: a possible association with gastroenteritis, lactose intolerance, and IgA deficiency. *Br. Med. J.* **1**: 1501−1504.

Hathaway MJ and Warner JO (1983) Compliance problems in the dietary management of eczema. *Arch. Dis. Child.* **58**: 463−464.

Katchburian A, Horn J and Bentley D (1986). Abdominal migraine in childhood: food intolerance and the IgE level. *Sixth International Migraine Symposium*, London.

Kilby A, Walker-Smith JA and Wood CBS (1975) Small intestinal mucosa in cows' milk allergy. *Lancet* i: 531.

King DS (1981) Can allergic exposure provoke psychological symptoms? A double-blind test. *Biol. Psychiatr.* **16**: 3−19.

Kuzemko JA and Simpson KR (1975) Treatment of allergy to cows' milk. *Lancet* i: 337−338.

Lebenthal E, Laor J, Lewitus Z, Matoth Y and Freier S (1970) Gastrointestinal protein loss in allergy to cows' milk β-lactoglobulin. *Isr. J. Med. Sci.* **6**: 506−510.

Lehman CW (1980a) A double-blind study of sublingual provocative food testing: a study of its efficacy. *Ann. Allergy* **45**: 144−149.

Lehman CW (1980b) The leucocytic food allergy test: a study of its reliability and reproducibility. Effect of diet and sublingual food drops on this test. *Ann. Allergy* **45**: 150−158.

Lessof MH (1984) *Update Postgraduate Centre Series, Allergy*, 3rd edn. *Intolerance to Food*, pp. 30−34.

Lessof MH, Wraith DG, Merrett TG, Merrett J and Buisseret PD (1980) Food allergy and intolerance in 100 patients—local and systemic effects. *Q. J. Med.* **49**: 259−271.

Littlewood JT, Glover V and Sandler M (1985) Red wine contains a potent inhibitor of phenolsulphotransferase. *Br. J. Clin. Pharmacol.* **19**: 275−278.

Littlewood J, Glover V, Sandler M, Petty R, Peatfield R and Rose FC (1982) Platelet phenolsulphotransferase deficiency in dietary migraine. *Lancet* i: 983−986.

McLaughlin P, Anderson KJ, Widdowson EM and Coombs RR (1981) Effect of heat on the anaphylactic-sensitising capacity of cows' milk and goat milk fed to guinea pigs. *Arch. Dis. Child.* **56**: 165−171.

Matthew DJ, Taylor B, Norman AP, Turner MW and Soothill JF (1977) Prevention of eczema. *Lancet* i: 321−324.

Matthews TS and Soothill JF (1970) Complement activation after milk feeding in children with cows' milk allergy. *Lancet* ii: 893−895.

Medina JL and Diamond S (1978) The role of diet in migraine. *Headache* **18**: 31−34.

Merrett TG, Gawel MJ and Peatfield RC (1980) Food allergy in migraine. *Lancet* ii: 532.

Monro J, Brostoff J, Carini C and Zilkha K (1980) Food allergy in migraine. Study of dietary exclusion and RAST. *Lancet* ii: 1−4.

Morin CL, Buts JP, Weber A, Roy CC and Brochu P (1979) One-hour blood-xylose test in diagnosis of cows' milk protein intolerance. *Lancet* i: 1102−1104.

NIH (1982) *Consensus Development Conference Draft Statement: defined diet and childhood hyperactivity*. National Institutes of Health, Washington.

Noone C, Menzies IS, Banatvala JE and Scopes JW (1986). Intestinal permeability and lactose hydrolysis in human rotaviral gastroenteritis assessed simultaneously by non-invasive differential sugar permeation. *Eur. J. Clin. Invest.* **16**: 217−225.

Ramage JK, Hunt RH and Perdue MH (1988) Changes in intestinal permeability and epithelial differentiation during inflammation in the rat. *Gut* **29**: 57−61.

Royal College of Physicians/British Nutrition Foundation (1984) Food intolerance and food aversion. A joint report of the Royal College of Physicians and the British Nutrition Foundation. *J. R. Coll. Phys. Lond.* **18**(2): 4.

Rutter M (1965) Classification and categorization in child psychiatry. *J. Child. Psychol. Psychiatr.* **6**: 71−83.

Sacks O. (1970) *Migraine: The Evolution of a Common Disorder.*, p. 71. University of California Press, Berkeley.

Safer D, Allen R and Barr E (1972) Depression of growth in hyperactive children on stimulant drugs. *N. Engl. J. Med.* **287**: 217−220.

Salfield SA, Wardley BL, Houlsby WT, Turner SL, Spaeton AP, Beckles-Wilson NR and Herber SM (1987) Controlled study of exclusion of dietary vasoactive amines in migraine. *Arch. Dis. Child.* **62**: 458−460.

Sandler M, Youdim MBH and Hanington E (1974) A phenylethylamine oxidising defect in migraine. *Nature* **250**: 335−337.

Savilahti E, Tainio VM, Salmenpera L, Siimes MA and Perheentup J (1987) Prolonged exclusive breast feeding and heredity as determinants in infantile atopy.

Am. J. Dis. Child. **62**: 269−273.

Shiner M, Ballard J and Smith ME (1975) The small-intestinal mucosa in cows' milk allergy. *Lancet* **i**: 136−140.

Speight JW and Atkinson P (1980) Food allergy in migraine. *Lancet* **ii**: 532.

Strobel S (1986) Allergenicity of feeds and gastrointestinal immunoregulation in man and experimental animals. *Hum. Nutr. Appl.* **40a**, Suppl 1: 45−54.

Swanson JM and Kinsbourne M (1980) Food dyes impair performance of hyperactive children on a laboratory learning test. *Science* **207**: 1485−1487.

Taitz LS and Armitage BL (1984) Goats' milk for infants and children *Br. Med. J.*, **288**: 428−429.

Tomasi TB Jr (1972) Secretory immunoglobulins. *N. Engl. J. Med.* **287**: 500−506.

Van Asperen PP, Kemp AS and Mellies CM (1983) Immediate food hypersensitivity reactions on the first known exposure to the food. *Arch. Dis. Child.* **58**: 253−256.

Visakorpi JK (1970) An international enquiry concerning the diagnostic criteria of coeliac disease. *Acta Paediatr. Scand.* **59**: 461−463.

Walker WA (1975) Antigen absorption from the small intestine and gastrointestinal disease. *Pediatr. Clins N. Am.* **22**: 731−746.

Walker WA and Hong R (1973) Immunology of the gastrointestinal tract. Part I. *J. Pediatr.* **83**: 517−530.

Walker-Smith JA (1984). Food allergies and bowel disease. *J. R. Soc. Med.* Suppl. No. 5, **78**: 3−6.

Weiss B, Williams JH, Margen S, Abrams B, Caan B, Citron LJ, Cox C, McKibben J, Ogar D and Schultz S (1980) Behavioral response to artificial food colors. *Science* **207**: 1487−1489.

Weiss G (1983) Long-term outcome: findings, concepts and practical implications. In: *Developmental Neuropsychiatry*. M. Rutter (ed.), pp. 422−436. Guildford Press, New York.

Williams JI and Cram DM (1978) Diet in the management of hyperkenesis. A review of the tests of Feingold's hypotheses. *Can. Psychiatr. Assoc. J.* **23**: 241−248.

Zametkin A, Rapoport JL, Murphy DL, Linnoila M and Ismond D (1985) Treatment of hyperactive children with monoamine oxidase inhibitors: 1. Clinical efficacy. *Arch. Gen. Psychiatr.* **42**: 962−966.

Chapter 11

Abrahamian FP and Lloyd-Still JD (1984) Chronic constipation in childhood: longitudinal study of 186 patients. *J. Pediatr. Gastroenterol. Nutr.* **3**: 460−467.

Apley J (1975) *The Child with Abdominal Pains*, 2nd edn, p. 7. Blackwell Scientific, Oxford.

Bain HW (ed.) (1974) Chronic vague abdominal pain in children. In: *Symposium on Chronic Disease in Children, Pediatr. Clin. N. Am.* **21**: 991−1000.

Barr RG, Levine MD and Watkins JB (1979) Recurrent abdominal pain of childhood due to lactose intolerance. *N. Engl. J. Med.* **300**: 1449−1452.

Bentley D, Katchburian A and Brostoff J (1984) Abdominal migraine and food sensitivity in children. *Clin. Allergy* **14**: 499−500.

Blumenthal I, Kelleher J and Littlewood JM (1981) Recurrent abdominal pain and lactose intolerance in childhood. *Br. Med. J.* **282**: 2013−2014.

Christensen MF (1980) Prevalence of lactose intolerance in children with recurrent abdominal pain. *Pediatrics* **65**: 681.

Davidson M, Kugler MM and Bauer CH (1963) Diagnosis and management in children with severe and protracted constipation and obstipation. *J. Pediatr.* **62**: 261−275.

Krishnamurthy S, Schuffler MD, Rohrmann CA and Pope CE (1985) Severe idiopathic constipation is associated with a distinctive abnormality of the colonic myenteric plexus. *Gastroenterology* **88**: 26−34.

Lebenthal E, Rossi TM, Nord KS and Branski D (1981) Recurrent abdominal pain and lactose absorption in children. *Pediatrics* **67**: 828−832.

Levine MD and Bakow H (1976) Children with encopresis: a study of treatment outcome. *Pediatrics* **58**: 845−852.

Liebman WM (1979). Recurrent abdominal pain in children: lactose and sucrose intolerance. A prospective study. *Pediatrics* **64**: 43−45.

Loening-Baucke VA (1984) Abnormal rectoanal function in children recovered from chronic constipation anf encopresis. *Gastroenterology* **87**: 1299−1304.

McCormick J (1980) Recurrent abdominal pain in childhood. *Br. Med. J.* **1**: 1377.

Meunier P, Marechal JM and Jaubert De Beaujeu M (1979) Rectoanal pressure and rectal sensitivity studies in chronic childhood constipation. *Gastroenterology* **77**: 330−336.

Meunier P, Louis D and Jaubert De Beaujeu M (1984) Physiologic investigation of primary chronic constipation in children: comparison with the barium enema study. *Gastroenterology* **87**: 1351−1357.

Oderda G and Ansaldi N (1988) Peptic ulcers in childhood. *Lancet* **i**: 302−303.

Pringle MLK, Butler NR and Davie R (1966) 11,000 seven year olds. *First Report of National Child Development (1958 Cohort)*. Longmans, London.

Sondheimer J (1986) Comment on chronic constipation. In *1986 Year Book of Pediatrics*, F.A. Oski and J.A. Stockman (eds), pp. 254−255. Year Book Medical Publishers Inc., London.

Wald A, Chandra R, Fisher SE, Gartner JC and Zitelli B (1982) Lactose malabsorption in recurrent abdominal pain of childhood. *J. Pediatr.* **100**: 65−68.

Weaver LT and Steiner H (1984) The bowel habit of young children. *Arch. Dis. Child.* **59**: 649−652.

Whytt R (1765) *Disorders commonly called nervous hypochondriac, or hysteric*. Edinburgh+ T. Becket, P. Du Hondt, J. Balfour.

Chapter 12

Alward CT, Hook JB, Helmrath TA, Mattson JC and Bailie MD (1978) Effects of asphyxia on cardiac output and organ blood flow in the newborn piglet. *Pediatr. Res.* **12**: 824–827.

Arulanantham K, Kramer MS and Gryboski JD (1980) The association of inflammatory bowel disease and X chromosomal abnormality. *Pediatrics* **66**: 63–67.

Bentley D, Lynn J and Laws JW (1985) Campylobacter colitis with intestinal aphthous ulceration mimicking obstruction. *Br. Med. J.* **291**: 634.

Cave DR, Mitchell DN and Brooke BN (1976) Evidence of an agent transmissible from ulcerative colitis tissue. *Lancet* **i**: 1311–1315.

Chong SKF, Bartram C, Campbell CA, Williams CB, Blackshaw AJ and Walker-Smith JA (1982) Chronic inflammatory bowel disease in childhood. *Br. Med. J.* **284**: 101–103.

Crohn BB (1967) Granulomatous disease of the small and large bowel. A historical survey. *Gastroenterology* **52**: 767–772.

Crohn BB, Ginzburg L and Oppenheimer GD (1932) Regional ileitis: a pathological and clinical entity. *J. Am. Med. Assoc.* **99**: 1323–1329.

Devroede GJ, Taylor WF, Sauer WG, Jackman RJ and Stickler GB (1971) Cancer risk and life expectancy of children with ulcerative colitis. *N. Engl. J. Med.* **285**: 17–21.

Dixon FJ (1963) The role of antigen—antibody complexes in disease. *Harvey Lecture* **58**: 21–52.

Drug and Therapeutic Bulletin (1986) The drug treatment of Crohn's disease. *Drug Ther. Bull.* **24**: 13–16.

Gerlach K, Morowitz DA and Kirsner JB (1970) Symptomatic hypomagnesemia complicating regional enteritis. *Gastroenterology* **59**: 567–574.

Girardet JP, Charritat JL, Mougenot JF, Borrongibod L, Navarro J and Fontaine JL (1981) A study of immunoglobulin producing cells in the colonic mucosa of children with Crohn's disease. *Nouv. Presse Méd.* **10**: 1803–1805.

Grace RH, Gent AE and Hellier MD (1987) Comparative trial of sodium cromoglycate enemas with prednisolone enemas in the treatment of ulcerative colitis. *Gut* **28**: 88–92.

Grady GF and Keusch GT (1971) Pathogenesis of bacterial diarrheas. Part II. *N. Engl. J. Med.* **285**: 891–900.

Greenstein AJ, Sachar DB, Pasternack BS and Janowitz HD (1975) Reoperation and recurrence in Crohn's colitis and ileocolitis. *N. Engl. J. Med.* **293**: 685–690.

Habal FM and Greenberg GR (1988). Treatment of ulcerative colitis with oral 5-aminosalicylic acid including patients with adverse reactions to sulphasalazine. *Am. J. Gastroenterol.* **83**, 15–19.

Halpin TC, Byrne WJ and Ament ME (1977) Colitis, persistent diarrhea, and soy protein intolerance. *J. Pediatr.* **91**: 404–407.

Jewell DP and Truelove SC (1972a) Reaginic hypersensitivity in ulcerative colitis. *Gut* **13**: 903–906.

Jewell DP and Truelove SC (1972b) Azathioprine in ulcerative colitis: an interim report on a controlled therapeutic trial. *Br. Med. J.* **1**: 709–712.

Kanto WP, Wilson R, Breart GL, Zieler S, Purohit DM, Peckham GJ and Ellison RC (1987) Perinatal events and necrotizing enterocolitis in premature infants. *Am. J. Dis. Child.* **141**: 167–169.

Lake AM, Whitington PF and Hamilton SR (1982) Dietary protein-induced colitis in breast-fed infants. *J. Pediatr.* **101**: 906–910.

Mani V, Lloyd G, Green FHY, Fox H and Turnberg LA (1976) Treatment of ulcerative colitis with oral disodium cromoglycate. *Lancet* **i**: 439–441.

Mayberry JF and Rhodes J (1984) Epidemiological aspects of Crohn's disease: a review of the literature. *Gut* **25**: 886–899.

Milla P (1986) Wyeth Nutrition symposium on Food intolerance—current research and paediatric practice. *Food-sensitive Colitis in Infants*, pp. 18–19.

Miller DS, Keighley AC and Langman MJS (1974) Changing patterns in epidemiology of Crohn's disease. *Lancet* **ii**: 691–693.

Mitchell DN, Rees RJW and Goswami KKA (1976) Transmissible agents from human sarcoid and Crohn's disease tissues. *Lancet* **ii**: 761–765.

O'Donoghue DP and Dawson AM (1977) Crohn's disease in childhood. *Arch. Dis. Child.* **52**: 627–632.

Pitt J (1975) In *Necrotizing Enterocolitis in the Newborn Infant*, Report of the Sixty-Eighth Ross Conference on Pediatric Research, T.D. Moore (ed.), pp. 53–60. Columbus, Ohio, Ross Laboratories.

Powell GK (1978) Milk-and soy-induced enterocolitis of infancy. *J. Pediatr.* **93**: 553–560.

Rotbart HA, Nelson WL, Glode MP, Triffon TC, Kogut SJH, Yolken RH, Hernandez JA and Levin MJ (1988). Neonatal rotavirus-associated necrotizing enterocolitis: Case control study and prospective surveillance during an outbreak. *J. Pediatr.* **112**: 87–93.

Sanderson IR, Udeen S, Davies PSW, Savage MO and Walker-Smith JA (1987) Remission induced by an elemental diet in small bowel Crohn's disease. *Arch. Dis. Child.* **61**: 123–127.

Saverymuttu SH, Camilleri M, Rees H, Lavender JP, Hodgson HJF and Chadwick VS (1986) Indium-111-granulocyte scanning in the assessment of disease extent and disease activity in inflammatory bowel disease. *Gastroenterology* **90**: 1121–1128.

Shorter RG, Spencer RJ, Huizenga KA and Hallenbeck GA (1968) Inhibition of in vitro cytotoxicity of lymphocytes from patients with ulcerative colitis and granulomatous colitis for allogeneic colonic epithelial cells using horse anti-human thymus serum. *Gastroenterology* **54**: 227–231.

Silverman A and Roy CC (1983) *Pediatric Clinical Gastroenterology*, 3rd edn, pp. 366–367. CV Mosby Co., St Louis.

Thomas DFM (1982) Pathogenesis of neonatal necrotizing enterocolitis. *J. R. Soc. Med.* **75**: 838–840.

Thornton JR, Emmett PM and Heaton KW (1979) Diet and Crohn's disease: characterictics of the pre-illness diet. *Br. Med. J.* **2**: 762–764.

Touloukian RJ, Posch JN and Spencer R (1972) The pathogenesis of ischemic gastroenterocolitis of the neonate: selective gut mucosal ischemia in asphyxiated neonatal piglets. *J. Pediatr. Surg.* **7**: 194–205.

Truelove SC (1961) Ulcerative colitis provoked by milk. *Br. Med. J.* **1**: 154–160.

Walker JEG (1978) Possible diagnostic test for Crohn's disease by use of buccal mucosa. *Lancet* **ii**: 759–760.

Waterlow JC (1972) Classification and definition of protein calorie malnutrition. *Br. Med. J.* **3**: 566–569.

Chapter 13

Aggett PJ, Thorn JM, Delves HT, Harries JT and Clayton BE (1979) Trace element malabsorption in exocrine pancreatic insufficiency. *Monogr. Paediatr.* **10**: 8–11.

Aggett PJ, Cavanagh NPC, Matthew DJ, Pincott JR, Sutcliffe J and Harries JT (1980) Shwachman's syndrome — A review of 21 cases. *Arch. Dis. Child.* **55**: 331–347.

Andersen DH (1938) Cystic fibrosis of the pancreas and its relation to celiac disease. A clinical and pathological study. *Am. J. Dis. Child.* **56**: 344–399.

Anon (1985) Prenatal diagnosis in cystic fibrosis *Lancet* **i**: 1199.

Anon (1988) Too many H$_2$ antagonists. *Lancet* **i**: 28–29.

Antonowicz I, Reddy V, Khaw K-T and Shwachman H (1968) Lactase deficiency in patients with cystic fibrosis. *Pediatrics* **42**: 492–500.

Azizi F, Bentley D, Vagenakis A, Portnay G, Shwachman H, Ingbar S and Braverman L (1974) Abnormal thyroid function and the response to iodides in cystic fibrosis (CF). *Clin. Res.* **22**: 556A.

Barry RE, Barry R, Ene MD and Parker G (1982) Fluorescein-dilaurate-tubeless test for pancreatic exocrine failure. *Lancet* **ii**: 742–744.

Beaudet AL, Spence JE, Montes M, O' Brien WE Estivill X, Farrall M and Williamson R (1988) Experience with new DNA markers for the diagnosis of cystic fibrosis. *N. Eng. J. Med.* **318**: 50–51.

Bentley D and Cline J (1970) Estimation of clubbing by analysis of shadowgraph. *Br. Med. J.* **3**: 43.

Bentley D, Moore A and Shwachman H (1976) Finger clubbing: a quantitative survey by analysis of the shadowgraph. *Lancet* **ii**: 164–167.

Bertrand JM, Morin CL, Lasalle R, Patrick J and Coates AL (1984) Short-term clinical, nutritional, and functional effects of continuous elemental enteral alimentation in children with cystic fibrosis. *J. Pediatr.* **104**: 41–46.

Bodian M, Sheldon W and Lightwood R (1964) Congenital hypoplasia of the exocrine pancreas. *Acta Paediatr. Scand.* **53**: 282–293.

Borgström B, Erlanson-Albertsson C and Wieloch T (1979) Pancreatic co-lipase: chemistry and physiology. *J. Lipid Res.* **20**: 805–816.

Bowling F, Cleghorn G, Chester A, Curran J, Griffin B, Prado J, Francis P and Shepherd R (1988) Neonatal screening for cystic fibrosis. *Arch. Dis. Child.* **63**: 196–198.

Braganza J, Critchley M, Howat HT, Testa HJ and Torrance HB (1973) An evaluation of ^{75}Se selenomethionine scanning as a test of pancreatic function compared with the secretin-pancreozymin test. *Gut* **14**: 383–389.

Brock DJH (1983) Amniotic fluid alkaline phosphatase isoenzymes in early prenatal diagnosis of cystic fibrosis. *Lancet* **ii**: 941–943.

Brueton MJ, Mavromichalis J, Goodchild MC and Anderson CM (1977) Hepatic dysfunction in association with pancreatic insufficiency and cyclic neutropenia. *Arch. Dis. Child.* **52**: 76–78.

Burke V, Colebatch JH, Anderson CM and Simons MJ (1967) Association of pancreatic insufficiency and chronic neutropenia in childhood. *Arch. Dis. Child.* **42**: 147–157.

Carbarns NJB, Gosden C and Brock DJH (1983) Microvillar peptidase activity in amniotic fluid: possible use in the prenatal diagnosis of cystic fibrosis. *Lancet* **i**: 329–331.

Carter EP, Barrett AD, Heeley AF and Kuzemko JA (1984) Improved sweat test method for the diagnosis of cystic fibrosis. *Arch. Dis. Child.* **59**: 919–922.

Congden PJ, Bruce G, Rothburn MM, Clarke PCN, Littlewood JM, Kelleher J and Losowsky MS (1981) Vitamin status in treated patients with cystic fibrosis. *Arch. Dis. Child.* **56**: 708–714.

Crossley JR, Berryman CC and Elliott RB (1977). Cystic fibrosis screening in the newborn. *Lancet* **ii**: 1093–1095.

Deren JJ, Arora B, Toskes PP, Hansell J and Sibinga MS (1973) Malabsorption of crystalline vitamin B$_{12}$ in cystic fibrosis. *N. Engl. J. Med.* **288**: 949–950.

Di Sant'Agnese PA, Darling RC, Perera GA and Shea E (1953) Abnormal electrolyte composition of sweat in cystic fibrosis of pancreas: clinical significance and relationship to disease. *Pediatrics* **12**: 549–63.

Dworki B, Newman LJ, *et al.* (1987) Low blood selenium levels in patients with cystic fibrosis compared to controls and healthy adults. *J. Parent. Ent. Nutr.* **11**: 38–42.

Editorial (1987) Omeprazole. *Lancet* **ii**: 1187–1188.

Ehrhardt P, Miller MG and Littlewood JM (1987) Iron deficiency in cystic fibrosis. *Arch. Dis. Child.* **62**: 185–187.

Farrall M, Law H-Y, Rodeck CH, Warren R, Stanier P, Super M, Lissens W, Scambler P, Watson E, Wainwright B and Williamson R (1986) First-trimester prenatal diagnosis of cystic fibrosis with linked DNA probes. *Lancet* **i**: 1402–1405.

Figarella C, Negri GA and Sarles H (1972) Presence of colipase in a congenital pancreatic lipase deficiency. *Biochim. Biophys. Acta* **280**: 205–210.

Gibson LE and Cooke RE (1959) A test for concentration of electrolytes in sweat in cystic fibrosis of the pancreas utilizing pilocarpine by iontophoresis. *Pediatrics* **23**: 545–549.

Gitlin N, McCullogh AJ, Smith JL, Mantell G and Berman (1987). A multicentre double blind, randomised placebo controlled comparison of nocturnal and twice a day famotidine in the treatment of active duodenal disease. *Gastroenterology* **92**: 49–53.

Gow R, Bradbear R, Francis P and Shepherd R (1981) Comparative study of varying regimens to improve steatorrhoea and creatorrhoea in cystic fibrosis: effectiveness of an enteric-coated preparation with and without antacids and cimetidine. *Lancet* **ii**: 1071–1074.

Hahn TJ, Squires AE, Halstead LR and Strominger DB (1979) Reduced serum 25-hydroxyvitamin D concentration and disordered mineral metabolism in patients with cystic fibrosis. *J. Pediatr.* **94**: 38–42.

Harries JT, Muller DPR, McCollum JPK, Lipson A, Roma E and Norman AP (1979) Intestinal bile salts in cystic fibrosis. *Arch. Dis. Child.* **54**: 19–24.

Hill RE, Durie PR, Gaskin KJ, Davidson GP and Forstner GG (1982) Steatorrhea and pancreatic insufficiency in Shwachman syndrome. *Gastroenterology* **83**: 22–27.

Hodson ME, Beldon I, Power R, Duncan FR, Bamber M and Batten JC (1983) Sweat test to diagnose cystic fibrosis in adults. *Br. Med. J.* **286**: 1381–1383.

Hodson ME, Roberts CM, Butland RJA, Smith MJ and Batten JC (1987) Oral ciprofloxacin compared with conventional intravenous treatment for *Pseudomonas aeruginosa* infection in adults with cystic fibrosis. *Lancet* **i**: 235–237.

Holsclaw DS and Shwachman H (1971) Increased incidence of inguinal hernia, hydrocele and undescended testicle in males with cystic fibrosis. *Pediatrics* **48**: 442–445.

Holsclaw DS, Rocmans C and Shwachman H (1971) Intussusception in patients with cystic fibrosis. *Pediatrics* **48**: 51–58.

Knowlton RG, Cohen-Haguenauer O, Cong NV, Frézal J, Brown VA, Barker D, Braman JC, Schumm JW, Tsui L-C, Buchwald M and Donis-Keller H (1985) A polymorphic DNA marker linked to cystic fibrosis is located on chromosome 7. *Nature* **318**: 380–382.

Kopito L, Mahmoodian A, Townley RRW, Khaw KT and Shwachman H (1965) Studies in cystic fibrosis: analysis of nail clippings for sodium and potassium. *N. Engl. J. Med.* **272**: 504–509.

Kopito L, Elian E and Shwachman H (1972) Sodium, potassium, calcium and magnesium in hair from neonates with cystic fibrosis and in amniotic fluid from mothers of such children. *Pediatrics* **49**: 620–624.

Kopito LE, Kosasky HJ and Shwachman H (1973) Water and electrolytes in cervical mucus from patients with cystic fibrosis. *Fertil. Steril.* **24**: 512–516.

Kulczycki LL and Schauf V (1978) Incidence of cystic fibrosis in black children—revisited. *Pediatrics* **92**: 855.

Kulczycki LL, Butler JS, McCord-Dickman D and Herer GR (1970) The hearing of patients with cystic fibrosis. *Arch. Otolaryngol.* **92**: 54–59.

Lester LA, Rothberg RM *et al.* (1986) Supplemental parenteral nutrition in cystic fibrosis. *J. Parent. Ent. Nutr.* **10**: 289–293

Lilibridge CB and Townes PL (1973) Physiologic deficiency of pancreatic amylase in infancy: a factor in iatrogenic diarrhea. *J. Pediatr.* **82**: 279–282.

Lloyd-Still JD, Johnson SB and Holman RT (1981) Essential fatty acid status in cystic fibrosis and the effect of safflower oil supplementation. *Am. J. Clin. Nutr.* **34**: 1–7.

Lindemans J, Neijens HJ, Kerrebijn KF and Abels J (1984) Vitamin B_{12} absorption in cystic fibrosis. *Acta Paediatr. Scand.* **73**: 537–540.

Littlewood JM (1986) The sweat test. *Arch. Dis. Child.* **61**: 1041–1043.

Lobeck CC and McSherry NR (1963) Response of sweat electrolyte concentrations to 9-alpha-fluorohydrocortisone in patients with cystic fibrosis and their families. *J. Pediatr.* **62**: 393–398.

Lowe CU and May CD (1951) Selective pancreatic deficiency. *Am. J. Dis. Child.* **82**: 459–464.

McCollum JPK, Muller DPR and Harries JT (1977) Test meal for assessing intraluminal phase of absorption in childhood. *Arch. Dis. Child.* **52**: 887–889.

McPartlin JF, Dickson JAS and Swain VAJ (1972) Meconium ileus immediate and long-term survival. *Arch. Dis. Child.* **47**: 207–210.

Mansell AL, Andersen JC, Muttart CR, Ores CN, Loeff DS, Levy JS and Heird WC (1984) Short-term pulmonary effects of total parenteral nutrition in children with cystic fibrosis. *J. Pediatr.* **104**: 700–705.

Mastella G, Pederzini F, Girella E, Righetti G, Zanchetta M and Rizzotti P (1984) Cystic fibrosis screening policy (letter). *Lancet* **ii**: 575–576.

Mearns MB (1985) Cystic fibrosis. *Arch. Dis. Child.* **60**: 272–277.

Miller M, Ward L, Thomas BJ, Cooksley WGE and Shepherd RW (1982) Altered body composition and muscle protein degradation in nutritionally growth-retarded children with cystic fibrosis. *Am. J. Clin. Nutr.* **36**: 492–499.

Mornet E, Simon-Bouy B, Serre JL, Estivill X, Farrall

M, Williamson R, Boue J and Boue A (1988) Genetic differences between cystic fibrosis with and without meconium ileus. *Lancet* i: 376–378.

Muller DPR, McCollum JPK, Trompeter RS and Harries JT (1975) Studies on the mechanism of fat absorption in congenital isolated lipase deficiency. *Gut* 16: 838.

Oppenheimer EH and Esterly JR (1970) Observation on cystic fibrosis of the pancreas. *J. Pediatr.* 77: 991–995.

Scott RB, O'Loughlin EV and Gall DG (1985) Gastro-esophageal reflux in patients with cystic fibrosis. *J. Pediatr.* 106: 223–227.

Sheldon W (1964) Congenital pancreatic lipase deficiency. *Arch. Dis. Child.* 39: 268–271.

Shmerling DH, Prader A, Hitzig WH, Giedion A, Hadorn B and Kuhni M (1969) The syndrome of exocrine pancreatic insufficiency neutropenia, metaphyseal dysostosis and dwarfism. *Helvet. Paediatr. Acta* 24: 547–575.

Shwachman H (1975) Gastrointestinal manifestations of cystic fibrosis. In: *Chronic Disease in Children*, H. W. Bain (ed.) *Pediatric Clinics of North America*, Vol. 22, No. 4, pp. 787–805. WB Saunders Co, Philadelphia.

Shwachman H and Holsclaw D (1972) Some clinical observations on the Shwachman syndrome (pancreatic insufficiency and bone marrow hypoplasia). *Birth defects: Original Article Series*, Vol. VIII, No. 3.

Shwachman H, Diamond LK, Oski FA and Khaw K-T (1964) The syndrome of pancreatic insufficiency and bone marrow dysfunction. *J. Pediatr.* 65: 645–63.

Solomons NW, Wagonfeld JB, Rieger C, Jacob RA, Bolt M, Horst JV, Rothberg R and Sandstead H (1981) Some biochemical indices of nutrition in treated cystic fibrosis patients. *Am. J. Clin. Nutr.* 34: 462–474.

Stephan U, Busch E-W, Kollberg H and Hellsing K (1975) Cystic fibrosis detection by means of a test-strip. *Pediatrics* 55: 35–38.

Super M (1975) Cystic fibrosis in the South-West African Afrikaner. *S. A. Med. J.* 49: 818–820.

Super M, Schwarz M, Elles RG, Ivinson A, Giles L, Read AP and Harris R (1987) Clinical experience of prenatal diagnosis of cystic fibrosis by use of linked DNA probes. *Lancet* ii: 782–784.

Tarlow MJ, Hadorn B, Arthurton MW and Lloyd JK (1970) Intestinal enterokinase deficiency. *Arch. Dis. Child.* 45: 651–655.

Wainwright BJ, Scambler PJ, Schmidtke J, Watson EA, Law H-Y, Farrall M, Cooke HJ, Eiberg H and Williamson R (1985) Localisation of cystic fibrosis locus to human chromosome 7cen-q22. *Nature* 318: 384–385.

White R, Woodward S, Leppert M, O'Connell P, Hoff M, Herbst J, Lalouel J-M, Dean M and Woude GV (1985) A closely linked genetic marker for cystic fibrosis. *Nature* 318: 382–384.

Wright SW and Morton NE (1968) Genetic studies on cystic fibrosis in Hawaii. *Am. J. Human Genet.* 20: 157–169.

Yassa JG (1983) Nutrition in cystic fibrosis. In: *Topics in Paediatric Nutrition*, J.A. Dodge (ed.), pp. 212–224. Pitman, London.

Chapter 14

Anon (1987a) Transplantation for acute liver failure. *Lancet* ii: 1248–1249.

Anon (1987b) α_1-Antitrypsin deficiency and prenatal diagnosis. *Lancet* i: 421–422.

Arasu TS, Wyllie R, Hatch TF and Fitzgerald JF (1979) Management of chronic aggressive hepatitis in children and adolescents. *J. Pediatr.* 4: 514–522.

Brandt NJ (1980) *Inherited Disorders of Carbohydrate Metabolism.* D. Burman, JB Holton and CA Pennock (eds), pp. 117–123. MTP Press, Lancaster.

Brunner RL, O'Grady DJ, Partin JC, Partin JS and Schubert WK (1979) Neuropsychologic consequences of Reye syndrome. *J. Pediatr.* 95: 706–711.

Campbell DP, Poley JR, Alaupovic P and Smith EI (1974) The differential diagnosis of neonatal hepatitis and biliary atresia. *J. Pediatr. Surg.* 9(5): 699–705.

Clothier CM and Davidson DC (1983) Galactosaemia workshop. *Human Nutr. Appl.* 37A: 483–490.

Cossack ZT (1988) The efficacy of oral zinc therapy as an alternative to penicillamine for Wilson's disease. *N. Eng. J Med.* 318: 322–323.

Crocker JFS, Renton KW, Lee SH, Rozee KR, Digout SC and Malatjalian DA (1986) Biochemical and morphological characterisation of a mouse model of Reye's syndrome induced by the interaction of influenza B virus and a chemical emulsifier. *Lab. Invest.* 54: 32–40.

Dick MC and Mowat AP (1986) Biliary scintigraphy with DISIDA. *Arch. Dis. Child.* 61: 191–192.

Donnell GN, Koch R, Fishler K and Ng WG (1980) In Clinical aspects of galactosaemia. In: *Inherited Disorders of Carbohydrate Metabolism.* D Burman, JB Holton and CA Pennock (eds), pp. 103–115. MTP Press, Lancaster.

Editorial (1982) Clouds over galactosaemia. *Lancet* ii: 1379–1380.

Fagerhol MK (1964) Quantitative studies on the inherited variants of serum alpha-1-antitrypsin. *Scand. J. Clin. Lab. Invest.* 23: 97–103.

Fagerhol MK and Laurell CB (1967) The polymorphism of 'prealbumin' and alpha-1-antitrypsin in human sera. *Clin. Chim. Acta* 16: 199–203.

Finch RG (1987). Time for action on hepatitis B immunisation. *Br. Med. J.* 294: 197–198.

Garrod A (1909) *Inborn Error of Metabolism.* Oxford: Oxford University Press

Jenkins JG, Glasgow JFT, Black GW, Fannin TF, Hicks EM, Keilty SR and Crean PM (1987) Reye's syndrome: assessment of intracranial monitoring. *Br. Med. J.* 294: 337–338.

Kidd VJ, Golbus MS, Wallace RB, Itakura K and Woo SLC (1984) Prenatal diagnosis of α_1-antitrypsin deficiency by direct analysis of the mutation site in the gene. *N. Engl. J. Med.* **310**: 639—642.

Konovalov NV, Muttel' Shtedt AA, Bauman LK and Gotovtseva EV (1957) Copper metabolism in hepatolenticular degeneration thiol therapy. *Zh. Nevropatol. Psikhiatr.* **57**: 39—48.

Kvittingen EA, Steinmann B, Gitzelmann R, Leonard JV, Andria G, Borresen AL, Mossman J, Micara G and Lindblad B (1985) Prenatal diagnosis of hereditary tyrosinemia by determination of fumarylacetoacetase in cultured amniotic fluid cells. *Pediatr. Res.* **19**: 334—337.

Landing BH (1974) Changing approach to neonatal hepatitis and biliary atresia. *Pediatrics* **53**: 647—648.

Lubin BH, Baehner RL, Schwartz E, Shohet SB and Nathan DG (1971) The red cell peroxide hemolysis test in the differential diagnosis of obstructive jaundice in the newborn period. *Pediatrics* **48**: 562—565.

Melhorn DK, Gross S and Izant RJ (1972) The red cell hydrogen peroxide hemolysis test and vitamin E absorption in the differential diagnosis of jaundice in infancy. *J. Pediatr.* **81**: 1082—1087.

Mowat AP (1980) Viral hepatitis in infancy and children. *Clin. Gastroenterol.* **9**: 191—212.

Mowat AP (1981) Current developments in chronic liver disease. In: *Recent Advances in Pediatrics*. No. 6, D Hull (ed.), pp. 137—156. Churchill Livingstone, Edinburgh.

Mowat AP (1987a) *Liver Disorders in Childhood*, 2nd edn. Butterworths, London.

Mowat AP (1987b) Liver transplantations—a role for all paediatricians. *Archs Dis. Child.* **62**: 325—326.

Novick DM and Thomas HC (1984) Antiviral treatment of chronic hepatitis B virus infection. *J. R. Soc. Med.* **77**: 998—1001.

Partin JS, Partin JC, Schubert WK and Hammond JG (1982) Serum salicylate concentrations in Reye's disease. *Lancet* **i**: 191—194.

Perman JA, Werlin SL, Grand RJ and Watkins JB (1979) Laboratory measures of copper metabolism in the differentiation of chronic active hepatitis and Wilson disease in children. *J. Pediatr.* **94**: 564—568.

Poley JR, Smith EI, Boon DJ and Bhatia M (1972) Lipoprotein-X and the double ^{131}I-Rose Bengal test in the diagnosis of prolonged infantile jaundice. *J. Pediatr. Surg.* **7**: 660—669.

Redeker AG (1981) Treatment of chronic active hepatitis. *N. Engl. J. Med.* **304**: 420—421.

Remington PL, Rowley D, McGee H, Hall WN and Monto AS (1986) Decreasing trends in Reye syndrome and aspirin use in Michigan, 1979 to 1984. *Pediatrics* **77**: 93—98.

Reye RDK, Morgan G and Baral J (1963) Encephalopathy and fatty degeneration of the viscera: a disease entity in childhood. *Lancet* **ii**: 749—752.

Rogers MF, Schonberger LB, Hurwitz ES and Rowley DL (1985) National Reye Syndrome Surveillance, 1982. *Pediatrics* **75**: 260—264.

Ryan NJ, Hogan GR, Hayes AW, Unger PD and Siraj MY (1979) Aflatoxin B_1: its role in the etiology of Reye's syndrome. *Pediatrics* **64**: 71—75.

Scheinberg IH and Sternlieb I (1988) The efficacy of oral zinc therapy as an alternative to penicillamine for Wilson's disease. *N. Eng. J. Med.* **318**: 323.

Shank RC, Bourgeois CH, Keschamras N and Chandavimol P (1971) Alfatoxins in autopsy specimens from Thai children with an acute disease of unknown aetiology. *Food Cosmet. Toxicol.* **9**: 501—507.

Sharp HL, Bridge RA, Krivit W and Freier EF (1969) Cirrhosis associated with alpha-1-antitrypsin deficiency: A previously unrecognized inherited disorder. *J. Lab. Clin. Med.* **73**: 934—939.

Silverberg M (1979) Chronic liver disease in children. In: *The Liver and Biliary System in Infants and Children* K Chandra (ed.), pp. 174—195. Churchill Livingstone, Edinburgh.

Sveger T (1976) Liver disease in alpha-1-antitrypsin deficiency detected by screening of 200 000 infants. *N. Engl. J. Med.* **294**: 1316—1321.

Sveger T (1984) Prospective study of children with α_1-antitrypsin deficiency: eight-year-old follow-up. *J. Pediatr.* **104**: 91—94.

Walshe JM (1969) Management of penicillamine nephropathy in Wilson's disease: a new chelating agent. *Lancet* **ii**: 1401—1402.

Wright K and Christie DL (1981) Use of γ-glutamyl transpeptidase in the diagnosis of biliary atresia. *Am. J. Dis. Child.* **135**: 134—136.

Yeung CY (1972) Serum 5'-nucleotidase in neonatal hepatitis and biliary atresia. Preliminary observations. *Pediatrics* **50**: 812—814.

Zeltzer PM, Neerhout RC, Fonkalsrud EW and Stiehm ER (1974) Differentiation between neonatal hepatitis and biliary atresia by measuring serum-alpha-fetoprotein. *Lancet* **i**: 373—375.

Chapter 15

Acosta PB, Wenz E and Williamson M (1977) Nutrient intake of treated infants with phenylketonuria. *Am. J. Clin. Nutr.* **30**: 198—208.

American Academy of Pediatrics (1983) Committee on Nutrition: Towards a prudent diet. *Pediatrics* **71**: 78—80.

Andersen GE and Friis-Hansen B (1976) Neonatal diagnosis of familial type II hyperlipoproteinemia. *Pediatrics* **57**: 214—220.

Anon (1987) Advice about milk for infants and young children. *Lancet* **i**: 843—844.

Anon (1988) Bile acid sequestrants and hyperlipidaemia. *Lancet* **i**: 220—221.

Baker SG, Joffe BI, Mendelsohn D and Seftel HC (1982) Treatment of homozygous familial hypercholesterolaemia with probucol. *S. A. Med. J.* **62**: 7−11.

Bickel H (1980) Phenylketonuria: past, present, future. Hudson Memorial Lecture, Leeds 1979. *J. Inher. Metab. Dis.* **3**: 123−132.

Bilheimer DW, Grundy SM, Brown MS and Goldstein JL (1983) Mevinolin and colestipol stimulate receptor-mediated clearance of low density lipoprotein from plasma in familial hypercholesterolemia heterozygotes. *Proc. Natl Acad. Sci. USA* **80**: 4124−4128.

Chalstrey LJ, Winder AF and Galton DJ (1982) Partial ileal bypass in treatment of familial hypercholesterolaemia. *J. R. Soc. Med.* **75**: 851−856.

Childs B, Nyhan WL, Borden M, Bard L and Cooke RE (1961) Idiopathic hyperglycinemia and hyperglycinuria: a new disorder of amino acid metabolism. *Pediatrics* **27**: 522−538.

Clayton BE, Heeley AF and Heeley M (1970) An investigation of the hyperaminoaciduria in phenylketonuria associated with the feeding of certain commercial low-phenylalarine preparations. *Br. J. Nutr.* **24**: 573−580.

Collins JE and Leonard JV (1985) The dietary management of inborn errors of metabolism. *Human Nutr. Appl. Nutr.* **39A**: 255−272.

DHSS (1984) Diet and cardiovascular disease. *Report on Health and Social Subjects*, No. 28, HMSO, London.

DHSS (1987) *Milk for infants and young children.* Committee on the Medical Aspects of Food Policy, Panel on Child Nutrition. HMSO, London.

Dhondt JL (1984) Tetrahydrobiopterin deficiencies: preliminary analysis from an international survey. *J. Pediatr.* **104**: 501−508.

Drash A (1972) Atherosclerosis, cholesterol, and the pediatrician. *J. Pediatr.* **80**: 693−696.

Drogan E, Smith I, Beasley M and Lloyd JK (1987) Timing of strict diet in relation to fetal damage in maternal phenylkotenuria. *Lancet* ii: 928−930.

Drug and Therapeutic Bulletin (1987) Management of hyperlipidaemia. *Drug Ther. Bull.* **25**: 89−92.

Farris RP, Frank GC, Webber LS, Srinivasan SR and Berenson GS (1982) Influences of milk source and serum lipids and lipoproteins during the first year of life: The Bogalusa heart study. *Am. J. Clin. Nutr.* **35**: 42−49.

Følling A (1934) Uber ausscheidung von Phenylbenztraubensäure in den Harn als Stoffwechselanomalie in Verbindung mit Imbezillität. *Hoffe-Seyler's Z. Physiol. Chem.* **227**: 169.

Fredrickson DS, Levy RI and Lees RS (1967) Fat transport in lipoproteins—an integrated approach to mechanisms and disorders. *N. Engl. J. Med.* **276**: 34−44, 94−103, 148−156, 215−224, 273−281.

Ghadimi H, Partington MW and Hunter A (1961) A familial disturbance of histidine metabolism. *N. Engl. J. Med.* **265**: 221−224.

Glueck CJ (1983) Therapy of familial and acquired hyperlipoproteinaemia in children and adolescents. *Prevent. Med.* **12**: 835−847.

Glueck CJ (1986) Pediatric primary prevention of atherosclerosis. *N. Engl. J. Med.* **314**: 175−177.

Glueck CJ, Mellies MJ, Dine M, Perry T and Laskarzewski P (1986) Safety and efficacy of long-term diet plus bile acid-binding resin cholesterol-lowering therapy in 73 children heterozygous for familial hypercholesterolemia. *Pediatrics* **78**: 338−348.

Godfrey RC, Stenhouse NS, Cullen KJ and Blackman V (1972) Cholesterol and the child: studies of the cholesterol of Busselton School children and their parents. *Austr. Paediatr. J.* **8**: 72−78.

Goldstein JL, Schrott HG, Hazzard WR, Bierman EL and Motulsky AG (1973) II. Genetic analysis of lipid levels in 176 families and delineation of a new inherited disorder, combined hyperlipidemia. *J. Clin. Invest.* **52**: 1544−1568.

Guthrie R and Susi A (1963) A simple phenylalanine method for detecting phenylketonuria in large populations of newborn infants. *Pediatrics* **32**: 338−343.

Hames CG and Greenberg BG (1961) A comparative study of serum cholesterol levels in school children and their possible relation to atherogenesis. *Am. J. Publ. Hlth* **51**: 374−385.

Hjermann I, Byre KV, Holme I and Leren P (1981) Effect of diet and smoking intervention on the incidence of coronary heart disease. *Lancet* ii: 1303−1310.

Kindt E, Motzfeldt K, Halvorsen S and Lie SO (1983) Protein requirements in infants and children: a longitudinal study of children treated for phenylketonuria. *Am. J. Clin. Nutr.* **37**: 778−785.

Koch R, Azen CG, Friedman EG and Williamson ML (1982) Preliminary report on the effects of diet discontinuation in PKU. *J. Pediatr.* **4**: 870−875.

Laskarzewski P, Morrison JA, de Groot I, *et al.* (1979) Lipids and lipoprotein tracking in children over a 4 year period. *Pediatrics* **64**: 584−591.

Lauer RM, Connor WE, Leaverton PE, Reitter MA and Clarke WR (1975) Coronary heart disease and risk factors in school-children: the muscatine study. *J. Pediatr.* **86**: 697−706.

Leonard JV, Daish P, Naughten ER and Bartlett K (1984) The Management and longterm outcome of organic acidaemas. *J. Inher. Metab. Dis.* **7**: 13−17.

Levy HL, Shih VE and Madigan PM (1974) Routine newborn screening for histidinemia: clinical and biochemical results. *N. Engl. J. Med.* **291**: 1214−1219.

Lipid Research Clinics Program (1984a) The Lipid Research Clinics Coronary Primary Prevention Trial Results. I. Reduction in incidence of coronary heart disease. *J. Am. Med. Assoc.* **251**: 351−364.

Lipid Research Clinics Program (1984b) The Lipid Research Clinics Coronary Primary Prevention Trial Results. II. The relationship of reduction in incidence of coronary heart disease to cholesterol lowering. *J. Am. Med. Assoc.* **251**: 365−374.

McGandy RB, Hall B, Ford C and Stare FJ (1972)

Dietary regulation of blood cholesterol in adolescent males: a pilot study. *Am. J. Clin. Nutr.* 25: 61–66.

Mahoney MJ and Bick D (1987) Recent advances in the inherited methylmalonic acidemias. *Acta Paed. Scand.* 76: 689–696.

Mellies M and Glueck CJ (1983) Lipids and the development of atherosclerosis in children. *J. Pediatr. Gastroenterol. Nutr.* 2 (Suppl.): S298–S303.

Mendoza S, Contreras C, Ineichen E, Fernandez M, Nucete H, Morrison JA, Gartside PS and Glueck CJ (1980) Lipids and lipoproteins in Venezuelan and American schoolchildren within and cross-cultural comparisons. *Pediatr. Res.* 14: 272–277.

Nutrition Committee of the Canadian Paediatric Society (1981) Children's diets and atherosclerosis. *Can. Med. Assoc. J.* 124: 1545–1548.

Pocock SJ, Shaper AG, Phillips AN, Walker M and Whitehead TP (1986) High density lipoprotein cholesterol is not a major risk factor for ischaemia heart disease in British men. *Br. Med. J.* 292: 515–519.

Rohr FJ, Doherty LB, Waisbren SE, Bailey IV, Anpola MG, Benacerrf B and Levy HL (1987) New England Maternal PKU project: prospective study of untreated and treated pregnancies and their outcome. *J. Pediatr.* 110: 391–398.

Sardharwalla IB (1980) The management of homocystinuria. In: *Topics in Paediatrics 2, Nutrition in Childhood.* B Wharton (ed.), pp. 110–118. Pitman Medical, London.

Scriver CR and Levy HL (1983) Histidinaemia Part I. Reconciling retrospective and prospective findings. *J. Inher. Metab. Dis.* 6: 51–53.

Shortland D, Smith I, Francis DEM, Ersser R and Wolff OH (1985) Amino acid and protein requirements in a preterm infant with classical phenylketonuria. *Arch. Dis. Child.* 60: 263–265.

Smith I (1985) The hyperphenylalaninaemias. In: *Genetic and Metabolic Disorders in Paediatrics*, JK Lloyd and CR Scriver (eds), pp. 166–182. Butterworths, London.

Smith I, Erdohazi M, Macartney FJ, Pincott JR, Wolff OH, Brenton DP, Biddle SA, Fairweather DVI and Dobbing J (1979) Fetal damage despite low-phenylalanine diet after conception in a phenylketonuric woman. *Lancet* i: 17–19.

Tamir I, Heiss G, Glueck CJ, Christensen B, Kwiterovich P and Rifkind BM (1981) Lipid and lipoprotein distributions in white children ages 6–19 years. The lipid research clinics program prevalence study. *J. Chron. Dis.* 34: 27–29.

Tanaka K, Budd MA, Efron ML and Isselbacher KJ (1966) Isovaleric acidemia: a new genetic defect of leucine metabolism. *Proc. Natl Acad. Sci. USA* 56: 236–242.

Taylor CJ, Moore G and Davidson DC (1984) The effect of treatment on zinc, copper and calcium status in children with phenylketonuria. *J. Inher. Metab. Dis.* 7: 160–165.

Thompson GR (1985) The hyperlipidaemias. In: *Genetic and Metabolic Disease in Paediatrics.* JK Lloyd and CR Scriver (eds), pp. 211–233. Butterworths, London.

Waisbren SE, Schnell RR and Levy HL (1980) Diet termination in children with phenylketonuria: A review of psychological assessment used to determine outcome. *J. Inher. Metab. Dis.* 3: 149–153.

Watchel L (1986) Review of current practices in management of inherited disorders of amino acid metabolism in western Europe. *Hum. Nutr. Appl.* 40A (suppl.): 61–69.

Weidman WH, Elveback LR, Nelson RA, Hodgson PA and Ellefson RD (1978) Nutrient intake and serum cholesterol in normal children 6–16 years of age. *Pediatrics* 61: 354–359.

West RJ and Lloyd JK (1979) Hypercholesterolemia in childhood. In: *Advances in Pediatrics*, LA Barness (ed.). Vol. 26, pp. 1–34. Year Book Medical Publishers, Inc., London.

West RJ, Lloyd JK and Leonard JV (1980) Long-term follow-up of children with familial hypercholesterolaemia treated with cholestyramine. *Lancet* ii: 873–875.

Wilcken DEL, Wilcken B, Dudman NPB and Tyrrell PA (1983) Homocystinuria — the effects of betaine in the treatment of patients not responsive to pyridoxine. *N. Engl. J. Med.* 309: 448–453.

Yamamoto A, Sudo H and Endo A (1980) Therapeutic effects of ML-236B in primary hypercholesterolemia. *Atherosclerosis* 35: 259–266.

Zavoral JH, Hannan P, Fields DJ, Hanson MN, Frantz ID, Kuba K, Elmer P and Jacobs DR (1983) The hypolipidemic effect of locust bean gum food products in familial hypercholesterolemic adults and children. *Am. J. Clin. Nutr.* 38: 285–294.

Chapter 16

Bayer LM and Robinson SJ (1969) Grown history of children with congenital heart defects. *Am. J. Dis. Child.* 117: 564–572.

Berg V, Boulin A-B and Aperia A (1987) Short term effect of low and high protein intake on renal function in children with renal disease. *Acta Paediatr. Scand.* 76: 288–292.

Betts PR and Magrath G (1974) Growth pattern and dietary intake of children with chronic renal insufficiency. *Br. Med. J.* 2: 189–193.

Brouhard BH (1986) The role of dietary protein in progressive renal diseases. *Am. J. Dis. Child.* 140: 630–637.

Chantler C, El Bishti M and Counahan R (1980) Nutritional therapy in children with chronic renal failure. *Am. J. Clin. Nutr.* 33, 1682–1689.

Chantler C, Jones RWA, Dalton N and Rigden SPA (1981) Nutritional management of chronic renal failure in childhood. *Acta Chir. Scand.* (Suppl. 507) 147: 330–339.

Feldt RH, Strickler GB and Weidman WH (1969) Growth of children with congenital heart disease. *Am. J. Dis. Child.* **117**: 573−579.

Fennell III RS, Orak JK, Hudson T, Garin EH, Iravani A, Van Deusen WJ, Howard R, Pfaff WW, Walker III D and Richard GA (1984) Growth in children with various therapies for end-stage renal disease. *Am. J. Dis. Child.* **138**: 28−31.

Fomon SJ (ed.) (1974) Protein. In: *Infant Nutrition*, pp. 118−151. WB Saunders Co., Philadelphia.

Fries ED (1976) Salt, volume and the prevention of hypertension. *Circulation* **53**: 589−595.

Guthrie HA (1986) Infant feeding practices — a predisposing factor in hypertension? *Am. J. Clin. Nutr.* **21**: 863−867.

James WPT (1980) Dietary fiber and mineral absorption. In: *Medical Aspects of Dietary Fiber* GA Spiller and R McPherson Kay (eds) pp. 239−259. Plenum Medical, New York.

Jones RWA, Dalton N, Start K, El-Bishti MM and Chantler C (1980) Oral essential amino acid supplements in children with advanced chronic renal failure. *Am. J. Clin. Nutr.* **33**: 1696−1702.

Jones RWA, Rigden SP, Barratt TM and Chantler C (1982) The effects of chronic renal failure in infancy on growth, nutritional status and body composition. *Pediatr. Res.* **16**: 784−791.

McCrory WW, Gertner JM, Burke TM, Pimental CT and Nemery RL (1987) Effects of dietary phosphate restriction in children with chronic renal failure. *J. Pediatr.* **111**: 410−414.

Maschio G, Tessitore N, D'Angelo A, Bonucci E, Lupo A, Valvo E, Loschiavo C, Fabris A, Morachiello P, Previato G and Fiaschi E (1980) Early dietary phosphorus restriction and calcium supplementation in the prevention of renal osteodystrophy. *Am. J. Clin. Nutr.* **33**: 1546−1554.

Menahem S (1972) The clinical growth of infants and children with ventricular septal defects. *Austr. Paediatr. J.* **8**: 1−15.

Nadas AS, Rosenthal A and Crigler JF (1981) Nutritional considerations in the prognosis and treatment of children with congenital heart disease. In *Textbook of Pediatric Nutrition.*, RM Suskind (ed.), pp. 537−544. Raven Press, New York.

Naeye RL (1965) Organ and cellular development in congenital heart disease and in alimentary malnutrition. *J. Pediatr.* **67**: 447−458.

Strife CF, Quinlan M, Mearsk K, Davey ML and Clardy C (1986) Improved growth of three uraemic children by nocturnal nasogastric feeding. *Am. J. Dis. Child.* **140**: 438−443.

Suoninen P (1971) Physical growth of children with congenital heart disease. Pre- and postoperative studies of 355 cases. *Acta Paediatr. Scand. (Suppl.)* **225**, 1−50.

Umansky R and Hauck AJ (1962) Factors in the growth of children with patent ductus arteriosus. *Pediatrics* **30**: 540−551.

Wassner SJ (1982) The role of nutrition in the care of children with renal insufficiency. In: *Symposium on Pediatric Nephrology, The Pediatric Clinics of North America*, vol. 29, No. 4, RN Fine (ed.), pp. 973−990. WB Saunders Co., Philadelphia.

Whitten CF and Stewart RA (1980) The effect of dietary sodium in infancy on blood pressure and related factors. *Acta Paediatr. Scand. (Suppl.)* **279**, 3−17.

Zilleruelo G, Hsia SL, Freundlich M, Gorman HM and Strauss J (1984) Persistence of serum lipid abnormalities in children with idiopathic nephrotic syndrome. *J. Pediatr.* **104**: 61−64.

Chapter 17

American Diabetes Association (1979) Principles of nutrition and dietary recommendations for individuals with diabetes mellitus. *Diabetes* **28**: 1027−1036.

Anon (1986) Serological markers for Type 1 diabetes. *Lancet* i: 1132−1133.

Anon (1987) Pancreatic transplantation in diabetes. *Lancet* i: 1015.

Baker JR, O'Connor JP, Metcalf PA, Lawson MR and Johnson RN (1983). Clinical usefulness of estimation of serum fructosamine concentration as a screening test for diabetes mellitus. *Br. Med. J.* **287**: 863−867.

Baumer JH, Edelsten AD, Howlett BC, Owens C, Pennock CA and Savage DCL (1982) Impact of home blood glucose monitoring on childhood diabetes. *Arch. Dis. Child.* **57**: 195−199.

British Diabetic Association (1982) Dietary recommendations for the 1980s. *J. Human Nutr. Appl. Nutr.* **36**: 379−394.

Brooks KE, Rawal N and Henderson AR (1986) Laboratory assessment of three new monitors of blood glucose: Accu-Chek II, Glucometer II, and Glucoscan 2000 *Clin. Chem.* **32**: 2195−2200.

Canadian Diabetes Association (1981) Guidelines for the nutritional management of diabetes mellitus. *J. Can. Diet. Assoc.* **42**: 110−118.

Castells S (1984) Symposium on juvenile diabetes. *Pediatr. Clin. N. Am.* **31** (3).

Diabetes Bulletin (1985) Transplantation for diabetes: a real possibility. May issue, 1.

Craig O (1981) *Childhood Diabetes and its Management*, 2nd edn, pp. 31−33. Butterworths, London.

Dornan TL, Ting A, McPherson CK, Peckar Co, Mann JI, Turner RC and Morris PJ (1982) Genetic susceptibility to the development of retinopathy in insulin dependent diabetes. *Diabetes* **31**: 226−231.

Earis JE, Greenway MW and Macaulay MB (1980) Blood glucose monitoring without a meter. *Lancet* i: 823−824.

Gamble DR and Taylor KW (1973) Coxsackie B virus and diabetes. *Br. Med. J.* **1**: 289−290.

Ginsberg-Fellner F, Witt ME, Franklin BH, Yagihashi S, Toguchi Y, Dobersen MJ, Rubinstein P and Notkins

AL (1985) Triad of markers for identifying children at high risk of developing insulin-dependent diabetes mellitus. *J. Am. Med. Assoc.* **254**: 1469–1472.

Golden MP, Russel BP, Ingersoll GM, Gray DL and Hummer KM (1985) Management of diabetes mellitus in children younger than 5 years of age. *Am. J. Dis. Child.* **139**: 448–452.

Hackett AF, Court S, McCowen C and Parkin JM (1986) Dietary survey of diabetics. *Arch. Dis. Child.* **61**: 67–71.

Hazra DK, Singh R, Wahal PK, Lahiri V, Gupta MK, Jain NK and Elhence BR (1980) Coxsackie antibodies in young Asian diabetics. *Lancet* i: 877.

Jenkins DJA (1982) Lente carbohydrate: a newer approach to the dietary management of diabetes. *Diabetes Care* **5**: 634–641.

Jenkins DJA, Wolever TMS, Nineham R, Taylor R, Metz GL, Bacon S and Hockaday TDR (1978) Guar crispbread in the diabetic diet. *Br. Med. J.* **2**: 1744–1746.

Jenkins DJA, Wolever TMS, Taylor RH, Barker HM, Fielden H, Baldwin JM, Bowling AC, Newman HC, Jenkins AL and Goff DV (1981) Glycemic index of foods: a physiological basis for carbohydrate exchange. *Am. J. Clin. Nutr.* **34**: 362–366.

Käär M-L, Åkerblom HK, Huttunen N-P, Knip M and Säkkinen K (1984) Metabolic control in children and adolescents with insulin-dependent diabetes mellitus. *Acta Paediatr. Scand.* **73**: 102–108.

Kinmonth AL (1987) Management of diabetes in childhood. *Prescribers' Journal* **27**: 1–12.

Kinmonth AL and Baum JD (1980) Timing of pre-breakfast insulin injection and postprandial metabolic control in diabetic children . *Br. Med. J.* **1**: 604–606.

Knowles Jr HC, Guest HM, Lampe J, Kessler M and Skillman TG (1961) The course of juvenile diabetes treated with an unmeasured diet. *Diabetes* **14**: 239–273.

Krane EJ (1987) Diabetic ketoacidosis. In: *Pediatric and Adolescent Edocrinology*, CP Mahoney (ed.), Vol. 34, pp. 935–960. WB Saunders, Philadelphia.

Leslie ND and Sperling MA (1986) Relation of metabolic control to complications in diabetes mellitus. *J. Pediatr.* **108**: 491–497.

Nakhooda AF, Like AA, Chappel CI, Murray FT and Marliss EB (1976) The spontaneously diabetic Wistar rat. *Diabetes* **26**: 100–112.

Peterson CM, Jovanovich-Peterson L and Formby P (eds) (1988) *Fetal Islet Transplantation: Implications for Diabetes*. Spring-verlag, Berlin.

Pickup JC, White MC, Keen H, Parsons JA and Alberti KGMM (1979) Long-term continuous subcutaneous insulin infusion in diabetics at home. *Lancet* ii: 870–873.

Schober E, Schernthaner G and Mayr WR (1981) HLA-DR antigens in insulin-dependent diabetes. *Arch. Dis. Child.* **56**: 227–229.

Tamborlane WV and Sherwin RS (1983) Diabetes control and complications: new strategies and insights. *J. Pediatr.* **102**: 805–811.

Travis LB, Brouhard BH and Schreiner B-J (1987) Diabetes Mellitus in children and adolescents. *Major Problems in Clinical Pediatrics*, Vol. 29. W. B. Saunders, Philadelphia.

Watkins PJ (1980) Insulin infusion systems, diabetic control, and microvascular complications. *Br. Med. J.* **1**: 350–352.

WHO (1980) Diabetes Mellitus. Second Report. *WHO Technical Report Series No. 646*, Geneva.

WHO (1985) Diabetes Mellitus: report of a study group *WHO Technical Report Series No. 727*, Geneva.

Wilkin TJ, Armitage M and Wood P (1987) Tests for childhood diabetes. *Update* **34**: 177–179.

Chapter 18

Anon (1870) Apepsia hysterica *Br. Med. J.* i: 39.

AMA (1980) *Diagnostic and Statistical Manual of Mental Disorders*, 3rd edition. American Psychiatric Association, Washington DC.

Blackburn GL and Greenberg I (1980) Multidisciplinary approach to obesity therapy. In: *Childhood Obesity*, 2nd edition, PJ Collipp, (ed.) PSG Publishing Company Inc., Boston.

Botvin GJ, Cantlon A, Carter BJ and Williams CL (1979) Reducing adolescent obesity through a school health program. *J. Pediatr.* **95**: 1060–1062.

Brook CGD (1980) Obesity. The fat child. *Br. J. Hosp. Med.* **24** (6): 517–522.

Brooke OG and Abernethy E (1985) Obesity in children. *Hum. Nutr. Appl. Nutr.* **39A** (4): 304–314.

Brownell KD and Kaye FS (1982) A school-based behavior modification, nutrition education, and physical activity program for obese children. *Am. J. Clin. Nutr.* **35**: 277–283.

Brownell KD and Stunkard AJ (1978) Behavioral treatment of obesity in children. *Am. J. Dis. Child.* **132**: 403–412.

Bryant-Waugh R, Knibbs J, Fosson A, Kaminski Z and Lask B (1988) Long term follow up of patients with early onset anorexia nervosa. *Arch. Dis. Child.* **63**: 5–9.

Casper RC, Offer D and Ostrov E (1981) The self-image of adolescents with acute anorexia nervosa. *J. Pediatr.* **98**: 656–661.

Crisp AH (1983) Anorexia nervosa. *Br. Med. J.* **287**: 855–858.

Crisp AH (1965) Clinical and therapeutic aspects of anorexia nervosa — a study of 30 cases. *J. Psychosom. Res.* **9**: 67–78.

Croner S, Larsson J, Schildt B and Symreng T (1985) Severe anorexia nervosa treated with total parenteral nutrition. *Acta Paediatr. Scand.* **74**: 230–236.

Drossman DA, Ontjes DA and Heizer WD (1979) Anorexia nervosa. *Gastroenterology* **77**: 1115–1131.

Epstein LH, Wing RR, Penner BC and Kress MJ (1985) Effect of diet and controlled exercise on weight loss in obese children. *J. Pediatr.* **107**: 358–361.

Fosson A, Kubbs J, Bryant-Waugh R and Lask B (1987) Early onset anorexia nervosa. *Arch. Dis. Child.* **62**: 114−118.

Freeman CPL, Barry F, Dunkeld-Turnbull J and Henderson A (1988) Controlled trial of psychotherapy for bulimia nervosa. *Br. Med. J.* **296**: 521−525.

Gull WW (1874). Anorexia nervosa (apepsia hysterica, anorexia hysterica). *Trans. Clin. Soc. Lon.* **7**: 22−28.

Hull D (1980) Thoughts on obesity. *Arch. Dis. Child.* **55**: 838−840.

Jenkins AP, Treasure J and Thompson RPH (1988) Crohn's disease presenting as anorexia nervosa. *Br. Med. J.* **296**: 699−700.

Jonas JM and Gold MS (1986) Cocaine abuse and eating disorders. *Lancet* i: 390−391.

Jonas JM and Gold MS (1986) Naltrexone reverses bulimic symptoms. *Lancet* i: 807.

Knittle JL and Hirsch J (1968) Effects of early nutrition on the development of rat epididymal fat pads: cellularity and metabolism. *J. Clin. Invest.* **47**: 2091−2098.

Kramer MS, Barr RG, Leduc DG, Boisjoly C, McVey-White L and Pless IB (1985) Determinants of weight and adiposity in the first year of life. *J. Pediatr.* **106**, 10−14.

Lacey JH (1983) Bulimia nervosa, binge eating, and psychogenic vomiting: a controlled treatment study and long term outcome. *Br. Med. J.* **286**: 1609−1613.

Laséque EC (1873) On hysterical anorexia. Cited by Gull (1874).

Lole-Harris CA, Dodge JA, Bowen-Jones CA and Penny GA (1983) Management of obese children. In: *Topics in Paediatric Nutrition*, JA Dodge (ed.). Pitman Books Ltd, London.

Lorber J (1966). Obesity in childhood. A controlled trial of anorectic drugs. *Arch. Dis. Child.* **41**: 309−312.

McWilliams M (1980) *Nutrition for the Growing Years*, 3rd edn. John Wiley & Sons Inc., New York.

Mason E (1970) Obesity in pet dogs. *Vet. Rec.* **86**: 612−616.

Mayer J, Marshall NB, Vitale JJ, Christensen JH, Mashayekhi MB and Starte FJ (1954a) Exercise, food intake and body weight in normal rats and in genetically obese adult mice. *Am. J. Physiol.* **177**: 544−548.

Mayer J, Roy P and Mitra K (1954b) Relation between caloric intake, body weight and physical work in an industrial male population in West Bengal. *Am. Clin. Nutr.* **4**: 169−175.

Merritt RJ and Batrus C (1980) The role of the dietitian in the treatment of pediatric obesity. In: *Childhood Obesity*, 2nd edn, PJ Collipp (ed.) PSG Publishing Inc., Boston.

Nylander I (1971) The feeling of being fat and dieting in a school population. *Acta Socio-Medica Scand.* **1**: 17−26.

Poskitt EM (1987) Management of obesity. *Arch. Dis. Child.* **62**: 305−310.

Russell G (1979) Bulimia nervosa: an ominous variant of anorexia nervosa. *Psychol. Med.* **9**: 429−448.

Stefanik PA, Heald FP Jr and Mayer J (1959) Caloric intake in relation to energy output of obese and non-adolescent boys. *Am. J. Clin. Nutr.* **7**: 55−62.

Sveger T, Lindberg T, Weibull B and Olsson UL (1975) Nutrition, overnutrition and obesity in the first year of life in Malmö, Sweden. *Acta Paediatr. Scand.* **64**: 635−640.

Taitz LS (1983) *The Obese Child*. Blackwell Scientific, Oxford.

Tanner JM and Whitehouse RH (1975) Revised standards for triceps and subscapular skinfolds in British children. *Arch. Dis. Child.* **50**: 142−145.

Warren MP and Wiele RLV (1973) Clinical and metabolic features of anorexia nervosa. *Am. J. Obstet. Gynecol.* **117**: 435−449.

Williams E (1958) Anorexia nervosa: a somatic disorder. *Br. Med. J.* **2**: 190−195.

Further reading

Additional information on the various conditions described in this book can be found in the following:

Francis DEM (1986) *Diets for Sick Children*, 4th edn. Blackwells, Oxford.

Gryboski J and Walker WA (1983) *Gastrointestinal Problems in the Infants*, 2nd edn. WB Saunders, Philadelphia.

Milla PJ and Muller DPR (1988) *Harries' Paediatric Gastroenterology*, 2nd edn. Churchill Livingstone, Edinburgh.

Mowat AP (1987) *Liver Disorders in Childhood*, 2nd edn. Butterworths, London.

Silverman A and Roy CC (1983) *Pediatric Clinical Gastroenterology*, 3rd edn. CV Mosby, St Louis, USA.

Walker-Smith JA, Hamilton JR and Walker WA (1983) *Practical Paediatric Gastroenterology*. Butterworths, London.

Walker WA and Watkins JB (1985) *Nutrition in Pediatrics*. Little, Brown & Co., Boston.

Index